Hot Topics in Acute Care Surgery and Trauma

Series Editors

Federico Coccolini
Pisa, Italy

Raul Coimbra
Riverside, USA

Andrew W. Kirkpatrick
Calgary, Canada

Salomone Di Saverio
Cambridge, UK

This series covers the most debated issues in acute care and trauma surgery, from perioperative management to organizational and health policy issues. Since 2011, the founder members of the World Society of Emergency Surgery's (WSES) Acute Care and Trauma Surgeons group, who endorse the series, realized the need to provide more educational tools for young surgeons in training and for general physicians and other specialists new to this discipline: WSES is currently developing a systematic scientific and educational program founded on evidence-based medicine and objective experience. Covering the complex management of acute trauma and non-trauma surgical patients, this series makes a significant contribution to this program and is a valuable resource for both trainees and practitioners in acute care surgery.

More information about this series at http://www.springer.com/series/15718

Massimo Sartelli · Raul Coimbra
Leonardo Pagani · Kemal Rasa
Editors

Infections in Surgery

Prevention and Management

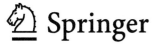
Springer

Editors
Massimo Sartelli
Department of Surgery
Macerata Hospital
Macerata
Italy

Raul Coimbra
Comparative Effectiveness and Clinical
Outcomes Research Center - CECORC
Riverside University Health System
Medical Center
Moreno Valley, CA
USA

Leonardo Pagani
Department of infectious diseases
Ospedale di Bolzano
Bolzano
Italy

Kemal Rasa
Department of Surgery
Anadolu Medical Centre
Kocaeli
Turkey

ISSN 2520-8284   ISSN 2520-8292   (electronic)
Hot Topics in Acute Care Surgery and Trauma
ISBN 978-3-030-62115-5   ISBN 978-3-030-62116-2   (eBook)
https://doi.org/10.1007/978-3-030-62116-2

This Springer imprint is published by the registered company Springer Nature Switzerland AG
The registered company address is: Gewerbestrasse 11, 6330 Cham, Switzerland

Foreword to the Series

Research is fundamentally altering the daily practice of acute care surgery (trauma, surgical critical care, and emergency general surgery) for the betterment of patients around the world. Management for many diseases and conditions is radically different than it was just a few years ago. For this reason, concise up-to-date information is required to inform busy clinicians. Therefore, since 2011 the World Society of Emergency Surgery (WSES), in partnership with the American Association for the Surgery of Trauma (AAST), endorses the development and publication of the "Hot Topics in Acute Care Surgery and Trauma," realizing the need to provide more educational tools for young in-training surgeons and for general physicians and other surgical specialists. These new forthcoming titles have been selected and prepared with this philosophy in mind. The books will cover the basics of pathophysiology and clinical management, framed with the reference that recent advances in the science of resuscitation, surgery, and critical care medicine have the potential to profoundly alter the epidemiology and subsequent outcomes of severe surgical illnesses and trauma.

Cesena, Italy
Riverside, USA
Calgary, Canada
Cambridge, UK

Federico Coccolini
Raul Coimbra
Andrew W. Kirkpatrick
Salomone Di Saverio

Preface

A Multidisciplinary Approach to Infections in Surgery

According to the World Health Organization (WHO), the simplest definition of patient safety is the prevention of errors and adverse effects to patients associated with health care. While health care has become more effective it has also become more complex, with greater use of new technologies, medicines and treatments, and estimates show that in high-income countries, as many as one in 10 patients is harmed while receiving hospital care, with nearly 50% of them considered preventable.

Improving patient safety in hospitals worldwide requires a systematic approach to combating healthcare-associated infections (HAIs) and antimicrobial resistance (AMR). The two go together.

The occurrence of HAIs, such as central line-associated bloodstream infections, catheter-associated urinary tract infections, surgical site infections, hospital-acquired/ventilator associated pneumonia, and *C. difficile* infection, continues to escalate at an alarming rate. These infections develop during health care and result in significant patient illnesses and deaths (morbidity and mortality); prolong the duration of hospital stays; and necessitate additional diagnostic and therapeutic interventions, which generate added costs to those already incurred by the patient's underlying disease. HAIs are considered an undesirable outcome, and as many are preventable, they are considered an indicator of quality of patient care, an adverse event, and a patient safety issue.

Patients in hospitals are often exposed to multiple risk factors for infection by multidrug-resistant bacteria. Acute care facilities are important sites for the development of antimicrobial resistance (AMR). The intensity of care, associated with populations highly susceptible to infection, creates an environment that facilitates both the emergence and transmission of resistant organisms.

Moreover, the surgical department represents one of the most critical challenges to infection prevention and control. Patients with medical devices (central lines, urinary catheters, ventilators) or who undergo surgical procedures are at risk of acquiring health care-associated infections (HAIs). Surgical site infections are the most common type of hospital-acquired infections in surgical departments worldwide.

Optimal infection control programs have been identified as important components of any comprehensive strategy to tackle AMR, primarily through prevention of HAIs and by limiting transmission of resistant organisms among patients.

The successful containment of AMR in acute care facilities requires also appropriate antibiotic use.

A growing body of evidence demonstrates that hospital-based programs dedicated to improving antibiotic use, commonly referred to as "Antibiotic Stewardship Programs" (ASPs), can both optimize the treatment of infections and reduce adverse events associated with antibiotic misuse.

Such programs significantly improve patients' outcomes by reducing the incidence of infections with antibiotic-resistant bacteria and *C. difficile* infections in hospitalized patients, making antimicrobial stewardship an important synergistic HAI prevention and control strategy. Infection prevention and antimicrobial stewardship share the common goal to keep patients safe and to improve clinical outcomes.

Leading international organizations, such as the WHO, acknowledge that a collaborative and concerted practice approach is essential for providing care that is bound to be the most appropriate to patients' needs, thus optimizing individual health outcomes and overall health care delivery services.

Collaborative, multidisciplinary efforts can help not only prevent HAIs, but also manage them more appropriately by making optimized antibiotic choice, at the right time, at the right dosing, with the right duration.

To be a champion in preventing and managing infections in surgery means creating a culture of collaboration in which infection prevention, antimicrobial stewardship and correct surgical management of infections are all crucial.

Macerata, Italy	Massimo Sartelli
Bolzano, Italy	Leonardo Pagani
Kocaeli, Turkey	Kemal Rasa
Moreno Valley, CA, USA	Raul Coimbra

Contents

The Burden of Surgical Site Infections: Pathophysiology and Risk Factors— Preoperative Measures to Prevent Surgical Site Infections

1

Francesco Di Marzo

A semantic approach to "the burden of surgical site infections" could give us an interesting and wide point of view on the topic.

A straight definition of burden is: a load, typically a heavy one, carried by someone or something.

In the context of Healthcare associated infections the use of this word is constantly rising, involving a wide group of "carriers" sharing the load with a different level of implications.

A very explicative figure is a trunk of pyramid with the number of patients affected by HAI at the lower base (high load in terms of morbidity-mortality-quality of life) and all the stakeholders in the upper part (reduced and different kind of load: professional responsibility, legal/insurance implications).

A relevant part, hidden and not even quantifiable, is under the pyramid and represents all the caregivers (part of social costs).

The smallest and actually missing part is the highest one representing the apex: politics, lawmakers, and industries' strategists.

The semantic and etymology of surgical site infections aids us in understanding almost everything in three words: to work with hands (from ancient Greek χειρ εργον) creating the opportunity for pathogenic microorganisms to spread into tissues and organs.

F. Di Marzo (✉)
UOC Chirurgia Generale, Ospedale Valtiberina - Sansepolcro, Azienda Usl Toscana Sud-est, Sansepolcro, Italy

1.1   History of Surgical Site Infections in a Nutshell

- Before the mid-nineteenth century fever, wound pus, sepsis, and death were routine sequelae of surgical procedures. Ignaz Semmelweis and Joseph Lister were the pioneers in infection control by introducing the principles of antisepsis and contributing to the clear reduction of post-surgical complications.
- In the 1980s, an infection increased the hospitalization period by approximately 10 days with an additional cost of 2000 dollars; in 1992, each SSI determined 7.3 additional days of hospitalization after the operation, with an additional charge of 3152 dollars.
- In the decade 1986–1996, the data of the National Nosocomial Infections Surveillance (NNIS), showed 15,523 SSI on 593,344 surgical operations (CDC). The SSIs were the most common HAIs (38% of the total): the two-thirds superficial or deep, one-third organ/space. 77% of deaths were attributable to infection most (93%) of which were organ/space.

1.2   Results Below Expectations

- In the last 30 years progress in the control of SSI has affected every aspect of assistance (from sterilization to the architecture of operating rooms) and the interventions applied are recognized as effective at the level of literature, yet the SSI remain a source of morbidity and mortality.

  Why

- The reasons are similar to those, more general, of HAI: antimicrobial resistant pathogens, increase in surgical patients, their age and comorbidities.
- Multiple factors have been identified in a patient's surgical path that contribute to the development of the infection.
- The prevention of surgical site infections is complex and requires a strategy that integrates a wide range of interventions before, during and after surgery, relating the different professionals involved in patient management.
- The implementation of these interventions is not standardized. National guidelines are available but there are discrepancies in the interpretation of scientific evidence, recommendations and in the application of good practices.

1.2.1   Burden

SSI data (and HAI's) are not included in the list of diseases for which the global burden is regularly evaluated by WHO or other international organizations working on global health.

The incidence of SSI varies worldwide (160,000 to 300,000 in the US and leading HAI reported in low-medium income countries) but numbers are understated, given the surveillance challenges. Despite the presence of robust data in some countries or regions, we lack accurate SSI rates and numbers about the economic effect (direct and indirect).

Use of SSI rates as a pay-for-performance metric, a target of quality-improvement efforts, a quality indicator and comparison benchmark for health-care facilities, countries and the public, is strictly linked to robust numbers to ensure valid comparisons. It's mandatory to have unique SSI definitions, strength and valid SSI data and to conduct sheer economic studies.

Surgical site infections (SSIs) are the most common and costly of all hospital-acquired infections (HAI), accounting for 20% of HAI. SSIs are associated with increased length of stay and morbidity, a 2- to 11-fold increase in the risk of mortality (77% of this is due to the infection itself); sequelae include prolonged antimicrobial treatment, redo-surgeries, reduced quality of life, post-hospital rehabilitation, lost work, and productivity [1].

The financial burden of SSI is considerable; it ranks as the third most costly of the hospital-acquired infections (doubled since 2005). The annual cost of SSI in the US is estimated at $3.5 to $10 billion.

Increased direct costs from SSIs are driven by prolonged length of stay, intensive care unit stay, reoperation, surgical techniques, emergency department visits, risk of readmission and medical resources erosion (diagnostic test, medical staff, operative, and treatment costs). Indirect costs are related to patients' quality of life, work absence, and earnings loss.

In addition to the economic burden, the development of an SSI and the subsequent prolonged hospitalization will likely have a negative impact on patient physical and mental health; patients who require absence from work constitute an economic cost in terms of lost income and reduced work productivity; infected patients diagnosed after their discharge from hospital may not have the same access to treatment with more distress than for in hospital diagnosed patients.

Furthermore infections detected after discharge may result in an underreporting, as well as the costs associated with community healthcare visits.

Medical costs, given variations across the globe, have been estimated to range from 15,800 to 43,900 $ per SSI.

SSI (in the US) extends hospital length of stay by 9.7 days and increases the cost of hospitalization by more than $20,000 per admission. More than 90,000 readmissions annually are attributed to SSIs, costing an additional $700 million per year. We have to consider that up to 60% of SSIs were estimated to be preventable with the use of evidence-based measures.

In a recent Centers for Disease Control and Prevention (CDC) report on the rates of national and state (US) HAIs based on data from 2018, 3345 acute care hospitals reported 21,265 SSI among 2,808,659 surgical procedures (all National Healthcare Safety Network—NHSN) performed in that year and an overall Standardized Infection Ratio (SIR) of 0.954 (95% CI 0.941–0.967) [2].

Of note, between 2017 and 2018, there was no significant change in overall SSI related to the 10 select procedures tracked in the CDC report (no changes in 336,585 performed abdominal hysterectomy and in 329,729 performed colon surgery).

Applying two different consumer price index adjustments to account for the rate of inflation in hospital resource prices, the CDC estimated that the attributable patient hospital costs for SSI is between $1087 and $29,443.

SSI is considered (using the consumer price index for urban consumers and inpatient hospital services) as the HAI with the largest range of annual costs (US$ 3.2–8.6 billion and US$ 3.5–10 billion, respectively).

The estimated economic costs of SSIs in Europe (in 2004) range between € 1.47–19.1 billion. It predicted also that the average patient stay would increase by approximately 6.5 days and cost three times as much. The analysis suggested that the SSI-attributable economic burden at that time was likely to be underestimated.

In 2017, 12 EU Member States and one EEA country reported SSIs for nine types of surgical procedure to ECDC. During this period, 10,149 SSIs were reported from a total of 648,512 surgical procedures. The percentage of SSIs varied from 0.5% to 10.1%. The incidence density of in-hospital SSIs per 1000 postoperative patient-days varied from 0.1 to 5.7. From 2014 to 2017, a statistically significant increasing trend was observed for both the percentage of SSIs and the incidence density of in-hospital SSIs following laparoscopic cholecystectomy (CHOL) [3].

Overall, 648,512 surgical procedures from 1639 hospitals were reported in 2017. Of these procedures, 622,999 were reported using patient-based surveillance, and 25,513 used the unit-based surveillance. The most frequently reported types of surgical procedure were HPRO operations, followed by KPRO operations and CSEC operations. 10,149 SSIs were reported using patient-based or unit-based surveillance. Of these, 4739 (47%) were superficial, 3088 (30%) deep, and 2274 (22%) organ/space SSIs. In 48 (0.5%) SSIs, the type of SSI was unknown. The proportion of deep or organ/space SSIs was 19% in CSEC operations, 42% in laparoscopic CHOL operations, 46% in open CHOL operations, 50% in open COLO operations, 53% in CABG operations, 54% in LAM operations, 61% in laparoscopic COLO, 71% in KPRO operations, and 77% in HPRO operations. Thirty-four per cent of the SSIs were diagnosed in hospitals, whereas 52% were detected after discharge; for 14% the discharge date was unknown. The proportion of SSIs diagnosed in hospital varied from 12% in KPRO operations to 67% in open COLO operations.

Detailed costs from five European countries (France, Germany, Italy, Spain, and the UK) were recently reviewed and published:

- France—following head and neck cancer surgery, patients who developed an SSI constitute a total per-patient medical cost €17,434 higher than those patients who did not develop an SSI
- Germany—matched case–control study demonstrated that total medical cost per patient was significantly elevated in SSI patients [$49,449 vs $18,218 (€36,261 vs €13,356)] and that intensive care unit (ICU) and ward-care costs accounted for the largest part (27.7% and 24.7%, respectively)
- Italy—in orthopedic and trauma surgery patients, SSI was associated to an average cost of €9560 ranging from 3411 to 22,273 (without specifications of resources and costs)

- Spain—across multiple surgical specialties, the sum of all costs (hospital, temporary and permanent incapacity for work, premature deaths and caregivers costs) per SSI patient is $97,433; healthcare costs only accounted for about 10% of the total financial burden
- UK—in general surgery an SSI constituted an additional financial burden of £10,523 per patient (operating theater and medical staff costs accounted for 11% and 18% of the total) [4].

1.3 Pathophysiology

Microbial contamination of the surgical site is a necessary precursor of SSI. The risk of SSI can be conceptualized according to the following relationship Dose of bacterial contamination x virulence / resistance of the host patient = Risk of SSI. Quantitatively, it has been shown that if a surgical site is contaminated with >10^5 microorganisms per gram of tissue, the risk of SSI is markedly increased [5]. However, the dose of contaminating microorganisms required to produce infection may be much lower when foreign material is present at the site (i.e., 100 staphylococci per gram of tissue introduced on silk sutures or mesh or prosthesis). Microorganisms may contain or produce toxins and other substances that increase their ability to invade a host, produce damage within the host, or survive on or in host tissue.

Pathogens' source is the endogenous flora of the patient's skin, mucous membranes or hollow viscera [6].

When mucous membranes or skin are incised, the exposed tissues are at risk for contamination with endogenous flora (aerobic gram-positive cocci, anaerobic bacteria, and gram-negative aerobes from fecal flora when incisions are close to the perineum or groin). When a gastrointestinal organ is opened during an operation and is the source of pathogens, gram-negative bacilli (e.g., *E. coli*), gram-positive organisms (e.g., enterococci), and sometimes anaerobes (e.g., *Bacillus fragilis*) are the typical SSI isolates.

Another SSI source is seeding from a distant focus of infection in patients who have prosthesis or other implant placed during the operation. Any device provides a nidus for attachment of the organism.

Exogenous sources include surgical personnel (members of the surgical team), the operating room environment (including air), tools, instruments and materials brought to the sterile field during a procedure. Exogenous flora are primarily aerobes (gram-positive organisms). Anal, vaginal, or nasopharyngeal carriage of group A streptococci by operating room personnel has been implicated as a cause of several SSI outbreaks. Carriage of gram-negative organisms on the hands has been shown to be greater among surgical personnel with artificial nails. Rarely, outbreaks or clusters of surgical site infections caused by unusual pathogens have been traced to contaminated dressings, bandages, irrigants, or disinfection solutions. Fungi (particularly *Candida albicans*) have been isolated from an increasing percentage of SSIs. This trend probably is due to the widespread use of prophylactic and empiric antibiotics, increased severity of illness, and greater numbers of immunocompromised patients undergoing surgical procedures.

Bacteria contaminate all surgical wounds; a minority of wounds actually demonstrates clinical infection. In most patients, infection does not develop because innate host defenses are efficient against contaminants at the surgical site.

Surgical incision activates 5 critical initiators of the human inflammatory response:

- Coagulation proteins and platelets (hemostatic mechanism)
- Mast cells and complement proteins
- Bradykinin (produced from its ubiquitous protein precursor).

The effect is vasodilation and increased local blood flow with velocity reduction in order to aid the margination of phagocytes. The increasing vascular permeability and local vasodilation facilitates the formation of edema, creating more space between endothelial cells and providing phagocytic access to the injured soft tissue and aqueous conduits for their navigation through the normally condensed extracellular tissues.

After this phase we have both nonspecific chemoattractant signals and specific chemokine signals (from mast cells) that "draw" neutrophil, monocyte and other leukocyte populations into the area of the surgical site.

"Phagocytes' recruitment" into the wound before bacterial contamination actually occurs from the procedure itself (innate host defenses) and gives the patient an advantage against infection as an outcome.

Chemoattractant signaling proteins bind to local vascular endothelial cells and upregulate selectin proteins on their endothelial surface.

Neutrophils move on the endothelial surface within the post-capillary venule. Further interaction between neutrophil and endothelial cell adhesion proteins link the neutrophil to endothelial cell's surface and the chemoattractant gradient leads neutrophil to the site of injury inducing systematic ingestion and digestion of any microbial contaminants.

During the first 24 h monocytes enter the surgical site. If microbial contamination has been minimal and the early arriving neutrophils have been able to adequately control the bacteria, then monocytes produce local chemical signals to regulate the wound-healing process. Myofibrocytes migrate into the fibrin matrix of the wound and collagen deposition displaces its fibrin latticework.

Otherwise, if microbial contamination and proliferation overwhelm the initial neutrophil infiltration, the monocyte becomes a proinflammatory cell with cytokines' release (Tumor necrosis factor—TNF—alpha). The effects are:

- Potent paracrine signal to upregulate neutrophil activity
- TNF-alpha-stimulated neutrophils consume microbes, and lysosomal vacuoles may release reactive oxygen intermediates and acid hydrolases into the extracellular space from its lysosomal vacuoles.

- The extracellular release of reactive oxygen intermediates and the acid hydrolases results in lipid peroxidation of the local environment, with further tissue injury and further activation of the initiator signals.
- The inflammatory response is further intensified.
- Interleukin (IL)-1, IL-6, and other proinflammatory signals are released by the activated monocyte and serve as endocrine signals responsible for fever, stimulation of acute-phase reactants, and other responses.
- The wound is, actually, a host-pathogen battlefield, filled with necrotic tissue, neutrophils, bacteria, and proteinaceous fluid that together constitute pus.

The viable tissues around exhibit the classic signs of inflammation:

- Rubor reflects local vasodilation.
- Calor is the warmth of the vasodilated tissues resulting in increased heat conduction.
- Tumor is due to edema.
- Dolor occurs from stimulation of nerve nociceptors by the numerous products of the inflammatory cascade and tissue injury and distension.
- Functio Laesa is the unavoidable inhibition of normal anatomical function.

Four different determinants lead to either uneventful wound healing or SSI: (1) inoculum of bacteria, (2) virulence of bacteria, (3) adjuvant effects of microenvironment, and (4) innate and acquired host defenses.

Contaminants may enter the wound from the air in the OR, from the instruments or surgeon(s). Skin bacteria are always present. The largest inoculum occurs when the operation involves a body structure heavily colonized by bacteria, such as the bowel (10^3–10^4 bacteria/mL distal in small bowel, 10^5–10^6 bacteria/mL in right colon, and 10^{10}–10^{12} bacteria/g of stool in rectosigmoid colon). Bacteria are also present in the stomach of older patients who have hypo or achlorhydria. Significant concentrations of bacteria are encountered in the biliary tract (patients older than 70 years of age, obstructive jaundice, common bile duct stones, acute cholecystitis). Procedures involving the female genital tract will encounter 10^6–10^7 bacteria/mL [7–9]

The more virulent the contaminant, the greater the probability of infection. Coagulase-positive staphylococci require a smaller inoculum than the coagulase-negative species. Uncommon but virulent strains of *Clostridium perfringens* or Group A streptococci require only a small inoculum to cause an especially severe necrotizing infection at the surgical site. *Escherichia coli* has endotoxin in its outer cell membrane that gives it a particular virulence. *Bacteroides fragilis* and other Bacteroides species are ordinarily organisms of minimal virulence as solitary pathogens, but when combined with other oxygen-consuming organisms, they will result in microbial synergism and cause very significant infection following operations of the colon or female genital tract. Due to the intrinsic features of this variable (related to procedure and patient's colonizing bacteria) it's difficult to control it by preventive strategies.

Adjuvant factors (secondary to the surgical procedure) in the microenvironment of the wound may result in clinical infection:

- Hemoglobin by the release of ferric iron during the degradation of red blood cells and stimulation of microbial proliferation
- Necrotic tissue can act as a haven for contaminants avoiding phagocytic action
- Foreign bodies (braided sutures)
- Dead space

Impaired host defenses could be innate or acquired.

In the first case is difficult to elaborate strategy based on the measure of differences between groups of patients (more or less "competent" against infections).

Otherwise, acquired impairment is linked to increased rates of SSI. Shock and hypoxemia are positively associated with SSI, especially in trauma patients. Transfusion appears to be immunosuppressive. Chronic illnesses, hypoalbuminemia (is the most robust predictor of infectious complications after major abdominal surgery) and malnutrition are significant factors. Hypothermia and hyperglycemia are also responsible.

Medications (especially corticosteroids) may also adversely affect the host and increase SSI rates.

The pathophysiology of SSI is complex, even more if we consider all the determinants in a common context focusing on specific causes of an infection (the so called "Aggregate Effect").

1.3.1   Risk Factors

Numerous risk factors have been identified for the development of an SSI and we can identify two broad categories affecting the outcome at three different levels:

intrinsic (patient related level, modifiable, or non-modifiable) factors
extrinsic (operative level and institutional level) factors

Patient related factors are:

- Individual characteristics (sex, age, frailty, dependence, socioeconomic status)
- Lifestyle (smoking, alcohol)
- Comorbidities (diabetes, chronic obstructive pulmonary disease, congestive heart failure, acute myocardial infarction, renal insufficiency, hypertension, osteoporosis, Charlson comorbidity score)
- Medications (immunosuppression)
- Prior environment (preoperative length of stay, admission from a long-term facility)
- Risk calculators—scoring system (NNIS, ASA)
- Operative level

- Procedure
  - Incision class
  - Type of surgery
  - Elective vs emergency procedure
  - Case complexity
  - Surgery duration
  - Blood loss / Transfusions
  - Medical device implant
- Institutional level
- Current environment
  - Safety culture
- Hospital
  - Size
- Experience
  - Physician
  - Facility

Potentially modifiable patient risk factors include glycemic control and pre-surgery diabetic evaluation, alcohol and smoking abuse, preoperative albumin <3.5 mg/dL, total bilirubin >1.0 mg/dL, obesity, and immunosuppression. Non-modifiable patient factors include increasing age, recent radiotherapy, and history of skin or soft tissue infection.

Procedure-related factors include emergency and more complex surgery and wound classification.

Facility risk factors include inadequate ventilation, increased operating room (OR) traffic, and appropriate sterilization of equipment. Preoperative risk factors include presence of a preexisting infection; inadequate skin preparation; hair removal; and antibiotic choice, administration, and duration. Intraoperative risk factors include duration of surgery, blood transfusion, maintenance of asepsis, poor-quality surgical hand scrubbing and gloving, hypothermia, and poor glycemic control.

Different surgical sites may contribute to the risk of developing clinical infection. Stratification into groups that have similar risks for infection is crucial to implement preventive strategies among similar patients and to identify infection rates variation from benchmark within an institution. Assessment of gross SSI rates without stratification is likely to be a reflection of patient risk rather than quality of performance. SSIs are a significant healthcare quality issue, resulting in increased morbidity, disability, length of stay, mortality, resource utilization, and costs. Identification of high-risk patients may improve preoperative counseling, inform resource utilization and allow modifications in perioperative management to optimize outcomes.

Many risk factors are beyond practitioner control, but optimizing perioperative conditions can certainly help decrease infection risk.

High-risk surgical patients may be identified on the basis of individual risk factors or combinations of them. In particular, statistical models and risk calculators may be useful in predicting infectious risks, both in general and for SSIs. These models differ in the number of variables; inclusion of preoperative, intraoperative or postoperative variables; ease of calculation and specificity for particular procedures. Furthermore, the models differ in their accuracy in stratifying risk.

Although multiple strategies exist for identifying surgical patients at high risk for SSIs, no one strategy is superior for all patients, and further efforts are necessary to determine if risk stratification in combination with risk modification can reduce SSIs in this patients' population [10].

Early evaluation of perioperative SSI risk factors and patient risk stratification could be of great value in the development of predictive risk models. Predictive risk models could, in turn, assist surgeons and their patients in the clinical decision-making process (e.g., counseling patients on the appropriateness and risks of surgery). In addition, risk models could be used to develop targeted perioperative prevention strategies and diagnostic care process models and improve risk adjustment for risk modeling used in the public reporting of SSI as a quality metric.

However, a study reviewing SSIs in patients undergoing colorectal resections (C-SSIs), identified from an institutional ACS-NSQIP dataset (2006–2014), showed that risk prediction models do not accurately predict C-SSI in their own independent institutional dataset.

Published C-SSI risk scores: the National Nosocomial Infection Surveillance (NNIS), Contamination, Obesity, Laparotomy, and American Society of Anesthesiologists (ASA) class (COLA), Preventie Ziekenhuisinfecties door Surveillance (PREZIES) and NSQIP-based models were compared with receiver operating characteristic (ROC) analysis to evaluate discriminatory quality.

There were 2376 cases included, with an overall C-SSI rate of 9% (213 cases). None of the models produced reliable and high quality C-SSI predictions. For any C-SSI, the NNIS c-index was 0.57 vs 0.61 for COLA, 0.58 for PREZIES, and 0.62 for NSQIP: all well below the minimum "reasonably" predictive c-index of 0.7. Predictions for superficial, deep, and organ space SSI were similarly poor.

Published C-SSI risk prediction models do not accurately predict C-SSI in their independent institutional dataset. Application of externally developed prediction models to any individual practice must be validated or modified to account for institution and case-mix specific factors. This questions the validity of using externally or nationally developed models for "expected" outcomes and interhospital comparisons.

1.3.2 Preop Measures

Thirteen recommendations (made by the WHO) were published on Lancet in 2016 covering the preoperative path of surgical patients and taking into account evidence quality, cost and resource use implications, patient values and preferences.

1.3.3 Perioperative Discontinuation of Immunosuppressive Agents

It's not indicate to discontinue immunosuppressive medication before surgery to prevent SSI (conditional recommendation, very low quality of evidence). The decision should be made on an individual basis, involving the prescribing physician, the patient, and the surgeon.

1.3.4 Enhanced Nutritional Support

It's possible to consider the administration of oral or enteral multiple nutrient-enhanced nutritional formulas to prevent SSI in underweight patients who undergo major surgical operations (conditional recommendation, very low quality of evidence). Multiple nutrient-enhanced formulas can be used to prevent SSIs in adult patients undergoing major surgery. However, it is expensive and requires additional work for clinical staff, including expertise from dietitians and pharmacists. When considering this intervention in the context of a priority assessment approach to reduce the SSI risk, resources and product availability should be carefully assessed, particularly in settings with limited resources.

1.3.5 Preoperative Bathing

Good clinical practice requires that patients bathe or shower before surgery. Both a plain or antimicrobial soap can be used for this purpose (conditional recommendation, moderate quality of evidence. Evidence was insufficient to formulate any recommendation on the use of chlorhexidine gluconate-impregnated cloths for the purpose of reducing SSIs.

Decolonization with mupirocin ointment with or without CHG body wash in nasal carriers of *Staphylococcus aureus* undergoing cardiothoracic and orthopedic surgery / other types of surgery

Patients undergoing cardiothoracic and orthopedic surgeries, who are known nasal carriers of *S. aureus*, should receive perioperative intranasal applications of mupirocin 2% ointment with or without a combination of chlorhexidine gluconate body wash (strong recommendation, moderate quality of evidence). It's to consider the use of the same treatment in patients with known nasal carriage of *S. aureus* undergoing other types of surgery (conditional recommendation, moderate quality of evidence). *S. aureus* is one of the most common health-care-associated pathogen worldwide with increased mortality when it has methicillin-resistance patterns.

S. aureus nasal carriage is a well-defined risk factor for subsequent infection in various patient groups. Mupirocin nasal ointment (usually applied twice daily for 5 days) is an effective, safe, and fairly cheap treatment for the eradication of *S. aureus* carriage and is generally used in combination with a whole body wash. A meta-regression analysis showed that the effect on the *S. aureus* infection prevalence did not differ between different types of surgery ($p = 0.986$). To avoid unnecessary treatment and resistance spread, this intervention should be done only on known *S. aureus* carriers. Therefore, these recommendations apply to facilities where screening for *S. aureus* is feasible, and indeed, studies were done mostly in high-income countries. There is no recommendation on the role of screening for *S. aureus* carriage or the surgical patient population that should undergo screening.

1.3.6 MBP with/without the Use of Oral Antibiotics

Preoperative oral antibiotics combined with mechanical bowel preparation (MBP) should be used to reduce the risk of SSI in adult patients undergoing elective colorectal surgery (conditional recommendation, moderate quality evidence) and MBP alone (without administration of oral antibiotics) should not be used (strong recommendation, moderate quality evidence). There is no recommendation on the preferred type of oral antibiotic, including the timing of administration and dosage, but an activity against both facultative Gram-negative and anaerobic bacteria should be guaranteed and non-absorbable antibiotics should be used preferably. The choice should be made according to local availability, updated resistance data within institutions and the volume of surgical activity. This intervention is for preoperative use only and should not be continued postoperatively. The use of oral antibiotics in association with MBP does not replace the need for intravenous surgical antibiotic prophylaxis.

1.3.7 Hair Removal

In patients undergoing any surgical procedure, hair should either not be removed or, if absolutely necessary, it should be removed only with a clipper. Shaving is strongly discouraged at all times, whether preoperatively or in the operating room (strong recommendation, moderate quality of evidence).

When hair is removed, clipping significantly reduces SSIs compared with shaving (OR 0.51; 0.29–0.91). Because they have similar potential to cause microscopic skin trauma, no hair removal and clipping were combined in an additional meta-analysis, which showed that they are associated with significantly reduced prevalence of SSIs compared with shaving (combined OR 0.51; 0.34–0.78). No recommendation regarding the timing of hair removal could be formulated as only one study assessed this question with no relevant results, but the panel suggested that removal by clipping shortly before surgery is the safest approach, if required.

1.3.8 Optimal/Precise Timing for Administration of SAP

Is suggested the administration of SAP before surgical incision, if indicated, depending on the type of operation (strong recommendation, low quality of evidence); it should be done within the 120 min before the incision, while considering the half-life of the antibiotic (strong recommendation, moderate quality of evidence).

Successful SAP requires delivery of the antimicrobial agent in effective concentrations to the operative site through intravenous administration at the appropriate time.

On the basis of the available evidence, a more precise timing of less than 120 min before incision cannot be defined, and the widely implemented recommendation of within 60 min before incision is not supported by evidence. The half-life of the agent used, the underlying condition(s) of the individual patient (e.g., body-mass index, or renal or liver function), the time needed to complete the procedure, and the protein binding of the antibiotic should be taken into account to achieve adequate serum and tissue concentrations at the surgical site at the time of incision and up to wound closure—in particular to prevent incisional SSI. Administration should be closer to the incision time (<60 min before) for antibiotics with a short half-life (cefazolin, cefoxitin, and penicillins in general). Most available guidelines recommend a single preoperative dose; intraoperative redosing is indicated if the duration of the procedure exceeds two half-lives of the drug, or if there is excessive blood loss during the procedure.

1.3.9 Surgical Hand Preparation

Surgical hand preparation should be done either by scrubbing with a suitable antimicrobial soap and water or using a suitable alcohol-based hand rub (ABHR) before donning sterile gloves (strong recommendation, moderate quality of evidence).

Is crucial to maintain the least possible contamination of the surgical field, especially in the case of sterile glove puncture during the procedure. Appropriate surgical hand preparation is recommended in the WHO guidelines on hand hygiene in health care issued in 2009 and in all other existing national and international guidelines for the prevention of SSIs.

When selecting an ABHR, health-care facilities should procure products with proven efficacy according to international standards and position no-touch or elbow-operated dispensers in surgical scrub rooms. In LMICs in which ABHR availability might be low, WHO strongly encourages facilities to undertake the local production of an alcohol-based formulation (feasible and low-cost).

Alternatively, antimicrobial soap, clean running water, and disposable or clean towels for each health-care worker should be available in the scrub room.

1.3.10 Surgical Site Preparation

Alcohol-based antiseptic solutions (based on chlorhexidine gluconate) should be used for surgical site skin preparation in patients undergoing surgical procedures (strong recommendation, low to moderate quality of evidence).

The aim is to reduce the microbial load on the patient's skin as much as possible before incision. The most common agents include chlorhexidine gluconate and povidone-iodine in alcohol-based solutions, but aqueous solutions are also widely used in LMICs, particularly those containing iodophors.

Operating room staff should be trained and informed about the potential harms associated with the solutions used for surgical site preparation. Alcohol-based solutions should not be used on neonates or come into contact with mucosa or eyes and caution should be exercised because of their flammable nature. Chlorhexidine gluconate solutions can cause skin irritation and must not be allowed to come into contact with the brain, meninges, eye or middle ear. Alcohol-based solutions might be difficult to procure and expensive in LMICs, particularly when combined with an antiseptic compound. Local production could be affordable and feasible in these settings, provided that adequate quality control is in place.

1.3.11 Antimicrobial Skin Sealants

Antimicrobial sealants should not be used after surgical site skin preparation for the purpose of reducing SSI (conditional recommendation, very low quality of evidence).

Antimicrobial skin sealants are sterile, film-forming cyanoacrylate-based sealants commonly applied as an additional antiseptic measure after using standard skin preparation on the surgical site and before skin incision. They are intended to remain in place and block the migration of flora from the surrounding skin into the surgical site by dissolving over several days postoperatively. To avoid unnecessary costs, antimicrobial sealants should not be used after surgical site skin preparation for the purpose of reducing SSIs.

References

1. Haque M, Sartelli M, McKimm J, Abu Bakar M. Health care-associated infections – an overview. Infect Drug Resist. 2018;11:2321–33. Published 2018 Nov 15. https://doi.org/10.2147/IDR.S177247.
2. Centers for Disease Control and Prevention. Acute care hospital surveillance for surgical site infections. http://www.cdc.gov/nhsn/acute-care-hospital/ssi/index.html
3. European Centre for Disease Prevention and Control. Healthcare-associated infections: surgical site infections. In: ECDC. Annual epidemiological report for 2017. Stockholm: ECDC; 2019.
4. Badia JM, Casey AL, Petrosillo N, Hudson PM, Mitchell SA, Crosby C. Impact of surgical site infection on healthcare costs and patient outcomes: a systematic review in six European countries. Journal of Hospital Infection. 2017;96(1):1–15. ISSN 0195-6701, https://doi.org/10.1016/j.jhin.2017.03.004
5. Raahave D. Wound contamination and postoperative infection. A review. Dan Med Bull. 1991;38(6):481–5.
6. Altemeier WA, Culbertson WR, Hummel RP. Surgical considerations of endogenous infections – sources, types, and methods of control. Surg Clin North Am. 1968;48:227–40.
7. Robson MC, Krizek TJ, Heggers JP. Biology of surgical infection. Curr Probl Surg. 1973;March:1–62.

8. Chetlin SH, Elliott DW. Biliary bacteremia. Arch Surg. 1971;102:303–7.
9. Onderdonk AB, Bartlett JG, Louie T, et al. Microbial synergy in experimental intra-abdominal abscess. Infect Immun. 1976;13:22–6.
10. Sartelli M, Pagani L, Iannazzo S, et al. A proposal for a comprehensive approach to infections across the surgical pathway. *World J Emerg Surg*. 2020;15(1):13. Published 2020 Feb 18. https://doi.org/10.1186/s13017-020-00295-3

Antibiotic Prophylaxis: When, How, and How Long?

2

Patrick Bishop O'Neal and Kamal M. F. Itani

2.1 Introduction

Surgical site infections (SSI) are common, morbid, and costly. SSI affects approximately 300,000 surgical patients annually in the United States thus affecting 2–5% of all patients undergoing inpatient surgery. Representing 20% of all hospital-acquired infections, SSIs are the most common of all hospital-acquired infections. In addition to increasing the length of stay by an average of about 10 days, surgical site infections are associated with a twofold to 11-fold increase in mortality. The annual cost of SSI in the United States is estimated between $3.5 billion and $10 billion [1].

The proper use of perioperative antibiotic prophylaxis has been shown to reduce the risk of SSI. In this chapter, we review evidence and recommendations for the use of perioperative antibiotic prophylaxis including indications and proper administration. We also explore trends and challenges to typical recommendations within special populations and with specific operations.

P. B. O'Neal
VA Boston Health Care System, Boston University, Boston, MA, USA
e-mail: Patrick.oneal2@va.gov

K. M. F. Itani (✉)
VA Boston Health Care System, Harvard Medical School, Boston University,
Boston, MA, USA
e-mail: Kamal.Itani@va.gov

© Springer Nature Switzerland AG 2021
M. Sartelli et al. (eds.), *Infections in Surgery*, Hot Topics in Acute Care Surgery
and Trauma, https://doi.org/10.1007/978-3-030-62116-2_2

17

2.2 General Principles and the Surgical Care Improvement Project

In an effort to encourage the proper use of perioperative antibiotic prophylaxis, Mangram, et al., outlined in 1999 four general principles that should guide the practitioner in the use of perioperative antibiotics:

- Antimicrobial agents should be used for all operations in which they have been shown to reduce SSI rates based on evidence from clinical trials or for those operations after which incisional or organ/space SSI would represent a catastrophe.
- Use an antimicrobial agent that is safe, inexpensive, and bactericidal with an in vitro spectrum that covers the most probable intraoperative contaminants for the operation.
- Time the infusion of the initial dose of antimicrobial so that a bactericidal concentration of the drug is established in serum and tissues by the time the skin is incised.
- Maintain therapeutic levels of the antimicrobial agent in both serum and tissues throughout the operation and until, at most, a few hours after the incision is closed in the operating room [2].

Given the high impact of SSI on patient safety and the overall associated healthcare costs, SSI has been a focus of the Surgical Care Improvement Project (SCIP). Formalized in 2006, SCIP set out to standardize care with the goal of reducing the incidence of multiple postoperative complications including SSI. Initially driven by the Centers for Medicare and Medicaid, SCIP draws from the expertise of numerous national health care organizations including the American College of Surgeons and the Joint Commission on Accreditation of Healthcare Organizations. The measures outlined by SCIP have served as metrics to quantify the quality of surgical care.

Although SCIP measures are not currently tracked for the purposes of influencing hospital reimbursement, they continue to be the foundation for SSI prevention. One of the most important measures in preventing SSI is the appropriate use of perioperative antibiotic prophylaxis. As such, three measures were established by SCIP for the appropriate use of perioperative antibiotic prophylaxis.

- SCIP Inf-1: Prophylactic antibiotic should be received within one hour prior to surgical incision.
- SCIP Inf-2: Appropriate choice of prophylactic antibiotic.
- SCIP Inf-3: Prophylactic antibiotics should be discontinued within 24 h of surgery end time.

Updates from the 2017 *Centers for Disease Control and Prevention Guideline for the Prevention of Surgical Site Infection* also clearly state that:

- For clean and clean-contaminated procedures, additional prophylactic antimicrobial agent should not be administered after the surgical incision is closed in the operating room, even in the presence of a drain [3].

2.3   Choice of Perioperative Antibiotic

In choosing the appropriate perioperative antibiotic, one must consider the classification of the wound, i.e., clean vs. clean-contaminated, the organisms likely to be present, and the typical microbial burden of the region or hospital. In considering clean cases, the predominant organisms present are skin flora including staphylococcus species. For these cases, a first-generation cephalosporin such as cefazolin is generally considered the agent of choice for perioperative antibiotic prophylaxis. This agent is effective against most Gram positive and many Gram-negative organisms and generally covers microorganisms in normal skin flora. Additionally, in the spirit of the principles outlined by Mangram, it is generally safe, inexpensive, and bactericidal. In patients with penicillin allergy, clindamycin is a good alternative for clean cases. Again, it covers normal skin flora, is inexpensive, and is generally safe. The accepted initial perioperative dose for clindamycin is 900 mg rather than the 600 mg typically given as maintenance doses for other purposes. In considering patients who are known to be colonized with methicillin-resistant *Staphylococcus aureus* (MRSA), vancomycin should be administered. Again, vancomycin is a relatively inexpensive drug compared to other MRSA-effective agents and is a relatively safe medication in most populations. One should note, however, that there is an increase in risk of acute kidney injury when vancomycin is used rather than cefazolin for perioperative antibiotic prophylaxis. One should weigh the risks and benefits when choosing this agent [4]. Cefazolin may be added with vancomycin as combination therapy, particularly in cardiac surgery, as it exhibits better tissue penetration and improved bactericidal effect on a host of organisms including methicillin-sensitive Staphylococcus aureus than does vancomycin. However, this combination therapy should be judiciously used as it has been shown to increase risk of perioperative acute kidney injury [5]. Clean-contaminated operations, particularly those involving enteric organisms, require anaerobic organism coverage. Although other agents such as second generation cephalosporins (i.e., cefoxitin and cefotetan) as well as ampicillin-sulbactam were commonly used in the past, their effectiveness has decreased with the emergence of resistant organisms. The combination of cefazolin and metronidazole remains efficacious and is generally the preferred perioperative antibiotic regimen for those clean-contaminated cases likely to require coverage for anaerobic organisms. This combination also honors the requirements of safety and cost-effectiveness. A list of common prophylactic antibiotics and dosing parameters is presented in Table 2.1.

Table 2.1 Suggested initial dose and time to redosing for antimicrobial drugs commonly utilized for surgical prophylaxis[a]

Antimicrobial	Standard dose[b]	Weight-based dose recommendation[c]	Recommended redosing interval,[d] in hours
Cefazolin	1–2 g iv	20–30 mg/kg (if <80 kg, use 1 g; if >80 kg, use 2 g)	2–5
Cefoxitin	1–2 g iv	20–40 mg/kg	2–3
Cefotetan	1–2 g iv	20–40 mg/kg	3–6
Ciprofloxacin	400 mg iv	400 mg	4–10
Clindamycin	900 mg iv	If <10 kg, use at least 37.5 mg; if >10 kg, use 3–6 mg/kg	3–6
Erythromycin base	1 g po 19, 18, and 9 h before surgery	9–13 mg/kg	NA
Neomycin	1 g po 19, 18, and 9 h before surgery	20 mg/kg	NA
Metronidazole	0.5–1 g iv	15 mg/kg initial dose (adult); 7.5 mg/kg on subsequent doses	6–8
Vancomycin	1 g iv	10–15 mg/kg (adult)	6–12

The intervals in the table were calculated for patients with normal renal function
[a]Adapted from Bratzler [26]
[b]Dose may vary with renal function
[c]Data are primarily from published pediatric recommendations
[d]For procedures of long duration, antimicrobials should be readministered at intervals of 1–2 times the half-life of the drug

2.4   Is the 60-Minute Timing Important?

It is important to ensure that adequate serum and tissue concentrations of antibiotic have been reached at the time of incision. This entails administration of perioperative antibiotic within one hour of incision. This is particularly true given the pharmacokinetics of most widely used prophylactic antibiotics including cefazolin. A two-hour infusion window is required for vancomycin and the quinolones in order to avoid the side effects of rapid administration of these agents. This principle of dosing within a one-hour window is the result of a sentinel study by Classen, et al., who reviewed 2847 patients that underwent a wide range of clean and clean-contaminated general, gynecologic, and orthopedic operations from which the timing of antibiotic administration was electronically reported. In this study, patients received antibiotic prophylaxis at a wide range of time points from several hours prior to incision to several hours after incision. It was noted that the frequency in which surgical wound infection was the lowest was in patients who received prophylaxis within an hour of incision [6]. A more recent study by Hawn and colleagues [7] suggests that the 60-min timing window may not be as critical and may be variable based on surgical specialty. Nonetheless, observing the 60-min metric facilitates standardization of care within a healthcare system and remains a good goal to achieve.

2.5 Weight-Based Dosing

Achieving minimal inhibitory concentrations within the serum and tissues may be a challenge in obese patients. For this reason, weight-based dosing of antimicrobials should be instituted to achieve optimal serum concentration in these patients. Studies as far back as the 1980s recognized that blood and tissue levels of cefazolin are consistently below the minimal inhibitory concentrations of the common pathogens responsible for causing surgical site infections in obese patients who received a 1 g versus a 2 g cefazolin dose [8]. In a 2016 study of bariatric operations that evaluated serum and tissue concentrations of perioperative antibiotic, it was found that weight-based dosing showed improved attainment of target concentrations than did fixed doses of antibiotic [9]. These data highlight the risk of under-dosing perioperative antibiotics in the obese patient and should raise awareness about proper dosing of each prophylactic antibiotic used. It should be noted as well that under-dosing perioperative antibiotics places patients at risk for the emergence of resistant organisms. Guidelines for weight-based dosing of common perioperative prophylactic antibiotics is presented in Table 2.1.

2.6 Importance of Redosing as a Function of Operative Duration

Not only is it important to achieve the minimum inhibitory concentration of the perioperative antibiotic at the time of incision, but it should also be maintained for the duration of the operation. As one would anticipate, during long cases, the serum and tissue concentration of perioperative antibiotic decay based on half-life. For this reason, it is recommended that the prophylactic antibiotic be redosed every two half-lives. The time for repeat doses should be measured from the time of initial dose and not from the time of incision [10]. To illustrate this principle, Zanetti, et al., retrospectively evaluated 1548 patients who received cefazolin as perioperative antibiotic prophylaxis during cardiac surgery. It was found that, in patients whose operations were over 400 min, antibiotic redosing had a beneficial effect. Surgical site infection occurred in 16.0% of patients who did not have their antibiotic redosed, whereas those who did have a repeat dose only had a 7.7% incidence of surgical site infection [11]. The half-life of the most common perioperative antibiotic, cefazolin is about 1.2–2.2 h. One should expect to redose cefazolin approximately every 3–4 h. Further guidelines for redosing intervals of various antibiotics can be found in Table 2.1.

2.7 Importance of Redosing as a Function of Blood Loss

Not only is it important to redose antibiotics as a function of operative time, it should also be recognized that operative cases with heavy blood loss or administration of a large amount of intravenous fluids are expected to have a more rapid decrease in serum and tissue concentrations of antibiotic. As such, antibiotics administered to patients under those circumstances should be redosed at earlier intervals. In support of this principle, Swoboda et al., evaluated serum and tissue samples from patients undergoing spinal surgery. Although serum concentrations of cefazolin were nonlinearly affected by blood loss, tissue concentrations were directly related to blood loss. Based on the pharmacokinetics of this decrease in tissue concentration, it was advised that cefazolin be redosed in patients with over 1500 ml intraoperative blood loss [12]. This recommendation has been further supported through joint guidelines created by American Society of Health-System Pharmacists, the Infectious Diseases Society of America, the Surgical Infection Society, and the Society for Healthcare Epidemiology of America [10].

2.8   Avoid Additional Antibiotic Once the Wound Is Closed

Over time, recommendations regarding the duration of perioperative antibiotic administration have become progressively shorter. Older guidelines recommended that perioperative antibiotic prophylaxis should not exceed 24 h. The Centers for Disease Control and Prevention Guideline for the Prevention of Surgical Site Infection 2017 no longer supports the administration of perioperative antibiotics for clean and clean-contaminated cases once the incision is closed [3]. Evidence in support of this more restrictive pattern of antibiotic prophylaxis include the lack of benefit of repeated postoperative dosing, the emergence of drug resistant bacteria, increased risk of *Clostridium difficile* infection with prolonged dosing regimens, and increased risk of acute kidney injury with prolonged dosing regimens [10, 13].

2.9   Perioperative Antibiotic Use in Special Populations

With the increasing concern about emergence of resistant organisms, *Clostridium difficile* infections, and side effects of antimicrobials, the universal use of prophylactic perioperative antibiotics, particularly in the setting of clean cases, has undergone scrutiny. The surgical community has identified various subgroups of clean cases that may not fit the mold and which may be better managed with less aggressive or even entire avoidance of perioperative antibiotic prophylaxis. On the other hand, other cases might be better served by a more aggressive perioperative antibiotic prophylaxis regimen.

2.9.1   Inguinal Hernia Repair

In 2018, The HerniaSurge Group, an international consortium of experts in the field of hernia repair surgery issued the International Guidelines for Groin Hernia Management [14]. One of the focuses of this Group was to outline recommendations regarding the appropriate use of perioperative antibiotics in inguinal hernia repair with mesh. The recommendations, which were based largely on data from a 2012 Cochrane Database meta-analysis [15], concluded that, in open inguinal hernia repair, administration of prophylactic antibiotics should be avoided in average-risk patients undergoing surgery in a low-risk environment. Conversely, the Group concluded that the use of perioperative antibiotic prophylaxis is warranted in high-risk patient undergoing open inguinal hernia surgery in a low-risk environment and in any patients undergoing open inguinal hernia surgery in a high-risk environment. They also acknowledge an increased risk of SSI in patients undergoing bilateral open inguinal hernia repair and in patients undergoing repair of recurrent inguinal hernias. The Group does not recommend perioperative antibiotic prophylaxis for patients undergoing laparoscopic inguinal hernia repair in any environment.

2.9.2   Breast Surgery

In 2014, prophylactic antibiotic use in the setting of surgery for breast cancer was analyzed and reported in a Cochrane review. This study concluded that perioperative antibiotic prophylaxis reduced the rate of surgical site infection in breast surgery [16].

2.9.3   Endocrine Surgery

Endocrine surgeons have long questioned the utility of perioperative antibiotics in open thyroid and parathyroid surgery often citing increased risk of antibiotic related complications such as *Clostridium difficile* infection, increased cost, and lack of efficacy in reducing surgical site infection. Although, practice patterns continue to vary, Fachinetti, et al., concluded in their 2017 literature review that antibiotic prophylaxis is not indicated in standard transcervical thyroid and parathyroid surgery. Rather, they highlight the importance of proper patient preparation, observation of strict sterile technique, and management of patient comorbidity as paramount in reducing perioperative surgical site infection [17].

2.9.4   Cardiac Surgery

Patients undergoing cardiac surgery have often received prolonged periods of antibiotic prophylaxis, often until all drains and chest tubes have been removed. Justification for this practice refers to the unique characteristics of cardiac surgery including the use of cardiopulmonary bypass and systemic cooling procedures, the use of invasive devices remaining after surgery, and the seriousness of complications associated with cardiac surgery resulting in substantial morbidity and mortality. For this reason, cardiac surgeons have advocated for 48 h of antibiotic prophylaxis in cardiac surgery. However, an extensive body of work challenges this practice, showing that periods of antibiotic prophylaxis past 48 h and often even past 24 h do not decrease the risk of surgical site infection and can often lead to an increase risk of antibiotic complications including *Clostridium difficile* and the emergence of resistant organisms. This has resulted in newer recommendations and consensus guidelines by multiple professional societies [18].

- The Society of Thoracic Surgeons
- There is evidence indicating that antibiotic prophylaxis of 48-hours duration is effective. There is some evidence that single-dose prophylaxis or 24-hour prophylaxis may be as effective as 48-hour prophylaxis, but additional studies are necessary before confirming the effectiveness of prophylaxis lasting less than 48 h. There is no evidence that prophylaxis administered for longer than 48 h is more effective than a 48-hour regimen even with tubes and drains in place.
- Paul-Ehrlich Society for Chemotherapy (Germany)
- Prophylaxis for 24 h or less may be appropriate for cardiothoracic procedures. This recommendation is based on consensus of the expert panel as no definitive data is available about the optimal duration of prophylaxis.
- Surgical Infection Prevention Guideline Writers Workgroup
- The consensus of the workgroup is that administration of prophylaxis for <24 h is acceptable and that there is no evidence that providing antimicrobials for longer periods will reduce surgical site infection rates.
- American College of Cardiology/American Heart Association Task Force
- Data suggest that a 1-day course of intravenous antimicrobials is as efficacious as the traditional 48-hour (or longer) regimen.
- American Society of Health-System Pharmacists Commission on Therapeutics
- Prophylaxis for 24 h or less may be appropriate for cardiothoracic procedures.

2.9.5 Joint Arthroplasty

Joint arthroplasty represents another field in which a surgical site infection would result in a devastating complication, often requiring extensive additional surgery and even removal of hardware. For this reason, it is recommended that prophylactic antibiotics, generally cefazolin (or vancomycin in MRSA colonized patients), be administered within 1 h of incision and tourniquet placement and be redosed as appropriate given the length of the operation and in response to unusual blood loss [19, 20]. Previous recommendations suggested that prophylaxis be administered for 24 h after surgery; however, current guidelines by the U.S. Centers for Disease Control and Prevention now recommend that, even in prosthetic joint arthroplasty, in clean and clean-contaminated cases, additional antimicrobial should not be administered after the incision is closed, even in the presence of a drain [3].

2.9.6 Tunneled Central Venous Catheter Placement

Historically, perioperative antibiotics have often been given to patients undergoing tunneled central venous catheter placement given the concern for implantation of a foreign body and the risk for catheter infection often requiring catheter removal. In 2011, a Cochrane Review was performed to evaluate this practice. The authors evaluated tunneled line placements performed in oncology patients and found that it is not beneficial to administer perioperative antibiotics prior to insertion of the catheter [21].

2.9.7 Colorectal Surgery

In addition to parenteral antibiotic prophylaxis, it is important to acknowledge the use of oral bowel preparation in colorectal surgery when considering reduction in SSI rates. Although the use of mechanical and oral antibiotic bowel preparation has seen variations over the decades, there is extensive literature supporting the use of bowel preparation in colorectal surgery. In 2012, data from the Veterans Administration revealed that oral antibiotic use resulted in a 67% decrease in SSI occurrence (OR = 0.33, 95% CI 0.21–0.53) [22]. After extensive literature review, guidelines by the American Society of Colon and Rectal Surgeons were released in 2019 with a strong recommendation endorsing the combined use of mechanical and oral antibiotic bowel preparation. In these guidelines, the use of antibiotic or mechanical bowel preparations alone as well as no preparation at all are not recommended [23]. See Table 2.1 for recommended dosing of erythromycin and neomycin oral bowel preparation combination.

2.10 Bundles

Despite some controversy between traditional guidelines such as SCIP and various evolving societal guidelines, it should be recognized that general antibiotic stewardship should be observed in an effort to reach the right balance of reducing surgical site infection while minimizing the adverse effects of antibiotic administration. In doing so, one cannot neglect other interventions that may also mitigate patient risk of surgical site infection. The use of care bundles is well recognized to decrease the risk of surgical site infection, and the synergistic effect of these interventions may decrease this risk better than perioperative antibiotic prophylaxis alone [24]. Keenan, et al., for example, evaluated 559 patient undergoing colorectal surgery. In addition to parenteral antibiotic prophylaxis and oral antibiotic bowel preparation, preventative measures observed included maintenance of strict normoglycemia and normothermia, wound dressings left in place for 48 h, changing of gown and gloves prior to fascial closure, dedicated wound closure tray, and minimizing superfluous operating room traffic. After implementation of the bundle, surgical site infection incidence decreased from 19.3% to 2.4% [25].

2.11   Conclusion

Appropriate use of perioperative antibiotic prophylaxis is paramount in the reduction of SSI. When appropriate, perioperative antibiotic prophylaxis should be used with the goal of achieving therapeutic serum and tissue levels while the incision is open. In order to achieve this, (1) the antibiotic must be administered at the appropriate time, traditionally within one hour of surgery, (2) the dose of antibiotic may need to be adjusted based on patient weight, (3) the antibiotic should be redosed at approximately every two half-lives, and (4) antibiotic should be redosed based on large volume resuscitations and heavy blood loss. The antibiotic used should be relatively safe, inexpensive, and efficacious against the probable organisms present at the time of surgery. The duration of perioperative antibiotic use has become progressively shorter and is sometimes not recommended at all. When used, most guidelines suggest stopping antibiotic prophylaxis once the incision is closed. A paradigm shift based on evidence and consensus is evolving toward no antibiotic usage in certain clean surgeries.

References

1. Ban KA, Minei JP, Laronga C, et al. American College of Surgeons and surgical infection society: surgical site infection guidelines, 2016 update. J Am Coll Surg. 2016;224:59–74.
2. Mangram AJ, Horan TC, Pearson ML, et al. Guideline for prevention of surgical site infection, 1999. Infect Control Hosp Epidemiol. 1999;20(4):250–80.
3. Berrios-Torres SI, Umscheid CA, Bratzler DW, et al. Centers for Disease Control and Prevention guideline for the prevention of surgical site infection, 2017. JAMA Surg. 2017;152(8):784–91.
4. Branch-Elliman W, O'Brien W, Strymish J, et al. Association of Duration and Type of surgical prophylaxis with antimicrobial-associated adverse events. JAMA Surg. 2019;154(7):590–8.
5. Branch-Elliman W, Ripollone JE, O'Brien WJ, et al. Risk of surgical site infection, acute kidney injury, and Clostridium difficile infection following antibiotic prophylaxis with vancomycin plus a beta-lactam versus either drug alone: a national propensity-score-adjusted retrospective cohort study. PLoS Med. 2017;14(7):e1002340. https://doi.org/10.1371/journal.pmed.1002340
6. Classen DC, Evans RS, Pestotnik SL, et al. The timing of prophylactic administration of antibiotics and the risk of surgical-wound infection. N Engl J Med. 1992;326:281–6.
7. Hawn MT, Richman JS, Vick CC, et al. Timing of surgical antibiotic prophylaxis and the risk of surgical site infection. JAMA Surg. 2013;148(7):649–57.
8. Forse RA, Karam B, MacLean LD, Christou NV. Antibiotic prophylaxis for surgery in morbidly obese patients. Surgery. 1989;106:750–6.
9. Moine P, Mueller SW, Schoen JA, et al. Pharmacokinetic and pharmacodynamic evaluation of a weight-based dosing regimen of cefoxitin for perioperative surgical prophylaxis in obese and morbidly obese patients. Antimicrob Agents Chemother. 2016 Oct;60(10):5885–93.
10. Bratzler DW, Dellinger EP, Olsen KM, et al. Clinical practice guidelines for antimicrobial prophylaxis in surgery. Am J Health Syst Pharm. 2013 Feb 1;70(3):195–283.
11. Zanetti G, Giardina R, Platt R. Intraoperative redosing of cefazolin and risk for surgical site infection in cardiac surgery. Emerg Infect Dis. 2001;7(5):828–31.
12. Swoboda SM, Merz C, Kostuik J, et al. Does intraoperative blood loss affect antibiotic serum and tissue concentrations? Arch Surg. 1996 Nov;131(11):1165–71.
13. Branch-Elliman W, O'Brien W, Strymish J, et al. Association of duration and type of surgical prophylaxis with antimicrobial-associated adverse events. JAMA Surg. 2019;154(7):590–8.

14. The HerniaSurge Group. International guidelines for groin hernia management. Hernia. 2018;22:1–165.

15. Sanchez-Manuel FJ, Lozano-Garcia J, Seco-Gil JL. Antibiotic prophylaxis for hernia repair. Cochrane Database Syst Rev. 2012 Feb 15;2:CD003769.

16. Jones DJ, Bunn F, Bell-Syer SV. Prophylactic antibiotics to prevent surgical site infection after breast cancer surgery. Cochrane Database Syst Rev. 2014 Mar 9;3:CD005360.

17. Fanchineti A, Chiappa C, Arlant V, et al. Antibiotic prophylaxis in thyroid surgery. Gland Surg. 2017 Oct;6(5):525–9.

18. Hamouda K, Oezkur M, Sinha B, et al. Different duration strategies of perioperative antibiotic prophylaxis in adult patients undergoing cardiac surgery: an observational study. J Cardiothorac Surg. 2015;10:25.

19. Bosco JA, Bookman J, Slover J, et al. Principles of antibiotic prophylaxis in total joint arthroplasty: current concepts. J Am Acad Orhop Surg. 2015 Aug;23(8):e27–35.

20. Yates AJ. Postoperative prophylactic antibiotics in total joint arthroplasty. Arthroplasty Today. 2018:130e131.

21. Van de Wetering MD, Van Woensel JBM. Prophylactic antibiotics for preventing early central venous catheter gram positive infections in oncology patients. Cochrane Database Syst Rev. 2007;24(1):Art. No.: CD003295.

22. Cannon JA, Altom LK, Deierhoi RJ, et al. Preoperative oral antibiotics reduce surgical site infection following elective colorectal resections. Dis Colon Rectum. 2012 Nov;55(11):1160–6.

23. Migaly J, Bafford A, Francone TD, et al. The American Society of Colon and Rectal Surgeons clinical practice guidelines for the use of bowel preparation in elective colon and rectal surgery. Dis Colon Rectum. 2019;62:3–8.

24. Itani MF. Care bundles and prevention of surgical site infection in colorectal surgery. JAMA Surg. 2015 July;314(3):289–90.

25. Keenan JE, Speicher PJ, Thacker JKM, et al. The preventive surgical site infection bundle in colorectal surgery. JAMA Surg. 2014;149(10):1045–52.

26. Bratzler DW, Houck PM. Antimicrobial prophylaxis for surgery: an advisory statement from the National Surgical Infection Prevention Project. Am J Surg. 2005;189(4):395–404.

Intraoperative Measures to Prevent Surgical Site Infections

S. W. De Jonge

3.1 Introduction

The intraoperative period is of great importance to surgical site infection (SSI) prevention. The period is characterized by the performance of the surgical procedure. This inevitably involves breach of the barrier function of the skin and, depending of the type of surgery, that of potentially contaminated hollow viscera. As a consequence, the patient is exposed to in- and external micro-organisms that may cause infection of the surgical site. In addition, consequences of general anesthesia and surgical stress such as hypothermia, hypovolemia, hypoxia, and hyperglycemia may compromise defense mechanisms against these microorganisms and further increase the risk of infection. Arguably the most importvant innovation in intraoperative surgical infection prevention remains the introduction of sterile technique or antisepsis as developed in the nineteenth century by Semmelweis, Lister, and Pasteur [1–3]. Since then, a range of innovations have contributed to further reduction of SSI. As with other innovations in medicine, marketing may precede evidence of effectiveness. Surgeons should therefore strive to stay up to date with scientific developments to ensure adequate resource allocation and optimal use of evidence-based practices. Guidelines issued by the World Health Organization, The Center for Disease Control and others summarized the current state of the art between 2016 and 2018 [4–6]. In this chapter, we will summarize the most important components of intraoperative SSI prevention measures at present time. Preoperative antibiotic prophylaxis is discussed seperately. Broadly, intraoperative measures can be categorized as aimed to minimize exposure to microorganisms, or to support the physiological response against these micro-organisms. Some of the intraoperative preventive measures require other expertise than that of a surgeon and close

S. W. De Jonge (✉)
Department of Surgery, Amsterdam UMC, University of Amsterdam, Amsterdam, The Netherlands
e-mail: s.w.dejonge@amsterdamumc.nl; s.w.dejonge@amc.uva.nl

© Springer Nature Switzerland AG 2021
M. Sartelli et al. (eds.), *Infections in Surgery*, Hot Topics in Acute Care Surgery and Trauma, https://doi.org/10.1007/978-3-030-62116-2_3

collaboration with anesthesiologists and microbiologist is strongly recommended for an effective intraoperative infection prevention strategy.

3.2 Measures to Minimize Exposure to Micro-Organisms

3.2.1 Surgical Hand Preparation

Surgical hand preparation is of vital importance to minimize contamination of the surgical field and is strongly recommended by professional organizations around the world [7]. The use of sterile gloves does not dismiss the need for surgical hand preparation as they regularly puncture unnoticed during surgery [8]. This leaves bodily fluids and other contamination free to transfer from surgeon to patient, and the other way around. Although the requirement of surgical hand preparation has never been proven by randomized controlled trials, there is an abundance of observational research and indirect evidence for its effect [9]. Surgical hand preparation can be performed either by classical scrubbing, using clean water and antimicrobial soap, or by rubbing with an alcohol-based hand rub [6, 7].

3.2.2 Surgical Site Preparation

There is no evidence that routine hair removal helps reduce the risk of SSI. If hair is removed for any other reason, a clipper should be used [6, 10]. Razors increase the risk SSI and should be avoided [6, 10]. To minimize the bacterial load before skin incision, the surgical site should be prepared with an alcohol-based chlorhexidine gluconate solution [6]. Alcohol alone is highly effective in the immediate period after application [11]. The addition chlorhexidine ensures longer antiseptic activity [11]. Povidone iodine in alcohol is a reasonable alternative when chlorhexidine gluconate in alcohol is unavailable or intolerable [6]. Care should be taken that the solution has completely dried before proceeding to surgery as diathermia may ignite the flammable solutions. There is no evidence that (antimicrobial) plastic adhesive skin drapes contribute to a reduction of the incidence of SSI [6]. In open abdominal surgery, a wound protector device may be installed after incision to create a barrier between the clean wound edge and potential contamination from the surgical field [6].

3.2.3 Prophylactic Wound Irrigation

Prophylactic wound irrigation is the application of a flow of solution across the surface of an open wound to remove or dilute bacteria and debris to help prevent infection. Antiseptic additives may provide a further bactericidal effect. As many as 97% of surgeons commonly use prophylactic wound irrigation [12, 13]. However, enormous heterogeneity exists in the solutions used, the surfaces irrigated and the technique of application [14]. There is very limited evidence on the effectiveness of these practices. Only irrigation of the incisional wound with an aqueous povidone iodine solution has been proven effective to help reduce the incidence of SSI in meta-analysis [14]. Notably there is no evidence of effectiveness of irrigation with antibiotic solutions [14]. Considering this, and the contribution to selective pressure, antimicrobial resistance, and other adverse effects, the use of antibiotic solutions for wound irrigation should be avoided [6].

3.2.4 Antimicrobial Coated Sutures

Sutures are used to approximate the skin and aid natural wound healing. However, they also form a potential nidus for infection [15]. Inspired by listers antisepsis, sterile sutures have been in use since the nineteenth century. To prevent colonization and further reduce the risk of SSI, sutures with an antimicrobial coating have been developed in recent years. Sutures with several different coatings are available [16–18]. Of these, triclosan-coated sutures have been studied most extensively. Although there remains controversy on the risk of bias of some of these studies, triclosan-coated sutures were proven effective in a recent meta-analysis of randomized controlled trials [6, 14]. Meta-regression indicated this effect was generalizable across wound contamination and suture types [6, 14].

3.2.5 Laminar Airflow Ventilation Systems

In an effort to reduce contamination from aerosols and other airborne particles, advanced ventilating systems have been developed for operating rooms. Conventional ventilation systems pass fresh air with a mixed or turbulent flow into the operating room. Laminar air flow systems create zones of steady, approximately parallel, streamlines of fresh air through which particles and aerosols are driven out of the operating field. Although these systems have shown to reduce bacterial and particle counts in the air, there is no evidence of a benefit in reducing SSI when compared to conventional ventilation systems [19]. Considering the substantial cost involved, and the lack of evidence of effect, the use of laminar air flow systems is not recommended [6].

3.3 Measures to Support Physiological Protection to Micro-Organisms

3.3.1 Perioperative Oxygenation

Perioperative low tissue oxygen tension is associated with a high risk of SSI [20]. This may be explained by the dependency of neutrophils on oxygen availability for bactericidal superoxide production in oxidative killing [21]. Conversely, increasing tissue tension has been shown to reduce the risk of SSI [22]. Increasing the fraction of inspired oxygen during anesthesia is a relatively easy intervention to achieve this, and early trials showed promising effects on SSI [22]. More recently, the practice became topic of debate due to concerns on potential harms, and doubts on the effectiveness on SSI after negative trials emerged [23]. To address this, the World Health Organization issued two separate systematic reviews; one into potential harms and one into the effect on SSI. The investigators found no evidence of harm of the perioperative use high fraction of inspired oxygen, but also no evidence of benefit overall [24, 25]. However, there was evidence that high perioperative FiO_2 helped reduce the risk of SSI in surgical patients under general anesthesia with tracheal intubation [24]. This effect was not seen in patients under neuraxial anesthesia who were awake, breathing normally or through a facemask [24]. Much has changed since the early promising results, and more variables than administration of oxygen alone are likely at play [26]. While additional research is needed to fully understand the effect of supplemental oxygen on SSI prevention, it remains a cheap and safe intervention worth considering [6].

3.3.2 Maintenance of Adequate Circulating Volume (Normovolemia)

Adequate circulating volume is an essential component of tissue perfusion and thus oxygenation [27]. Delivery of oxygen, but also immune cells and antibiotics, all rely on adequate circulation to be transported to the wound. However, patients undergoing surgery are prone to both hypovolemia and fluid overload due to preoperative fasting, bowel preparation, blood loss, evaporation from the wound surface, or excessive intravenous infusion [28]. Comorbidity may exacerbate these conditions. Both hypo- and hypervolemia lead to poor postoperative outcomes [29, 30]. Trends toward both restricted and aggressive hydration regimens have led to disappointment [31, 32]. Goal directed fluid therapy is a promising new approach that individualizes fluid regimen and titration of vasopressors and inotropics based on dynamic hemodynamic parameters [33]. A wide variety of algorithms using a range of hemodynamic parameters have shown to help reduce the risk of SSI and other adverse events [33]. This broad effectiveness indicates that having a goal-directed algorithm at all may be more important for the reduction of SSI than any specific algorithm in particular [6, 33]. Local expertise and available resources should be taken in to consideration when selecting an algorithm for goal-directed fluid therapy to help prevent SSI [6].

3.3.3 Maintaining Normal Body Temperature (Normothermia)

Adequate body temperature is of vital importance for wound healing and coagulation but unintended perioperative hypothermia is common [34–37]. Patients are inevitably exposed to cold during the operative procedure. Even when the operating room is thoroughly heated to 26 degrees Celsius, this is still 11 degrees colder than the patient's body. In addition, general anesthesia impairs thermoregulation by leading to vasodilatation, redistribution of circulating volume, and eventually accelerated heat loss [38]. In addition to the immediate effects, hypothermia also leads to postoperative peripheral vasoconstriction when patients regain autonomous thermo-regulation [38]. This vasoconstriction in turn impairs tissue oxygen tension and transport of immune cells and antibiotics to the wound site. Active pre-, intra-, and postoperative warming is an easy and effective intervention to help prevent hypothermia and reduce the risk of SSI [6]. Active warming may include the use of forced air heating devices, warming mattresses, warming of intravenous fluids, or ordinary warm blankets depending on resources and availability [6]. Although a target temperature > 36 is generally accepted, no clear evidence exists on the optimal target temperature or the preferred warming method [6].

3.3.4   Use of Protocols for Intensive Perioperative Blood Glucose Control

Surgical stress results in a rise in blood glucose and potentially hyperglycemia through the release of catabolic hormones, impaired insulin production and inhibition of insulin function [39]. Hyperglycemia impairs wound healing through a host of negative effects on normal immune function and consequently increases the risk of SSI [40–42]. Observational research indicates that both diabetic and non-diabetic patients suffer from these perioperative hyperglycemic episodes and the corresponding increased risk of SSI [41, 42]. Glucose control and treatment when indicated may mitigate these risks but concerns on the risk of hypoglycemic episodes have caused controversy about this practice [43, 44]. In particular on the ideal glucose target to balance the risks and benefits. A recent systematic review sought out to identify the optimal perioperative glucose target and found that intensive protocols with glucose target levels <150 mg/dl (8.3 mmol/L) where most effective in reducing SSI with an inherent risk of hypoglycemic events but without an increase in serious adverse events [45].

References

1. Lister J. On the antiseptic principle in the practice of surgery. Br Med J. 1867;2(351):246–8.
2. Semmelweis IP. Die Aetiologie, der Begriff und die Prophylaxis des Kindbettfiebers. Pest, Wien & Leipzig: C. H. Hartleben; 1861.
3. Pasteur L. Recherches sur la putréfaction. Paris: Mallet-Bachelier; 1863.
4. Berrios-Torres SI, Umscheid CA, Bratzler DW, Leas B, Stone EC, Kelz RR, et al. Centers for Disease Control and Prevention guideline for the prevention of surgical site infection, 2017. JAMA Surg. 2017;152(8):784–91.
5. Ban KA, Minei JP, Laronga C, Harbrecht BG, Jensen EH, Fry DE, et al. American College of Surgeons and surgical infection society: surgical site infection guidelines, 2016 update. J Am Coll Surg. 2017;224(1):59–74.
6. Global Guidelines for the Prevention of Surgical Site Infection. WHO Guidelines Approved by the Guidelines Review Committee. Geneva 2018.
7. WHO Guidelines on Hand Hygiene in Health Care: First Global Patient Safety Challenge Clean Care Is Safer Care. WHO Guidelines Approved by the Guidelines Review Committee. Geneva 2009.

8. Misteli H, Weber WP, Reck S, Rosenthal R, Zwahlen M, Fueglistaler P, et al. Surgical glove perforation and the risk of surgical site infection. Arch Surg. 2009;144(6):553–8. discussion 8

9. Tanner J, Dumville JC, Norman G, Fortnam M. Surgical hand antisepsis to reduce surgical site infection. Cochrane Database Syst Rev. 2016;1:CD004288.

10. Tanner J, Norrie P, Melen K. Preoperative hair removal to reduce surgical site infection. Cochrane Database Syst Rev. 2011;11:CD004122.

11. Larson E. Guideline for use of topical antimicrobial agents. Am J Infect Control. 1988;16(6):253–66.

12. Pivot D, Tiv M, Luu M, Astruc K, Aho S, Fournel I. Survey of intraoperative povidone-iodine application to prevent surgical site infection in a French region. J Hosp Infect. 2011;77(4):363–4.

13. Whiteside OJ, Tytherleigh MG, Thrush S, Farouk R, Galland RB. Intra-operative peritoneal lavage – who does it and why? Ann R Coll Surg Engl. 2005;87(4):255–8.

14. de Jonge SW, Boldingh QJJ, Solomkin JS, Allegranzi B, Egger M, Dellinger EP, et al. Systematic review and meta-analysis of randomized controlled trials evaluating prophylactic intra-operative wound irrigation for the prevention of surgical site infections. Surg Infect. 2017;18(4):508–19.

15. Elek SD, Conen PE. The virulence of staphylococcus pyogenes for man; a study of the problems of wound infection. Br J Exp Pathol. 1957;38(6):573–86.

16. Matl FD, Zlotnyk J, Obermeier A, Friess W, Vogt S, Buchner H, et al. New anti-infective coatings of surgical sutures based on a combination of antiseptics and fatty acids. J Biomater Sci Polym Ed. 2009;20(10):1439–49.

17. Obermeier A, Schneider J, Wehner S, Matl FD, Schieker M, von Eisenhart-Rothe R, et al. Novel high efficient coatings for anti-microbial surgical sutures using chlorhexidine in fatty acid slow-release carrier systems. PLoS One. 2014;9(7):e101426.

18. Diener MK, Knebel P, Kieser M, Schüler P, Schiergens TS, Atanassov V, et al. Effectiveness of triclosan-coated PDS plus versus uncoated PDS II sutures for prevention of surgical site infection after abdominal wall closure: the randomised controlled PROUD trial. Lancet. 2014;384(9938):142–52.

19. Bischoff P, Kubilay NZ, Allegranzi B, Egger M, Gastmeier P. Effect of laminar airflow ventilation on surgical site infections: a systematic review and meta-analysis. Lancet Infect Dis. 2017;17(5):553–61.

20. Hopf HW, Hunt TK, West JM, Blomquist P, Goodson WH 3rd, Jensen JA, et al. Wound tissue oxygen tension predicts the risk of wound infection in surgical patients. Arch Surg. 1997;132(9):997–1004. discussion 5

21. Allen DB, Maguire JJ, Mahdavian M, Wicke C, Marcocci L, Scheuenstuhl H, et al. Wound hypoxia and acidosis limit neutrophil bacterial killing mechanisms. Arch Surg. 1997;132(9):991–6.

22. Greif R, Akça O, Horn EP, Kurz A, Sessler DI. Supplemental perioperative oxygen to reduce the incidence of surgical-wound infection. N Engl J Med. 2000;342(3):161–7.

23. Akca O, Ball L, Belda FJ, Biro P, Cortegiani A, Eden A, et al. WHO needs high FIO2? Turk J Anaesthesiol Reanim. 2017;45(4):181–92.

24. de Jonge S, Egger M, Latif A, Loke YK, Berenholtz S, Boermeester M, et al. Effectiveness of 80% vs 30–35% fraction of inspired oxygen in patients undergoing surgery: an updated systematic review and meta-analysis. Br J Anaesth. 2019;122(3):325–34.

25. Mattishent K, Thavarajah M, Sinha A, Peel A, Egger M, Solomkin J, et al. Safety of 80% vs 30–35% fraction of inspired oxygen in patients undergoing surgery: a systematic review and meta-analysis. Br J Anaesth. 2019;122(3):311–24.

26. de Jonge SW, Hollmann MW. Perioperative use of high fraction of inspired oxygen: another null result? Anesth Analg. 2019;128(6):1071–3.

27. Jonsson K, Jensen JA, Goodson WH 3rd, West JM, Hunt TK. Assessment of perfusion in postoperative patients using tissue oxygen measurements. Br J Surg. 1987;74(4):263–7.

28. Voldby AW, Brandstrup B. Fluid therapy in the perioperative setting-a clinical review. J Intensive Care. 2016;4:27.

29. Shin CH, Long DR, McLean D, Grabitz SD, Ladha K, Timm FP, et al. Effects of intraoperative fluid management on postoperative outcomes: a hospital registry study. Ann Surg. 2018;267(6):1084–92.
30. Thacker JK, Mountford WK, Ernst FR, Krukas MR, Mythen MM. Perioperative fluid utilization variability and association with outcomes: considerations for enhanced recovery efforts in sample US surgical populations. Ann Surg. 2016;263(3):502–10.
31. Myles PS, Bellomo R, Corcoran T, Forbes A, Peyton P, Story D, et al. Restrictive versus Liberal fluid therapy for major abdominal surgery. N Engl J Med. 2018;378(24):2263–74.
32. Kabon B, Akca O, Taguchi A, Nagele A, Jebadurai R, Arkilic CF, et al. Supplemental intravenous crystalloid administration does not reduce the risk of surgical wound infection. Anesth Analg. 2005;101(5):1546–53.
33. Pearse RM, Harrison DA, MacDonald N, Gillies MA, Blunt M, Ackland G, et al. Effect of a perioperative, cardiac output-guided hemodynamic therapy algorithm on outcomes following major gastrointestinal surgery: a randomized clinical trial and systematic review. JAMA. 2014;311(21):2181–90.
34. Rajagopalan S, Mascha E, Na J, Sessler DI. The effects of mild perioperative hypothermia on blood loss and transfusion requirement. Anesthesiology. 2008;108(1):71–7.
35. Kurz A, Sessler DI, Lenhardt R. Perioperative normothermia to reduce the incidence of surgical-wound infection and shorten hospitalization. Study of wound infection and temperature group. N Engl J Med. 1996;334(19):1209–15.
36. Melling AC, Ali B, Scott EM, Leaper DJ. Effects of preoperative warming on the incidence of wound infection after clean surgery: a randomised controlled trial. Lancet. 2001;358(9285):876–80.
37. Wong PF, Kumar S, Bohra A, Whetter D, Leaper DJ. Randomized clinical trial of perioperative systemic warming in major elective abdominal surgery. Br J Surg. 2007;94(4):421–6.
38. Sessler DI. Mild perioperative hypothermia. N Engl J Med. 1997;336(24):1730–7.
39. McAnulty GR, Robertshaw HJ, Hall GM. Anaesthetic management of patients with diabetes mellitus. Br J Anaesth. 2000;85(1):80–90.
40. Turina M, Fry DE, Polk HC Jr. Acute hyperglycemia and the innate immune system: clinical, cellular, and molecular aspects. Crit Care Med. 2005;33(7):1624–33.
41. Kotagal M, Symons RG, Hirsch IB, Umpierrez GE, Dellinger EP, Farrokhi ET, et al. Perioperative hyperglycemia and risk of adverse events among patients with and without diabetes. Ann Surg. 2015;261(1):97–103.
42. Kiran RP, Turina M, Hammel J, Fazio V. The clinical significance of an elevated postoperative glucose value in nondiabetic patients after colorectal surgery: evidence for the need for tight glucose control? Ann Surg. 2013;258(4):599–604. discussion -5
43. Vriesendorp TM, DeVries JH, van Santen S, Moeniralam HS, de Jonge E, Roos YB, et al. Evaluation of short-term consequences of hypoglycemia in an intensive care unit. Crit Care Med. 2006;34(11):2714–8.
44. Griesdale DE, de Souza RJ, van Dam RM, Heyland DK, Cook DJ, Malhotra A, et al. Intensive insulin therapy and mortality among critically ill patients: a meta-analysis including NICE-SUGAR study data. CMAJ. 2009;180(8):821–7.
45. De Vries FE, Wallert ED, Solomkin JS, Allegranzi B, Egger M, Dellinger EP, et al. A systematic review and meta-analysis including GRADE qualification of the risk of surgical site infections after prophylactic negative pressure wound therapy compared with conventional dressings in clean and contaminated surgery. Medicine (Baltimore). 2016;95(36):e4673.

Infection in Surgery: How to Manage the Surgical Wound

4

Domitilla Foghetti

A proper postoperative management of surgical wound can reduce Surgical Site Infection (SSI) rate, when preoperative and intra-operative measures have been applied. The aim of the surgical team should be to protect surgical incision from external environment contamination, to remove any obstacle to the completion of the healing process and to identify precociously any sign of complications, according to patient comfort and a good aesthetic result.

4.1 Surgical Wounds Healing Process

Surgical wounds are considered acute wounds that heal through *primary intention*. If dehiscence occurs, healing will be reached by *secondary intention*, through granulation and epithelization process, or *tertiary intention*, if advanced topical treatment or closure with approximation, grafting or flaps are chosen [1]. The healing process includes three overlapping phases: the inflammatory phase, the proliferative phase and the remodelling phase that culminates to scar formation, and four physiological events: haemostasis, inflammation, repair and scar remodelling. While the inflammatory and proliferative phases are faster than a standard process of wound healing when there is a suture, as in the surgical wounds, the remodelling phase takes 1 to 2 years to be completed. In a surgical scar, the maximal tensile strength is only 80% of the original skin and it can be reached after 2 months after the surgical operation.

In a surgical wound, after the achievement of haemostasis, during the inflammatory phase, the wound bed venules dilate and inflammation cells migrate to promote healing. A correct moisture balance atmosphere favours migration and matrix formation, leading to a complete healing 40% faster than a wound exposed to air. A moist wound healing can also reduce tenderness and pain and can produce better

D. Foghetti (✉)
General Surgery Department, Azienda Ospedaliera Marche Nord, Pesaro, Italy

© Springer Nature Switzerland AG 2021
M. Sartelli et al. (eds.), *Infections in Surgery*, Hot Topics in Acute Care Surgery and Trauma, https://doi.org/10.1007/978-3-030-62116-2_4

cosmetic outcomes, so dressing that offer protection and a balanced moisture environment can be suggested [1].

4.2   Surgical Wounds Dressing

At the end of surgical intervention, the incision created with a scalpel or other cutting device, is closed by suture, staple or glue and usually protected with a dressing. Wound dressing applied after skin closure can absorb exudate, maintaining the skin dry, can provide physical support and can protect wound from contamination from the external environment [2, 3].

Dressing should be sterile and should be applied with an aseptic technique. Traditionally the wound is covered with gauze and tape or gauze and a transparent dressing. The dressing should be left on the wound a minimum of 48 h: during this time a natural barrier is formed and the protective role of the dressing from the external environment can be considered completed. A 2015 Cochrane Review showed no significant differences between dressing removing within or beyond 48 h on surgical site infection from clean or clean-contaminated surgical wounds, even if the quality of evidence is low [4]. Early dressing removal may result in significant reduced costs and a shorter hospital stay.

Dressing should be changed if wet or saturated with blood or serum before 48 h: it allows to evaluate the surgical wound, to prevent bacterial contamination from environment and to avoid the gauze sticking to the suture line [1]. It is necessary to evaluate surgical wound even if patients have signs or symptoms of infection, as unusual pain or fever or if there is evidence of dehiscence, excessive exudate, leakage or peri-wound skin blisters [5].

A particular care is needed also for peri-wound skin: if an excess of drainage occurs, moisture associated damage could happen, when not highly absorbent gauze or transparent dressing is applied over surgical wound.

To manage particular situations many different dressing types are available but it is still not clear whether one type of dressing is better than any other for surgical wound.

An ideal dressing for acute and chronic wounds should possess these following attributes:

- ability to absorb and to contain exudate;
- impermeability to external environment (fluids, microorganism);
- thermal insulation;
- comfort and lack of trauma or pain on dressing removal;
- cosmesis and effect on scar formation;
- lack of dressing particulate contaminants left in the wound;
- transparency for visualizing the wound.

In 2016, a Cochrane Review examined RCTs comparing standard dressing (absorbent gauze) with different *interactive dressing* (films, hydrocolloids, polyurethane matrix, hydroactive dressing, antimicrobials as silver-containing or polyhexamethylene biguanide (PHMB) dressing, topical skin adhesives) [3]. The evidence to support that advanced dressings are more advantageous than standard dressings and that one dressing is better than others in preventing SSI, is insufficient. The use of any type of advanced dressing on primarily closed surgical wounds, with the aim to prevent infection, can't be suggested. However, the low quality of evidence of RCTs made the strength of the recommendation conditional [2].

National Institute for Health and Care Excellence (NICE) guideline (2019) suggests covering surgical incisions with an appropriate *interactive dressing* at the end of operations [6]. An interactive dressing promotes the healing process through the creation and maintenance of a moist environment. Some advanced dressings include the term *"surgical"* in their name: they usually contain long active antimicrobials, provide greater absorption than standard gauze (containing a hydrofiber/alginate or foam layer) and are designed to stay several days (from 5 to 7 days) on surgical wounds, protecting them from trauma and external contamination (Figs. 4.1 and 4.2). Their borders are made of hydrocolloid or silicone, to minimize surrounding skin damage. Some surgical dressings are semi-transparent, to consent surgical wound inspection without removing the dressing (Fig. 4.3).

Fig. 4.1 Postsurgical dressing: hydrocolloid protective and waterproof barrier is joined with an *hydrofiber* soft absorbent material layer with ionic silver, that transforms into a gel on contact with wound fluid. It can be use with a contemporary ostomy to protect wound from environment contamination

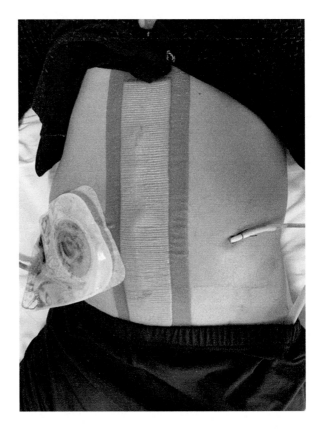

Fig. 4.2 Postsurgical
dressing: atraumatic
conformable contact layer,
easy to remove without
damaging the skin, joined
with *flex technology*
absorbent pad that can
reduce peri-wound
blistering

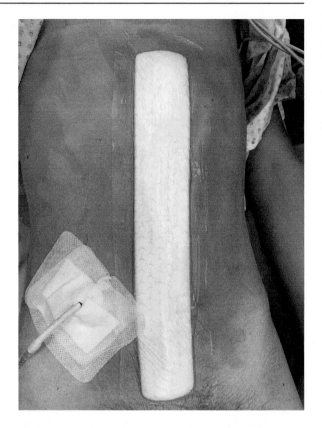

Fig. 4.3 Postsurgical
dressing: waterproof and
conformable, this
semi-transparent
honeycomb dressing
can manage exudate and
consents a constant
monitoring on the wound
and peri-wound area

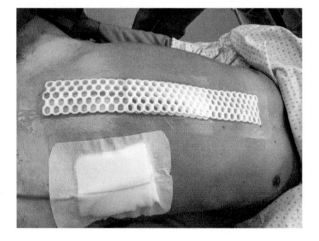

Other outcomes can be evaluated during the choice of different types of advanced
dressing on surgical wound, as patient comfort and desire for wound coverage, cosmetic result, reduction of frequency of dressing change, protection from external
contamination when the wound is near to a stoma. Other items to be considered are

availability and cost of advanced dressings, ease of application and nursing time consuming.

Patients' experiences and feelings about surgical wounds and dressings begin to be considered by surgical team too, even if data produced from patient interviews need to be supplemented and integrated by further randomized controlled trials (RCT) [7].

4.3   Topical Antibiotics and Antiseptics

NICE 2019 guidelines suggest do not use topical antimicrobial agents to reduce the risk of surgical site infection, for surgical wounds that are healing by primary intention [6].

Topical antibiotics use may increase antibiotics resistance, may cause additional skin injuries and tend not to be broad spectrum, so they shouldn't be used routinely to prevent SSI (1). A Cochrane Review (2016) has analyzed the role of topical antibiotics in the form of ointments, creams, lotions, solutions, gels, tinctures, foams, pastes and powders applied with or without a dressing, and impregnated dressings, applied after the wound closure by primary intention, with single or multiple applications in the postoperative period, in reducing SSI. Antibiotics irrigation and washouts, antibiotic-coated sutures, subcutaneous infiltration of antibiotics and any topical treatment applied only prior to closure of the wounds were excluded. The type of topical antibiotic applied varied: chloramphenicol, neomycin, bacitracin, rifamycin, soframycin, fusidic acid and neomycin/bacitracin/polymixin B were considered. The selected studies involved clean, clean-contaminated and contaminated surgery (class 1 to 3); in clean surgery (class 1) the absolute SSI risk reduction is probably smaller, so the instruction for topical antibiotics use is weaker. The review concluded that the use of topical antibiotics on surgical wounds, healing by primary intention, may reduce the risk of SSI if compared with no antibiotics and no topical antiseptics use (moderate quality of evidence) [8]. The relative effects of different antibiotics are unclear and definitive data are not available about topical antibiotics on adverse outcomes, as allergic contact dermatitis or their impact on antibiotic resistance development. Rationalizing the use of antibiotics is important in order to reduce the risk of antibiotic resistance and the evidence for use of topical antibiotics on surgical close wound is still conflicting. A cost analysis should be conducted in further studies, too.

4.4   Prophylactic Negative Pressure Wound Therapy

There is a rapidly emerging literature on the effect of incisional Negative Pressure Wound Therapy (iNPWT). The evidence from single-use NPWT device applied on closed surgical wound for preventing surgical site events (infection and dehiscence) is accumulating [9].

Single-use NPWT system is an evolution of standard device: the pump is smaller, lighter and more portable and the dressing system is easier to apply and remove and less painful, allowing greater utilization [10]. The device is composed of a closed sealed system connected to a battery-powered vacuum pump, which maintains a level of negative pressure between 75 mmHg and 125 mmHg on the wound surface. Exudate can be managed predominantly by evaporation (approximately 80%), through a multilayer easy-to-place dressing: the wound contact layer is a perforate flexible silicone, bonded to a lower airlock layer and a upper fluid absorption layer that delivers negative pressure, removes wound exudate and aids evaporation of fluid through the highly breathable film layer [10]; this kind of device is canister-free (Fig. 4.4). Another type of device is connected to a multilayer layer dressing, peel-and-place or customizable, made of a non-adherent interface layer with silver and a foam layer [11]; it is equipped with a small canister (range from 45 to 150 ml) (Fig. 4.5). The application time range is between 1 and 14 days. Ideal properties of

Fig. 4.4 IncisionalNPWT: canisterless single-use device

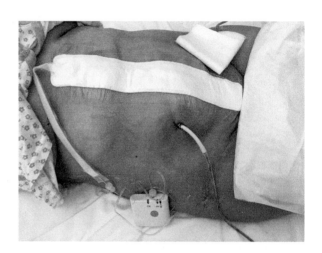

Fig. 4.5 IncisionalNPWT: single-use device with a small canister

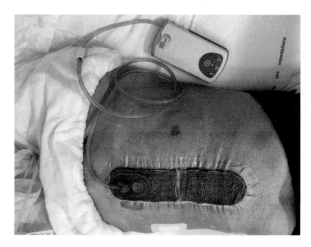

iNPWT system are: single-use/disposable, safe, affordable and cost-effective device, from 5 to 14 days use. As far as dressing features they include good adhesivity, hypoallergenicity, flexibility, a good range of sizes and shapes and readiness of removing without damage to skin. NPWT device should possess an imperfect seal or leak detector and low battery indicator [12].

Animal studies and clinical experiences reported that iNPWT can reduce lateral tension on incision line (the breaking strengths of wounds is increased), increase blood flow [13], decrease oedema (increasing the activity of lymphatic drainage) and risk of haematoma and seroma [9–14]. The reduction of collections of blood and serum in sub-incisional tissue, may reduce the risk both infection and dehiscence of surgical wound and improve the speed, strength and quality of scarring [9]. INPWT has also a positive effect on oxygen saturation and tissue perfusion, which are both associated with the wound healing process [15].

Incisional NPWT has been used on a variety of different type of closed surgical wounds, including abdominal, vascular [16], cardiothoracic, obstetric, orthopaedic, plastic/breast and trauma surgery [12]. Even if the clear benefits of standard NPWT are described in literature, the evidence for iNPWT compared with standard dressing is still low or very low, due to studies at high risk of bias [17]. Several recent studies [18, 19] and a 2019 Cochrane Review claim that the role of iNPWT remains uncertain about reduction of incidence of seroma or haematoma, wound dehiscence and wound-related readmission to hospital within 30 days [17], even if there is an association between NPWT and reduction in SSI rates [13–20], especially in general and colorectal surgery [21, 22].

World Health Organization (WHO) global guidelines for the prevention of surgical site infection (2016) suggest the use of prophylactic NPWT on primarily closed surgical incisions only in high-risk wounds, for the purpose of preventing SSI, considering available resources (2) (*conditional recommendation, low quality of evidence*), because NPWT devices are expensive and may not to be available in low-resources settings.

Incisional NPWT should be considered preoperatively when major patient-related risk factors are identified (BMI < 18 or > 40 kg/m^2, uncontrolled insulin dependent diabetes mellitus, renal dialysis, smoking) or when surgery has a higher risk (prolonged surgical time, high perioperative blood loss, hypothermia, reoperation, emergency operation) and/or a higher consequence of surgical site complications or when patient have two or more other patient-related or procedure-specific major or moderate risk factor for SSI [23, 24]. Surgical team can also reconsider iNPWT application if risk factors arise during surgery.

Surgical risk calculators were developed to identify high-risk patients basing on the results of preoperative assessment (ASA score), surgical wounds classification (from clean to dirty-infected) and duration of operation (National Nosocomial Infection Surveillance-NNIS, Risk Index) [24]. A limitation of NNIS risk Index score is that it does not consider details of different surgical procedures, as far as the placement of implant. A risk calculator should be developed for every different surgical speciality and it should be used for preoperative patient education and counselling and to identify the required interventions to reduce SSI risk [12]. Some calculators may be accessed via internet as www.riskcalc.sts.org by Society of Thoracic Surgeons (STS), www.brascore.org by Breast Reconstruction Risk Assessment (BRA) Score and www.riskcalculator.facs.org by American College of Surgeons (ACS).

When the decision to apply iNPWT is taken preoperatively, the aim and method of use of the device can be described to patient or caregiver. During surgery there are some tips that must be considered for an effective application of iNPWT:

- Consider placement of incision, ostomy (colostomy, ileostomy, urostomy) and surgical drains to accommodate NPWT dressing. The dressing should not be placed over drains or wires.
- Ensure drains are placed in a lower position; iNPWT does not replace the need for surgical drains were indicated.
- Consider placing of the port and tubing to avoid pressure damage.
- Ensure patient's skin is dry and hair free before dressing application to reach a good adhesion and sealing. In difficult areas gel or hydrocolloid strips may be used.
- Apply the dressing under aseptic condition and according to the manufacturer's instruction.

After surgery:

- Inspect the dressing, canister (if present) and power unit regularly.
- Leave the dressing in place for 5–7 days, unless there are concerns about the incision or dressing change is required. If a dressing changing is required, an aseptic technique must be used.
- If surgical wound is closed and dry when the dressing is removed, there is no need to reapply iNPWT or any other standard dressing.
- If patient is discharged from hospital with iNPWT dressing, written information about NPWT system care and when and how to contact a healthcare professional are required [12].

It is necessary to find health economic evidence to show that investing in prevention delivers advantages for patients and healthcare systems. To verify the cost effectiveness of iNPWT, the cost analysis can't be carried out just with a comparison with standard dressing unit cost and iNPWT device, but it should be performed regarding the SSI treating costs that can be avoided (further dressings, laboratory or diagnostic exams, length of hospital stay or readmission rate, antibiotic and analgesic drugs, etc.), without considering the human suffering costs, social costs and delate in adjuvant therapies in oncological patients. Studies regarding economic and organizational sustainability of iNPWT for SSI prevention are in progress [25].

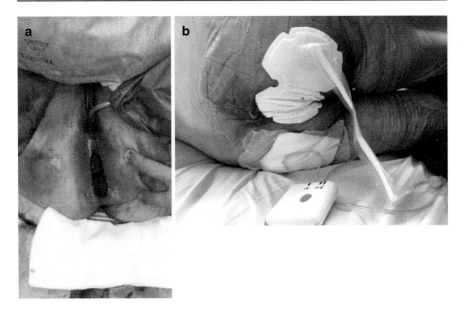

Fig. 4.6 (**a**) Perineal wound in abdominoperineal resection for rectal cancer. (**b**) IncisionalNPWT

4.5   Incisional NPWT in High-Risk Surgical Wounds

Incisional NPWT may be considered in high-risk surgical wounds as far as sternotomies or vascular surgical operations (to prevent the risk of wound infection that remains a devastating complication, decreasing short-term and long-term survival [26, 27]), ventral hernia repair [28] or major limb amputation [29], surgical operations associated with significant wound complication rates. In general surgery, some types of contaminated surgical wound have a high risk of surgical site infection, as far as perineal wound in abdominoperineal resection for rectal cancer [30], or in reversal of temporary ileostomy [31] or colostomy, or after pilonidal cyst removal. The application of surgical technical tips, as a projected incisional wound finalized to easier iNPWT application, and the position of a subcutaneous drainage that can be cut and covered by iNPWT dressing, could reduce the rates or the severity of wound infections (Figs. 4.6, 4.7, 4.8, and 4.9).

4.6   Surgical Wounds Healing by Secondary Or Tertiary Intention

When surgical wounds are left open to heal by secondary intention, i.e. abscesses or contaminated-dirty wounds or when dehiscence occur, proper and gentle dressings are required. Standard gauzes can cause trauma to healthy granulation tissue and pain when removed, can leave remnants in wound bed and, if the absorption power

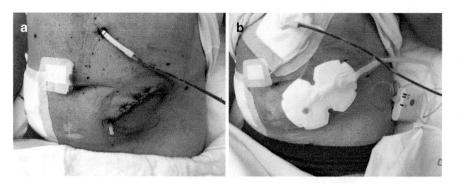

Fig. 4.7 (**a**) Colostomy reverse. (**b**) IncisionalNPWT over subcutaneous drain

Fig. 4.8 IncisionalNPWT: major lower limb amputation

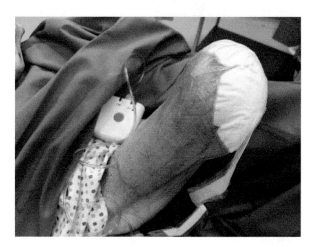

is not sufficient, peri-wound skin damage may occur. Interactive dressing or NPWT may be chosen considering the wound bed and the exudate characteristic (quantity and density). A surgical wound that is left open with the intent to be closed by tertiary intention, also requires interactive dressing or standard NPWT with foam or gauze filler as a *bridge* to subsequent closure [1].

4.7 Postoperative Care of Surgical Wound

As far as caring for a patient with a postoperative wound, international guidelines [3, 4] suggest:
- to avoid unnecessary touching of the postoperative wound site, including by the patient;
- don't touch dressing for at least 48 h after surgery, unless leakage or other complications occur;
- wear gloves if contact with body fluids is anticipated;
- to use aseptic non-touch technique for removing or changing wound dressing and for any wound-related procedures;

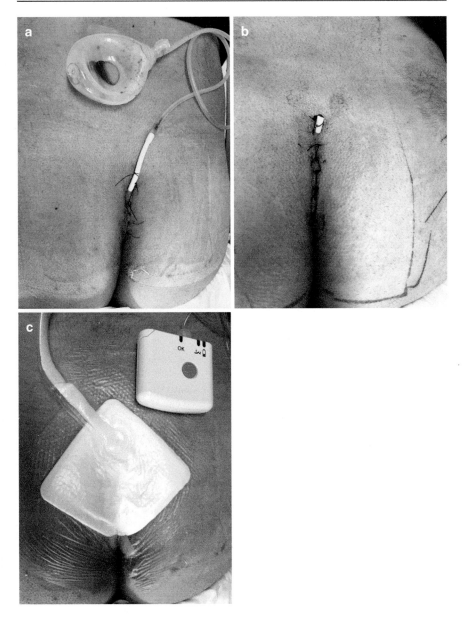

Fig. 4.9 (**a**) Surgical wound closed by primary intention after pilonidal cyst removal, with subcutaneous aspirative drain. (**b**) Surgical drain cut 1 cm from skin. (**c**) INPWT applied over surgical wound and drain for 7 days

- to use sterile saline for wound cleansing up to 48 h after surgery; tap water can be used after 48 h. Antiseptic agents are considered unnecessary for general wound cleansing, they can be considered in case of infected wound [5].
- to advise patients that they may shower safely 48 h after surgery.

As far as hands hygiene during postoperative wound care, WHO defines 5 moments:

1. Before touching a patient.
2. Before clean/aseptic procedure, immediately before touching the postoperative wound dressing/site:
   - **2a** before physically examining the postoperative wound site, including before taking wound samples for microbiological investigations, if required;
   - **2b** before touching the wound to remove stitches/clips;
   - **2c** before preparing the necessary items for replacing the wound dressing;
   - **2d** before replacing the actual postoperative wound dressing.
3. After body fluid exposure risk, immediately after any task involving potential body fluid exposure:
   - **3a** after postoperative wound examination/sample collection;
   - **3b** after removing stitches/clips;
   - **3c** after undertaking a postoperative wound dressing change.
4. After touching a patient.
5. After touching patient surroundings.

4.8 Monitoring Surgical Wounds for Infection After Hospital Discharge

As a consequence of the reduction of postoperative hospitalization, the number of post-discharge SSI diagnosed continues to rise. A large study in US identified SSI as the most common reason for readmission to hospital (19.5%) [12]. The improvement of post-discharge surveillance and the development of a high-quality homecare programme can contribute to achieve an accurate and efficient system to better measure surgical outcomes and to estimate the human, social and financial impact of complications [32]. To improve the quality of education and discharge instructions, a simple leaflet with information for patients regarding surgical wound infection, monitoring and symptoms, may be delivered [33]. Patients with suspected SSI may contact the hospital, allowing a timely diagnosis. A direct patient contact, with a telephone survey or questionnaire at 30 days, can be used to collect data prospectively [12]. Collecting data may be used to calculate rates of surgical wound infection and to improve standard of care. A specialist wound care service should be useful to guarantee a structured approach to improve management of surgical wounds [6].

References

1. Delmore B, Cohen JM, Chu A, Pham V, Chiu E. Reducing postsurgical wound complication: a critical review. Advanced Skin & Wound Care. 2017;30(6):272–85.
2. Global guidelines for the prevention of surgical site infection. WHO World Health Organization 2016.
3. Dumville JC, Gray TA, Walter CJ, Sharp CA, Page T, Macefield R, Blencowe N, Milne TKG, Reeves BC, Blazeby J. Dressing for the prevention of surgical site infection. Cochrane Database Syst Rev. 2016 Dec;12.

4. Toon CD, Lusuku C, Ramamoorthy R, Davidson BR, Gurusamy KS. Early versus delayed dressing removal after primary closure of clean and clean-contaminated surgical wounds. Cochrane Database Syst Rev. 2015 Sep 3;(9).
5. Milne J, Vowden P, Fumarola S, Leaper D. Postoperative incision management made easy. Wounds UK. 2012;(suppl. 8):4.
6. Surgical Site Infection: prevention and treatment. NICE (National Institute for Health and Care Excellence) guideline 2019.
7. Elliott D, The Bluebelle Study Group. Developing outcome measures assessing wound management and patient experience: a mixed methods study. BMJ Open. 2017;7.
8. Heal CF, Banks JL, Lepper DP et al. Topical antibiotics for preventing surgical site infection in wounds healing by primary intention. Cochrane Systematic Review. 2016.
9. Karlakki S, Brem M, Giannini S, et al. Negative pressure wound therapy for management of the surgical incision in orthopaedic surgery. Bone Join Res. 2013;2:276–84.
10. Malmsjo M, Huddlestone E, Martin R. Biological effects of a disposable, canisterless negative pressure wound therapy system. Eplasty.com. 2014;2:113–27.
11. Stannard JP, Gabriel A, Lehner B. Use of negative pressure wound therapy over clean, closed surgical incisions. Wound J. 2012;9(Suppl 1):32–9.
12. World Union of Wound Healing Societies. Consensus Document. Close surgical incision management: understanding the role of NPWT. 2016.
13. Hykdig N, Birke-Sorensen H, Kruse M, et al. Meta-analysis of negative-pressure wound therapy for closed surgical incisions. BJS. 2016;103:477–86.
14. Strugala V, Martin R. Meta-analysis of comparative trials evaluating a prophylactic single-use negative pressure wound therapy for the prevention of surgical site complications. Surg Infect. 2017;18(7):810–9.
15. Renno I, Boos AM, Horch RE, Ludolph I. Changes of perfusion patterns of surgical wounds under application of closed incision negative pressure wound therapy in postbariatric patients. Clin Hemorheol Microcirc. 2019;72(2):139–50.
16. Hasselman J, Bjork J, Svensson-Bjork R, Acosta S. Inguinal vascular surgical wound protection by incisional negative pressure wound therapy: a randomized controlled trial-INVIPS trial. Ann Surg. 2019;271:48–53.
17. Webster J, Liu Z, Norman G, Dumville JC, Chiverton L, Schuffham P, et al. Negative pressure wound therapy for surgical wounds healing by primary closure. Cochrane Database Syst Rev. 2019. Mar 26;3:CD009261.
18. Ingargiola MJ, Daniali LN, Lee ES. Does the application of incisional negative pressure therapy to high-risk wounds prevent surgical site complication? A systematic review. Eplasty.com. 2013;20:413–24.
19. Webster J, Schuffham P, Stankiewicz M, Chaboyer WP. Negative pressure wound therapy for skin grafts and surgical wounds healing by primary intention. Cochrane Database Syst Rev. 2014 Oct 7.
20. Sandy-Hodgetts K, Watts R. Effectiveness of negative pressure wound therapy/closed incision management in the prevention of post-surgical wound complication: a systematic review and meta-analysis. JBI Database System Rv Implement Rep. 2015 Feb 23;13(1):253–303.
21. Sahebally SM, McKevitt K, Stephens I, et al. Negative pressure wound therapy for closed laparotomy incision in general and colorectal surgery: a systematic review and meta-analysis. JAMA Surg. 2018 Nov 1;153(11):e183467.
22. Pellino G, Sciaudone G, Selvaggi F, Canonico S. Prophylactic negative pressure wound therapy in colorectal surgery. Effects on surgical site events: current status and call to action. Updat Surg. 2015 Sep;67(3):235–45.
23. Willy C, Agarwal A, Andresen CA, De Santis G et al. Closed incision negative pressure therapy: international multidisciplinary consensus recommendations. Int Wound J. 2016 published by Medicalhelplines.com.
24. Culver DH, Horan TC, Gaynes RP, et al. Surgical wound infection rates by wound class, operative procedure and patient risk index. Am J Med. 1991;91:152–7.

25. Foglia E, Ferrario L, Garagiola E, Signoriello G, Pellino G, Croce D, Canonico S. Economic and organizational sustainability of a negative-pressure portable device for the prevention of surgical-site complication. ClinicoEconomics and Outcomes Research. 2017(9):343–51.
26. Broadus ZA. Does negative pressure wound therapy have a role in preventing post-sternotomy wound complication? Surg Innov. June 2009;16(2):140–6.
27. Pleger SP, Nink N, Elzien M, et al. Reduction of groin wound complications in vascular surgery patients using closed incision negative pressure therapy (ciNPT): a prospective, randomised, single-institution study. Int Wound J. 2018 Feb;15(1):75–83.
28. Swanson EW, Cheng HT, Susarla SM, et al. Does negative pressure therapy applied to closing incisions following ventral hernia repair prevent wound complications and hernia recurrence? A systematic review and meta-analysis. Plast Surg. 2016;24:113–8.
29. Zayan NE, West JM, Schulz SA, et al. Incisional negative pressure wound therapy: an effective tool for major limb amputation and amputation revision site closure. Adv Wound Care. 2019;8(8):368–73.
30. Van der Valk M, De Graaf E, Doornebosch P, Vermaas M. Incisional negative-pressure wound therapy for perineal wounds after abdominoperineal resection for rectal cancer, a pilot study. Adv Wound Care. 2017;6(12):425–9.
31. Poehnert D, Hadeler N, Schrem H, et al. Decreased superficial surgical site infection, shortened hospital stay, and improved quality of life due to incisional negative pressure wound therapy after reversal of double loop ileostomy. Wound Rep Reg. 2017;25:994–1001.
32. Smith RL. Jamie K. Bohl, Shannon T, McElearney et al. wound infection after elective colorectal resection. Ann Surg. 2004;239:599–604.
33. Monitoring surgical wounds for infection: information for patients. Public Health England. 2018.

Guidelines for the Prevention of Surgical Site Infections. How to Implement Them

5

Massimo Sartelli

5.1 Introduction

Healthcare-associated infections (HAIs) are infections that occur while receiving health care. Patients with medical devices (central lines, urinary catheters, ventilators) or who undergo surgical procedures are at risk of acquiring HAIs [1, 2]. HAIs continue to be a tremendous issue today. Surgical site infections (SSIs) are the most common healthcare-associated infections among surgical patients. SSIs remain a major clinical problem in terms of morbidity, mortality, length of hospital stay, and overall direct and not-direct costs in all regions of the world.

Both the World Health Organization (WHO) [3, 4] and the Centers for Disease Control and Prevention (CDC) [5] have published guidelines for the prevention of SSIs. However, knowledge, attitude, and awareness of infection prevention and control (IPC) measures among surgeons are often inadequate and a great gap exists between the best evidence and clinical practice with regards to SSIs prevention.

5.2 The Global Guidelines for the Prevention of Surgical Site Infections

The 2016 WHO Global guidelines for the prevention of surgical site infections are evidence-based including systematic reviews presenting additional information in support of actions to improve practice [3, 4]. The guidelines include 13 recommendations for the preoperative period, and 16 for preventing infections during and after surgery. They range from simple precautions such as ensuring that patients bathe or shower before surgery, appropriate way for surgical teams to clean their hands, guidance on when to use prophylactic antibiotics, which disinfectants to use before incision, and which sutures to use. The proposed recommendations are as follows:

M. Sartelli (✉)
Department of Surgery, Macerata Hospital, Macerata, Italy

© Springer Nature Switzerland AG 2021
M. Sartelli et al. (eds.), *Infections in Surgery*, Hot Topics in Acute Care Surgery
and Trauma, https://doi.org/10.1007/978-3-030-62116-2_5

- "Strong"—Expert panel was confident that benefits outweighed risks, considered to be adaptable for implementation in most (if not all) situations, and patients should receive intervention as course of action.
- "Conditional"—Expert panel considered that benefits of intervention probably outweighed the risks; a more structured decision-making process should be undertaken, based on stakeholder consultation and involvement of patients and healthcare professionals.

Importantly, the guidelines recommend that antibiotic prophylaxis should be used to prevent infections before and during surgery only. Antibiotics should not be used after surgery, as is often done. Antibiotic prophylaxis should be administered for operative procedures that have a high rate of postoperative surgical site infection, or when foreign materials are implanted. Antibiotic prophylaxis should be administered within 120 min prior to the incision. However, administration of the first dose of antibiotics is dependent on its pharmacological characteristics. Underlying patient factors may also affect drug disposition (e.g., malnourishment, obesity, cachexia, and renal disease with protein loss may result in suboptimal antibiotic exposure through increased antibiotic clearance in the presence of normal or augmented renal function). Additional antibiotic doses should be administered intraoperatively for procedures >2–4 h (typically where duration exceeds two half-lives of the antibiotic). There is no evidence to support the use of postoperative antibiotic prophylaxis. The key evidence-based recommendations outlined in these guidelines should be adopted by all healthcare staff that care for surgical patients throughout all stages of that patient's surgical care.

5.3 How to Improve Healthcare Workers' Behavior in Preventing SSIs

Despite clear evidence and guidelines to direct SSIs prevention strategies, compliance is uniformly poor and major difficulties arise when introducing evidence and clinical guidelines into routine daily practice. Improving practices frequently implies modifying healthcare workers' (HCWs) behavior. There are generally three primary levels of influence related to behavior modification and infection control in healthcare facilities [6]:

1. Intrapersonal factors.
2. Interpersonal factors.
3. Institutional or organizational factors.

Intrapersonal factors are individual characteristics that influence behavior such as knowledge and skills. Knowledge can be taught formally in the classroom and informally on the job. Skills are practical tasks, ranging from very simple procedures to complex investigative techniques. Training and development in healthcare has historically focused on development of knowledge and competency in skill delivery. However, increasing knowledge and skills alone may not be sufficient to effect sustained change especially considering the multifactorial nature of HAIs.

HCWs can be influenced by or are influential in their social environments. Behavior is often influenced by peer group pressure. Peer-to-peer role modeling, and champions [7] on an interpersonal level have been shown to positively influence improvement of best practice in infection control practices. Many practitioners use educational materials or didactic continuing medical education sessions to keep up-to-date. However, these strategies might not be very effective in changing practice, unless education is interactive and continuous, and includes discussion of evidence, local consensus, feedback on performance (by peers), making personal and group learning plans, etc.

Identifying a local opinion leader to serve as a champion may be important because the "champion" may integrate best clinical practices and drive the colleagues in changing behaviors, working on a day-to-day basis, and promoting a culture in which infection prevention and control is of high importance. Surgeons with satisfactory knowledge in surgical infections may provide feedback to the prescribers, integrate the best practices among surgeons and implement change within their own sphere of influence interacting directly with IPC team [6].

Organizational obstacles may influence infection prevention and control implementation.

The institutional administration should openly support the creation of a multidisciplinary task force within the hospital. By this, it mandates representative members of the multidisciplinary institutional team to come together to identify the problem and to develop strategies to resolve it, endorses the choices and options taken, and mobilizes the hospital resources needed to implement the strategies.

Many different hospital disciplines are typically involved in IPC, making collaboration, coordination, communication, teamwork, and efficient care logistics essential [8]. IPC teams have been shown to be both clinically effective improving patient outcome, and cost-effective providing important cost savings in terms of fewer HAIs, reduced length of hospital stay, less antimicrobial resistance and decreased costs of treatment for infections. Raising awareness of IPC to stakeholders is a crucial factor in changing behaviors. Probably clinicians are more likely to comply with guidelines when they have been involved in developing the recommendations. One way to engage health professionals in guideline development and implementation is to translate practice recommendations into a protocol or pathway that specifies and coordinates responsibilities and timing for particular actions among a multidisciplinary team. There is now a substantial body of evidence that effective teamwork in health care contributes to improved quality of care. Leading international organizations, such as the WHO [8], acknowledge that collaborative practice is essential for achieving a concerted approach to providing care that is appropriate to meet the needs of patients, thus optimizing individual health outcomes and overall service delivery of health care. The use of such approaches reinforces the concept that each one brings with them their particular expertise and is responsible for their respective contributions to patient care. In this context the direct involvement of surgeons may be crucial.

5.4 Conclusion

The occurrence of HAIs continues to escalate at an alarming rate. However, the perception of the phenomenon is not yet sufficiently high both among healthcare workers and among patients, thus resulting in a low level of intervention request and relative adequate responses.

Guidelines for the prevention of SSIs can support healthcare workers to develop or strengthen infection prevention and control programs, with a focus on surgical safety, as well as antimicrobial resistance action plans. We recommend that all healthcare workers adopt evidence-based recommendations in their clinical practice.

Successful strategies to improve best practice in infection control practices result from their multidimensional aspect. Based on behavioral theories and reported experiences, multimodal intervention strategies have more chance of success than single approaches or promotion programs focusing on one or two elements alone.

References

1. Haque M, Sartelli M, McKimm J, Abu Bakar M. Health care-associated infections—an overview. Infect Drug Resist. 2018;11:2321–33.
2. Report on the Burden of Endemic Health Care-Associated Infection Worldwide. https://apps.who.int/iris/bitstream/handle/10665/80135/9789241501507_eng.pdf;jsessionid=94FBA716108FB235665EC4FA621901B4?sequence=1.
3. Allegranzi B, Zayed B, Bischoff P, Kubilay NZ, de Jonge S, de Vries F, et al. New WHO recommendations on intraoperative and postoperative measures for surgical site infection prevention: an evidence-based global perspective. Lancet Infect Dis. 2016;16:e288–303.
4. Allegranzi B, Bischoff P, de Jonge S, Kubilay NZ, Zayed B, Gomes SM, et al. New WHO recommendations on preoperative measures for surgical site infection prevention: an evidence-based global perspective. Lancet Infect Dis. 2016;16:e276–87.
5. Berríos-Torres SI, Umscheid CA, Bratzler DW, Leas B, Stone EC, Kelz RR, et al. Centers for disease control and prevention guideline for the prevention of surgical site infection, 2017. JAMA Surg. 2017;152:784–91.
6. Sartelli M, Kluger Y, Ansaloni L, Coccolini F, Baiocchi GL, Hardcastle TC, et al. Knowledge, awareness, and attitude towards infection prevention and management among surgeons: identifying the surgeon champion. World J Emerg Surg. 2018;13:37.
7. Pittet D. The Lowbury lecture: behaviour in infection control. J Hosp Infect. 2004;58(1):1–13.
8. Framework for Action on Interprofessional Education & Collaborative Practice. https://apps.who.int/iris/bitstream/handle/10665/70185/WHO_HRH_HPN_10.3_eng.pdf?sequence=1.

The Infected Mesh: How to Treat it

6

Ines Rubio-Perez and Estibaliz Alvarez-Peña

6.1 Introduction

Both primary hernia repair and ventral hernia repair are some of the most common operations performed by surgeons. In the United States over 350,000 ventral hernia repairs are performed each year, with increasing numbers [1]. The repair of the defect with a prosthetic mesh has demonstrated to be the most cost-effective treatment. Despite multiple techniques have been historically described for hernia repair, mesh reinforcement is now considered the gold standard [2]. However, it implies the introduction of a foreign material that must be integrated by the patient's tissues. In ventral hernia repair, this also implies the manipulation of previous scar tissue, as the defect is the consequence of a previous operation. The risk of infection in abdominal hernia repair seems higher than other clean interventions, with published incidence ranging from 1–10%, depending on the type of mesh, surgical technique and patient's characteristics [3].

The use of mesh can lead to a series of complications that have recently been classified by the Ventral Hernia Working Group (VHWG) as Surgical Site Occurrences (SSO). These include seromas, hematomas, wound dehiscence, mesh migration, infection or fistulas [4]. The VHWG proposes a classification of risk factors that can lead to these SSO in 4 categories, later simplified by Berger et al. [5] in 3 main risk groups, as can be seen in Table 6.1. Among them, the most relevant is surgical infection that can present in up to 1–8% of cases (depending on published series). As all surgical infections, they can have an important impact in patient's

I. Rubio-Perez (✉)
Department of General Surgery, Colorectal Surgery Unit, La Paz University Hospital, Madrid, Spain
e-mail: i.rubio@aecirujanos.es

E. Alvarez-Peña
Department of General Surgery, Abdominal Wall & Upper GI Unit, La Paz University Hospital, Madrid, Spain

© Springer Nature Switzerland AG 2021
M. Sartelli et al. (eds.), *Infections in Surgery*, Hot Topics in Acute Care Surgery and Trauma, https://doi.org/10.1007/978-3-030-62116-2_6

Table 6.1 Ventral Hernia Working Group classification of risk based on patient and wound characteristics, and the modified grading system from VHWG (2010) and Berger et al. (2013)

VHWG classification			
Grade 1	Grade 2	Grade 3	Grade 4
Low risk	Comorbid	Potentially contaminated	Infected
• Low risk of complications • No history of wound infection	• Obesity • Smoking • Diabetes • Immunosuppression	• Previous wound infection • Presence of ostomy • Violation of the GI tract	• Grossly infected mesh • Septic dehiscence
Modified VHWG grading system		
Grade 1	Grade 2	Grade 3
Low risk	Comorbid	Contaminated
• Low risk of complications • No history of wound infection	• Obesity • Smoking • Diabetes • Immunosuppression • Previous wound infection	A. Clean-contaminated B. Contaminated C. Active infection

quality of life, morbidity and increased costs. As in other prosthetic-related infections, the presence of mesh can perpetuate the local infection, leading to a prolonged treatment, reoperations and even fistulisation and other major complications, that can have a great impact on the patient. An important effort must be made in the prevention and early treatment of any mesh-related complications to avoid potentially severe consequences.

6.2   Risk Factors for Mesh Infection

There are numerous risk factors for mesh infection that would be the same for any surgical infection, but some have been associated specifically with mesh infection in recent meta-analyses [3, 6]. A way of classifying them would be as (a) preoperative: mainly patient's comorbidities and other factors, some of them potentially modifiable; (b) intraoperative factors: dependant on surgical technique and incidents during the intervention or on the type of mesh used; and (c) postoperative: related to early complications of the wound that can lead to an infection. Some of these risk factors for mesh infection are presented in Table 6.2.

One of the main strategies to try and reduce complication rates after ventral hernia repair is to act on preoperative factors [3]. In many cases, the operation can be performed electively, so patients may be asked by the surgeon for smoking cessation, weight loss (achievable goals) an exhaustive glycaemic control in case of diabetics and the optimization of any other chronic conditions, in order to perform a safer operation. These preoperative modifications have shown to have the most impact on patient's outcomes and costs.

Table 6.2 Classification of risk factors for mesh infection

Preoperative	Intraoperative	Postoperative
• Active smoking • Diabetes (poor glucose control) • Obesity • Skin conditions • Reintervention (previous scar tissue) • Advanced age • ASA score > 3 • Chronic obstructive pulmonary disease • Immunosuppression, steroids	• Type of surgical approach • Increased dissection • Operative time • Emergency operation (vs elective) • Grade of contamination • Type of mesh • Concomitant intestinal surgery/enterotomy/stoma • Location of mesh (plane of placement)	• Poor wound management • Wound complications, including dehiscence • Mesh exposure • Surgical site infection

Another important strategy is to confirm that adequate infection prevention practices are observed across the entire surgical pathway. It is important to do a correct preoperative skin preparation, administer antibiotic prophylaxis and maintain an adequate tissue oxygenation and sterile conditions with careful management of prosthesis throughout the surgical procedure.

In the postoperative period, unnecessary wound manipulation should be avoided, and the patient should be instructed for proper wound care and have an adequate support system for follow-up and early detection of complications. All preoperative factors (smoking, diabetes, etc.) should continue to be properly controlled after the procedure.

A useful tool for risk factor identification and assessment is Carolinas equation for the determination of associated risks (CeDAR) [7]. It is available as a smartphone application and can help surgeons inform patients appropriately about their individualized risk, and institute preoperative interventions (weight loss, smoking cessation, etc.). Factors most significantly associated with wound complications are preoperative HbA1c >7.2 with an odds ratio (OR) of 2.01, prior hernial repair (OR: 2.64), enterotomy (OR: 2.65), or an infected surgical field (OR: 2.07).

6.3   Presentation of Mesh Infection

A superficial SSI or wound infection may not (or not yet) involve the underlying mesh. If treated timely, contamination of the mesh can be avoided.

The contamination of the mesh may occur:

1. At the time of surgery (non-sterile conditions, patient's flora, caregivers).
2. Secondary hematogenous contamination of a residual fluid collection.
3. Contiguous contamination (direct extension from an adjacent focus).

Acute presentations happen in the early postoperative period, usually related to wound infections or other surgical site occurrences. The infection can present with the classical signs of tenderness, erythema, warmth or drainage. If a deep SSI occurs or there is an undrained collection, systemic symptoms such as fever, chills, malaise, pain and blood test alterations can appear.

In more chronic presentations, the infection can result from an incision that doesn't heal, an open wound with fibrin or chronic discharge or the formation of sinuses. Deep prosthetic infections are more frequent in ventral hernias (1–4%) compared to inguinal hernias (0–3.5%). In many cases, infection can present remotely from the initial operation site. Up to 50% of cases can present after 6 months of the operation, and even one third of infections can present >1 year after the operation [8].

Considering the surgical approach, minimally invasive techniques have shown a lower rate of infection when compared to open (3.6% vs 10%) in published literature. However, this must be considered with caution, as there can be complications of laparoscopic repairs that have late presentations or are not detected by examination (deep collections) and only visualized by imaging. Imaging techniques such as Ultrasound and CT tomography may be essential to study deep set fluid collections and their relationship with the mesh, rule out intra-abdominal complications or fistulas and help to plan the best treatment approach [9].

6.4   Biofilm

The pathogenesis of mesh infection can be a complex process. Apart from the patient's risk factors that can facilitate infections, there are other important factors such as virulence of the infective bacterial species, biomechanical and chemical properties of the mesh itself and host-pathogen interactions. Biofilms are one of the great concerns regarding mesh infections [10].

Biofilms develop rapidly, in just hours. Free unattached bacteria reach a surface (the mesh) where they attach and start growing in a single layer. If they are not eradicated by antibiotics or the host's immune system, they continue growing into a colony, where bacteria secrete extracellular polymeric substances and create a gel-like protective barrier around them, becoming inaccessible for antibiotics or host's immune cells (Fig. 6.1). *Staphylococcus aureus* and *Enterobacteriaceae* are some

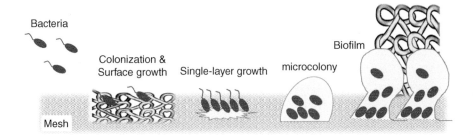

Fig. 6.1 Process of biofilm formation

of the most common bacteria found in mesh infections, and some have the capacity of producing biofilms [11].

Early antibiotics and mechanical scrubbing or irrigation to remove the biofilm are both important treatment strategies when the mesh is infected.

6.5   Types of Mesh and Infection Rates

Different types of prosthetic mesh are used for repairing hernias, the selection of which depends on the size and characteristics of the hernia, surgical technique and approach (open or laparoscopic). To date, there is no gold standard or "ideal" mesh [12].

Amid [13] proposed a classification of abdominal wall prosthetic mesh into four categories:

- Type I: Macroporous (Prolene).
- Type II: Microporous (expanded PTFE).
- Type III: Macro-microporous woven (Mersilene).
- Type IV: Impermeable (Silastic).

Synthetic meshes (usually polypropylene) are the most commonly used meshes: they are easily handled, cost-effective and usually well tolerated, but being completely prosthetic they can be contaminated and lead to chronic infections. The possibilities of salvaging a mesh are very different depending on material, porosity and structure. Pore size plays a major role in the integration of the prosthesis. Macroporous meshes allow for fibroblast migration and host defences to act if bacteria contaminate the mesh. Woven fibres or braided sutures may favour bacterial colonization. PTFE meshes have the highest reported infection rates (up to 10%) in published series [14]. Biological meshes can increase costs and have less favourable long-term results regarding hernia recurrence, but they have the benefit of a better tissue integration and a higher resistance to infections. Type II (microporous) meshes allow bacteria to penetrate the pores, but the host's macrophages cannot penetrate to dislodge them. Bacteria can nest in woven fibre meshes and remain inaccessible to the host's defences; this would also apply for braided suture material used for mesh fixation [8].

Mesh placement is also important: the more superficial (onlay) the mesh is located, the higher risk of infection.

Figure 6.2 shows different examples of mesh complications.

6.6   Treatment Options for the Infected Mesh

There are no clear guidelines on the management of infected mesh. Some studies have reported success of mesh salvage in selected cases, by using debridement and Negative Pressure Wound Therapy (NPWT). In other cases, complete mesh removal

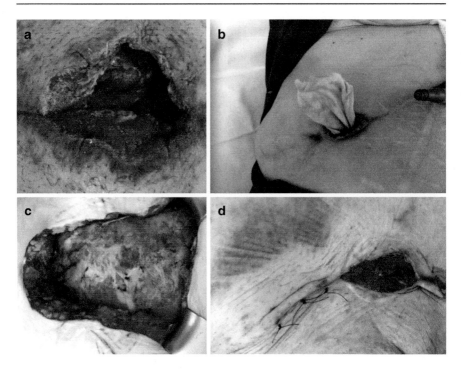

Fig. 6.2 Different examples of mesh-related complications: (**a**) chronic granulating open wound in an obese patient (mesh at the bottom), (**b**) rejected and completely detached mesh protruding from surgical wound, (**c**) surgical field after debridement of infected wound, partially integrated large-pore mesh, (**d**) NPWT treatment of partially opened wound after evacuation of hematoma

seems the only curative option, with the open question of when to perform repair (immediate or staged) [15].

Figure 6.3 shows a proposal for a treatment algorithm for mesh infection management.

6.7   Mesh Excision

There are some cases of acute infection where the mesh detaches completely from the surrounding tissue with abundant suppuration, as there has not been time for integration (for example in Type II or III meshes) and removal is easily performed. However, the most common scenario is a chronic infection where the mesh is partially integrated and only some of it is exposed or conditions persistent suppuration of a wound. Chronic sinuses or wounds with intermittent suppuration and fibrosis can be challenging and difficult to manage [8].

Surgical removal of the mesh involves opening the previous incision (or elsewhere in the abdomen), followed by extirpation of the mesh and any fixations (sutures, tacks, etc.) trying to respect as much tissue as possible to avoid a big

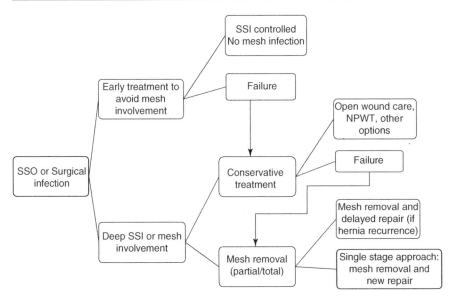

Fig. 6.3 Proposal for a treatment algorithm for mesh infection management

defect. In some cases, where the mesh is partially exposed in a determined area but the rest of the wound seems established, a partial removal can be attempted, followed by adequate wound care. The worst-case scenario is when the infection affects a large area and the whole mesh must be explanted, including the already established fibrosis with the tissues and conditioning a large abdominal wall defect that must be repaired.

In some cases, after the mesh removal, liberation of surrounding tissue, fascial release or component separation can suffice to achieve closure of the fascia. This repair might be enough to avoid recurrence. In other cases, a staged approach, with a new repair after 6–9 months is necessary. If the mesh explant is not followed by any repair, recurrence rate may be as high as 23% for ventral hernias [16].

The removed mesh might be replaced by a synthetic or biologic mesh. In a study by Birolini et al. [17] explanted polypropylene (PP) meshes were replaced with a new one, also PP. Despite being a small series of only 41 patients and the onlay position of the mesh, short-term results showed around 20% of infections that could mostly be managed conservatively and 95% of patients were considered cured from the chronic infection in a 74 months follow-up.

Finally, the use of biologic mesh, considering its resistance to infection has been advocated. There is evidence supporting that bridging of the defect is the one factor significantly associated with hernia recurrence [18]. Despite previous recommendations of the possibility of biologic meshes for immediate repair in infected or contaminated fields, recent findings are controversial. In a recent meta-analysis by Atema et al. [19] evaluating the repair of potentially contaminated and contaminated abdominal wall defects, biologic mesh repair of contaminated defects showed considerable higher rates of surgical site complication rates and a hernia recurrence rate of 30%. There was only one study on the use of synthetic mesh on contaminated fields, so conclusions cannot be drawn yet, as quality evidence is limited.

An interesting proposal for a partial and controlled mesh excision in case of infections with a chronic sinus or fistula tract was proposed by Boullenois et al. [20]. Indigo-carmine blue is injected in the fistula tract with a small catheter, and an oval incision is made, following the coloured areas until the mesh is reached. A "blue-ectomy" is performed, removing all the mesh stained blue, and leaving the rest in place (already embedded). If an underlying intestinal fistula is found, resection and repair are mandatory. The remaining abdominal wall can be either closed primarily, repaired with Vicryl mesh and interrupted sutures (placed retromuscularly) and a NPWT device is used for second-intention wound healing.

6.8   Mesh Salvage

Conservative management of mesh infection can consist of different approaches:

1. Percutaneous drainage of pus/fluid collections.
2. Drainage and instillation of saline and/or antiseptics.
3. Opening of the wound with local debridement and wound dressings.
4. Application of different NPWT devices (foam of sponge).

The studies reporting mesh salvage are limited and usually include a small number of patients. In a recent systematic review by Shubinets et al. [21] reporting studies on mesh salvage, limited conclusions could be obtained. Overall, polypropylene or other synthetic or composite meshes were more likely to be salvaged than PTFE meshes. Also, partially absorbed or incorporated meshes seemed to respond better (Greenberg 2010; [22]), and limited infections could be better controlled than meshes that were completely infected (Paton 2007; [23]). Berrevoet et al. [24], in a prospective observational study of 63 patients treated with NPWT for superficial and deep mesh infections after ventral hernia repair, reported that all meshes in the retromuscular mesh group were salvaged with a median of five dressing changes. Intraperitoneal meshes needed complete or partial excision in three cases. Mean duration to complete wound closure was 44 days.

Novel NPWT instillation systems and the development of new sponges and foams have proven to be effective in the management of contaminated wounds in other settings, including some preliminary studies with mesh infections, so could be a promising option for infected mesh treatment in the near future [25].

Successful prosthetic salvage also depends on an adequate management of the wound by specialized personnel, with adequate dressing changes and strict follow-up that can be time consuming and long to achieve, requiring patience from both the patient and the medical and nursing team.

6.9   Intestinal Fistulas

Mesh infection can affect deep tissues and result in a communication with the peritoneal cavity. Infection or the mesh itself can erode viscera and increase complications. Also, partial mesh removal and repeated manipulation and dressings of the wound can lead to a weakened abdominal wall, contact with the bowel and eventually fistula formation. Early diagnosis is essential to achieve a good control of the infection and avoid the involvement of bowel. Also, management of these complex wounds must be performed by a specialist team and trained surgical nurses to avoid complications. An underlying undetected fistula can also be the cause of a chronic infection, and diagnostic investigation or imaging should be performed accordingly to rule out this complication. If an intestinal fistula is diagnosed, treatment should be performed by specialized surgeons and abdominal wall reconstruction together with the fistula repair might be feasible in one stage [26].

Figure 6.4 shows a chronic PTFE mesh infection and rejection secondary to an undetected underlying intestinal fistula.

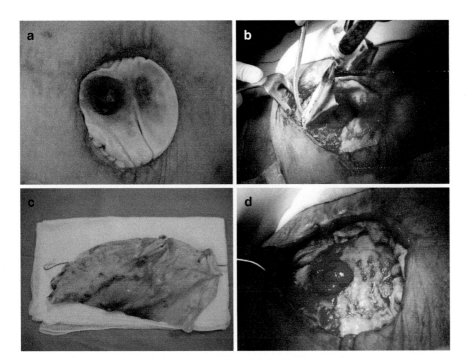

Fig. 6.4 Chronic PTFE mesh infection and rejection secondary to an undetected underlying intestinal fistula: (**a**) exposed mesh with chronic suppuration, (**b**) surgical removal of exposed mesh, (**c**) removed mesh, (**d**) underlying intestinal fistula

The updated (2018) **WSES/SIS-E consensus conference recommendations for the management of skin and soft-tissue infections** [27], made the following recommendations regarding treatment of infected meshes:

- Respect prevention strategies to avoid surgical site infection and prosthetic contamination (recommendation 1A).
- We suggest avoidance of mesh contamination following incisional SSI by an early and adequate local source control as well as antibiotic treatment (recommendation 1C).
- In chronic sinuses and infected meshes, we suggest a complete surgical removal of the mesh which remains the only way to eradicate infection (recommendation 1C).
- No clear recommendation on the benefit of biologic versus synthetic mesh in potentially contaminated fields can be proposed (recommendation 1C).

References

1. Poulose BK, Shelton J, Phillips S, Moore D, Nealon W, Penson D, Beck W, Holzman MD. Epidemiology and cost of ventral hernia repair: making the case for hernia research. Hernia. 2012;16(2):179–83. https://doi.org/10.1007/s10029-011-0879-9. Epub 2011 Sep 9
2. Luijendijk RW, Hop WC, van den Tol MP, et al. A comparison of suture repair with mesh repair for incisional hernia. N Engl J Med. 2000;343:392–8.
3. Mavros MN, Athanasiou S, Alexiou VG, Mitsikostas PK, Peppas G, Falagas ME. Risk factors for mesh-related infections after hernia repair surgery: a meta-analysis of cohort studies. World J Surg. 2011;35(11):2389–98. https://doi.org/10.1007/s00268-011-1266-5. Review
4. Ventral Hernia Working Group, et al. Incisional ventral hernias: review of the literature and recommendations regarding the grading and technique of repair. Surgery. 2010;148(3):544–58.
5. Berger RL, et al. Development and validation of a risk-stratification score for surgical site occurrence and surgical site infection after open ventral hernia repair. J Am Coll Surg. 2013;217(6):974–82.
6. Bueno-Lledó J, Torregrosa-Gallud A, Sala-Hernandez A, Carbonell-Tatay F, Pastor PG, Diana SB, Hernández JI. Predictors of mesh infection and explantation after abdominal wall hernia repair. Am J Surg. 2017;213(1):50–7. https://doi.org/10.1016/j.amjsurg.2016.03.007. Epub 2016 Jun 1
7. Augenstein V, Colavita PD, Wormer BA, et al. CeDAR: Carolinas equation for determining associated risks. J Am Coll Surg. 2015;221:S65–6. https://doi.org/10.1016/j.jamcollsurg.2015.07.145.
8. Gillion JF, Palot JP. Abdominal wall incisional hernias: infected prosthesis: treatment and prevention. J Visc Surg. 2012;149(5 Suppl):e20–31. https://doi.org/10.1016/j.jviscsurg.2012.04.003. Epub 2012 Nov 4
9. Narkhede R, Shah NM, Dalal PR, Mangukia C, Dholaria S. Postoperative mesh infection-still a concern in laparoscopic era. Indian J Surg. 2015;77(4):322–6. https://doi.org/10.1007/s12262-015-1304-x. Epub 2015 Jun 27. Review. PubMed PMID: 26702240; PubMed Central PMCID: PMC4688277
10. Kathju S, Nistico L, Melton-Kreft R, Lasko LA, Stoodley P. Direct demonstration of bacterial biofilms on prosthetic mesh after ventral herniorrhaphy. Surg Infect. 2015;16(1):45–53. https://doi.org/10.1089/sur.2014.026.

11. Blatnik JA, Krpata DM, Jacobs MR, Gao Y, Novitsky YW, Rosen MJ. In vivo analysis of the morphologic characteristics of synthetic mesh to resist MRSA adherence. J Gastrointest Surg. 2012;16:2139–44.

12. Baylón K, Rodríguez-Camarillo P, Elías-Zúñiga A, et al. Past, present and future of surgical meshes: a review. Membranes (Basel). 2017;7(3):pii: E47. https://doi.org/10.3390/membranes7030047. Review

13. Amid PK. Classification of biomaterials and their related complications in abdominal wall hernia surgery. Hernia. 1997;1:15–27.

14. Stremitzer S, Bachleitner-Hofmann T, Gradl B, Gruenbeck M, Bachleitner-Hofmann B, Mittlboeck M, Bergmann M. Mesh graft infection following abdominal hernia repair: risk factor evaluation and strategies of mesh graft preservation. A retrospective analysis of 476 operations. World J Surg. 2010;34(7):1702–9. https://doi.org/10.1007/s00268-010-0543-z.

15. Augenstein VA, Cox TA, Hlavacek C, Bradley T, Colavita PD, Blair LJ, et al. Treatment of 161 consecutive synthetic mesh infections: can mesh be salvaged? American Hernia Society Annual Meeting, Washington, DC; 2015.

16. Tolino MJ, Tripoloni DE, Ratto R, Garcia MI. Infections associated with prosthetic repairs of abdominal wall hernias: pathology, management and results. Hernia. 2009;13:631–7.

17. Birolini C, de Miranda JS, Utiyama EM, Rasslan S. A retrospective review and observations over a 16-year clinical experience on the surgical treatment of chronic mesh infection. What about replacing a synthetic mesh on the infected surgical field? Hernia. 2015;19(2):239–46. https://doi.org/10.1007/s10029-014-1225-9. Epub 2014 Feb 9

18. Montgomery A, Kallinowski F, Köckerling F. Evidence for replacement of an infected synthetic by a biological mesh in Abdominal Wall hernia repair. Front Surg. 2016;2:67. https://doi.org/10.3389/fsurg.2015.00067. eCollection 2015. Review. PubMed PMID: 26779487; PubMed Central PMCID: PMC4705815

19. Atema JJ, de Vries FE, Boermeester MA. Systematic review and meta-analysis of the repair of potentially contaminated and contaminated abdominal wall defects. Am J Surg. 2016;212(5):982–995.e1. https://doi.org/10.1016/j.amjsurg.2016.05.003. Epub 2016 Jun 12. Review

20. Boullenois H, Moszkowicz D, Poghosyan T, Bouillot JL. Surgical management of chronic mesh infection following incisional hernia repair. J Visc Surg. 2016;153(6):461–4. https://doi.org/10.1016/j.jviscsurg.2016.09.007. Epub 2016 Nov 15

21. Shubinets V, Carney MJ, Colen DL, Mirzabeigi MN, Weissler JM, Lanni MA, Braslow BM, Fischer JP, Kovach SJ. Management of infected mesh after abdominal hernia repair: systematic review and single-institution experience. Ann Plast Surg. 2018;80(2):145–53. https://doi.org/10.1097/SAP.0000000000001189.

22. Greenberg JJ. Can infected composite mesh be salvaged? Hernia. 2010;14(6):589–92. https://doi.org/10.1007/s10029-010-0694-8. Epub 2010 Jun 20

23. Paton BL, Novitsky YW, Zerey M, Sing RF, Kercher KW, Heniford BT. Management of infections of polytetrafluoroethylene-based mesh. Surg Infect. 2007;8(3):337–41.

24. Berrevoet F, Vanlander A, Sainz-Barriga M, Rogiers X, Troisi R. Infected large pore meshes may be salvaged by topical negative pressure therapy. Hernia. 2013;17:67–73.

25. Baharestani MM, Gabriel A. Use of negative pressure wound therapy in the management of infected abdominal wounds containing mesh: an analysis of outcomes. Int Wound J. 2011;8(2):118–25. https://doi.org/10.1111/j.1742-481X.2010.00756.x. Epub 2010 Dec 23

26. Hodgkinson JD, Maeda Y, Leo CA, Warusavitarne J, Vaizey CJ. Complex abdominal wall reconstruction in the setting of active infection and contamination: a systematic review of hernia and fistula recurrence rates. Color Dis. 2017;19(4):319–30. https://doi.org/10.1111/codi.13609. Review

27. Sartelli M, Guirao X, Hardcastle TC, Kluger Y, Boermeester MA, Raşa K, et al. 2018 WSES/SIS-E consensus conference: recommendations for the management of skin and soft-tissue infections. World J Emerg Surg. 2018;13:58. https://doi.org/10.1186/s13017-018-0219-9. eCollection 2018. Review. PubMed PMID: 30564282; PubMed Central PMCID: PMC6295010

Hospital-Acquired Pneumonia and Ventilator-Associated Pneumonia

7

Massimo Sartelli

7.1 Introduction

Nosocomial pneumonia is the second most common nosocomial infection and the leading cause of death from nosocomial infections in critically ill patients. Its incidence ranges from 5 to more than 20 cases per 1000 hospital admissions [1]. Approximately one-third of nosocomial pneumonia cases, with the majority being VAP, are acquired in the Intensive care unit (ICU). US epidemiological studies report an incidence of VAP of 2–16 episodes per 1000 ventilator-days [2].

In recent years, two different sets of guidelines for the management of hospital-acquired pneumonia (HAP) and ventilator-associated pneumonia (VAP) were published: 2016 Clinical Practice Guidelines by the Infectious Diseases Society of America (IDSA) and the American Thoracic Society (ATS) [3] and 2017 Guidelines of the European Respiratory Society (ERS), European Society of Intensive Care Medicine (ESICM), European Society of Clinical Microbiology and Infectious Diseases (ESCMID) and Asociación Latinoamericana del Tórax (ALAT) [4].

Nosocomial pneumonias are generally classified into hospital-acquired pneumonia (HAP) and ventilator-associated pneumonia (VAP).

Hospital-acquired pneumonia (HAP) is defined as pneumonia occurring at least 48 h after hospital admission, excluding any infection incubating at the time of admission.

Ventilator-associated pneumonia (VAP) is defined as a pneumonia occurring in patients under mechanical ventilation for at least 48 h. It is a frequent issue in intensive care units, with a great impact on morbidity, mortality, and cost of care. Treating VAP is a difficult task, as initial antibiotics have to be appropriate and prompt.

The term healthcare-associated pneumonia (HCAP) was included in the previous guidelines to identify patients coming from community settings at risk for multidrug-resistant (MDR) bacteria. HCAP referred to pneumonia acquired in healthcare

M. Sartelli (✉)
Department of Surgery, Macerata Hospital, Macerata, Italy

© Springer Nature Switzerland AG 2021
M. Sartelli et al. (eds.), *Infections in Surgery*, Hot Topics in Acute Care Surgery and Trauma, https://doi.org/10.1007/978-3-030-62116-2_7

facilities including nursing homes, hemodialysis centers and outpatient clinics or acquired in patients with previous hospitalization within the past 90 days. However, HCAP was not included in recent guidelines because there is increasing evidence that etiology in HCAP patients is similar to that of community-acquired pneumonia and that many patients with HCAP are not at high risk for multidrug-resistant (MDR) bacteria with the highest rates in immunocompromised, surgical, and elderly patients [3, 4].

7.2   Risk Factors

The pathogenesis of nosocomial pneumonia is multifactorial [5]. The concomitant illnesses of hospitalized patients may be a risk for nosocomial infections. in hospitalized patients, alterations in immune function make patients more susceptible to invasive infections that would not occur in healthy individuals. Many hospitalized patients are in poor nutritional status, increasing their risk of infection. Severe illness and hemodynamic compromise are associated with increased rates of nosocomial pneumonia. Aspiration of oropharyngeal secretions may play a significant role in the development of nosocomial pneumonia. In hospitalized patients, the combination of altered immune function, impaired mucocilliary clearance of the respiratory tract, and oropharynx colonization by enteric gram-negative pathogens make aspiration an important contributor to pneumonia. Moreover, supine positioning contributes greatly to the aspiration risk.

Risk factors are also prolonged hospital length of stay, cigarette smoking, increasing age, uremia, alcohol consumption, coma, major surgery, malnutrition, multiple organ-system failure, and neutropenia. Importantly, the use of stress ulcer prophylaxis, such as proton pump inhibitors commonly used in critically ill patients, is associated with risk of nosocomial pneumonia. Finally, foreign bodies, such as endotracheal and nasogastric tubes, may provide a source for further colonization allowing migration of pathogens to the lower respiratory. Specifically, the endotracheal tube is a foreign body that forms a direct conduit from the heavily colonized oropharynx to the normally sterile trachea. The presence of an endotracheal tube allows biofilm formation and promotes entrapment and adherence of bacteria to the biofilm, where antibiotics are not able to penetrate.

7.3   Diagnosis

The method of establishing the diagnosis of HAP remains controversial and no method has emerged as the gold standard.

The Centers for Disease Control and Prevention and the National Healthcare Safety Network have developed criteria for the diagnosis of nosocomial pneumonia, taking into account clinical factors, such as fever and leukocytosis, as well as radiological criteria, including persistent new findings on chest radiograph [5, 6].

7.3.1 Radiology

Two or more serial chest radiographs with at least one of the following:

New or progressive and persistent infiltrate.
Consolidation.
Cavitation.

7.3.2 Signs/Symptoms/Laboratory

At least one of the following:

- Fever (>38C or > 100.4F) with no other recognized cause.
- Leukopenia (<4000 white blood cell count per microliter [WBC/mL] or leukocytosis).
- (>12,000 WBC/mL).
- For adults 70 years old or older, mental status changes with no other recognized cause.

And at least two of the following:

- New onset of purulent sputum, or change in character of sputum, or increased respiratory.
- Secretions, or increased suctioning requirements.
- New onset or worsening cough, or dyspnea, or tachycardia.
- Rales or bronchial breath sounds.
- Worsening gas exchange (PaO2/fraction of inspired oxygen [FIO2] %240), increased oxygen.
- Requirements, or increased ventilation demand.

In clinical practice, it is difficult to determine the likelihood of pneumonia, and antibiotics are frequently used when pneumonia is not present. These results call into question the physician's ability to diagnose pneumonia based solely on clinical findings. The Clinical Pulmonary Infection Score (CPIS) was developed by Pugin et al. [7, 8] to help quantify clinical findings and minimize either the initiation of antibiotic therapy or to influence its duration.

CPIS scoring was based on measurement of six clinical parameters: Temperature, total leucocyte count, quality of tracheal aspirate, oxygenation, radiographic findings, and semiquantitative culture of the tracheal aspirate. Point values are assigned to each criteria and a sum is calculated. Traditionally, a threshold score of more than six has been used to diagnose pneumonia. Obtaining cultures of respiratory secretions and blood cultures from all patients with suspected HAP or VAP in order to guide antibiotic treatment are always recommended. Noninvasive techniques such as endotracheal aspiration can be done more rapidly than invasive sampling, with fewer complications and resources, however may led to an over-identification of bacteria by initial direct examination of samples. Invasive bronchoscopic techniques such as bronchoalveolar lavage (BAL) or protected specimen brush (PSB) require the participation of qualified clinicians, may compromise gas exchange during the procedure and may be associated with higher direct costs.

Microbiology can be confirmed by both semiquantitative culture results [4] (with growth of microorganism(s) reported as light/few, moderate, or abundant/many) and quantitative culture results [5] (growth thresholds considered significant at 10^3 colony-forming units [CFU]/mL for PSB or 10^4 CFU/mL for BAL). However, there is no still consensus in the clinical microbiology community as to whether these specimens should be cultured quantitatively, using the aforementioned designated bacterial cell count to designate infection, or by a semiquantitative approach.

7.4 Antibiotic Therapy

The most important factor influencing the mortality of HAP is prompt and adequate empiric treatment. Multiple studies have demonstrated that delays in appropriate antibiotic therapy are associated with increased mortality.

Once HAP or VAP is suspected clinically, antibiotic therapy should be started. In patients with sepsis or septic shock, antibiotics should be started as soon as possible (within 1 h).

Delaying empiric antibiotic treatment and failing to give an appropriate regimen are both associated with higher mortality rates.

Choice of a specific regimen for empiric therapy should be based on:

- Patient's clinical conditions,
- Knowledge of the prevailing pathogens within the healthcare setting, and,
- The individual patient's risk factors for multidrug resistance.

Knowledge of the predominant bacteria, and particularly their susceptibility patterns, should greatly impact the choice of empiric therapy. Awareness and knowledge of local resistance patterns is critical to decide empiric antibiotic therapy for HAP and VAP.

A narrow-spectrum empiric antibiotic therapy with activity against non-resistant gram-negative and methicillin-sensitive *S. aureus* (MSSA) is suggested in low risk patients and early-onset HAP/VAP. Low risk patients are those who present HAP/VAP without septic shock, with no other risk factors for MDR bacteria and those who are not in hospitals with a high background rate of resistant pathogens.

Conversely, broader-spectrum initial empiric therapy covering resistant gram-negative bacteria and include antibiotic coverage for MRSA is suggested in high-risk patients. High-risk patients are those with septic shock and/or who have the following risk factors for potentially resistant bacteria including hospital settings with high rates of MDR bacteria, previous antibiotic use, recent prolonged hospital stay, and previous colonization with MDR bacteria.

The traditional intermittent dosing of each agent for VAP may be replaced with prolonged infusions of certain beta-lactam antibiotics to optimize pharmacokinetic/ pharmacodynamic principles, especially in critically ill patients with infections caused by gram-negative bacilli and overall for those patients with infections caused by gram-negative bacilli that have elevated but susceptible MICs to the chosen agent.

Longer treatment course increases the risks of both *Clostridium difficile* infections and antimicrobial resistance. A 7–8 day course of antibiotic therapy in patients with HAP/VAP without immunodeficiency, cystic fibrosis, empyema, lung abscess, cavitation, or necrotizing pneumonia and with a good clinical response to therapy is generally suggested. In these patients prolonged regimens do not improve patients' outcome.

7.5 Conclusions

Hospital-acquired pneumonia (HAP) is an infection of the pulmonary parenchyma caused by pathogens that are present in hospital settings. It develops in patients admitted to the hospital for >48 h. Ventilator-associated pneumonia (VAP) develops in intensive care unit (ICU) patients who have been mechanically ventilated for at least 48 h.

HAP and, most prominently, VAP increase duration of hospitalization and healthcare costs.

To best prevent and treat HAP and VAP, it is important to have an understanding of the risk factors and pathophysiology causing them and to know the varying diagnostic and treatment regimens leading to improvements in patient care and outcomes.

References

1. American Thoracic Society Infectious Diseases Society of America. Guidelines for the management of adults with hospital-acquired, ventilator-associated, and healthcare-associated pneumonia. Am J Respir Crit Care Med. 2005;171:388–416.
2. Rosenthal VD, Bijie H, Maki DG, et al. International Nosocomial Infection Control Consortium (INICC) report, data summary of 36 countries, for 2004–2009. Am J Infect Control. 2012;40:396–407.
3. Kalil AC, Metersky ML, Klompas M, Muscedere J, Sweeney DA, Palmer LB, Napolitano LM, O'Grady NP, Bartlett JG, Carratalà J, El Solh AA, Ewig S, Fey PD, File TM Jr, Restrepo MI, Roberts JA, Waterer GW, Cruse P, Knight SL, Brozek JL. Management of adults with hospital-acquired and ventilator-associated pneumonia: 2016 clinical practice guidelines by the Infectious Diseases Society of America and the American Thoracic Society. Clin Infect Dis. 2016;63(5):e61–e111.
4. Torres A, Niederman MS, Chastre J, Ewig S, Fernandez-Vandellos P, Hanberger H, Kollef M, Li Bassi G, Luna CM, Martin-Loeches I, Paiva JA, Read RC, Rigau D, Timsit JF, Welte T, Wunderink R. International ERS/ESICM/ESCMID/ALAT guidelines for the management of hospital-acquired pneumonia and ventilator-associated pneumonia: guidelines for the

management of hospital-acquired pneumonia (HAP)/ventilator-associated pneumonia (VAP) of the European Respiratory Society (ERS), European Society of Intensive Care Medicine (ESICM), European Society of Clinical Microbiology and Infectious Diseases (ESCMID) and Asociación Latinoamericana del Tórax (ALAT). Eur Respir J. 2017;50(3):1700582.

5. Kieninger AN, Lipsett PA. Hospital-acquired pneumonia: pathophysiology, diagnosis, and treatment. Surg Clin North Am. 2009;89(2):439–61.
6. Andrews CP, Coalson JJ, Smith JD, et al. Diagnosis of nosocomial bacterial pneumonia in acute, diffuse lung injury. Chest. 1981;80:248–54.
7. Pugin J, Auckenthaler R, Mill N, et al. Diagnosis of ventilator-associated pneumonia by bacteriologic analysis of bronchoscopic and non-bronchoscopic "blind" bronchoalveolar lavage. Am Rev Respir Dis. 1991;143:1121–9.
8. Luyt CE, Chastre J, Fagon JY, et al. Value of the clinical pulmonary infection score for the identification and management of ventilator-associated pneumonia. Intensive Care Med. 2004;30:844–52.

How to Prevent and Treat Catheter-Associated Urinary Tract Infections

8

Belinda De Simone, Massimo Sartelli, Luca Ansaloni, and Fausto Catena

Abbreviations

CA-ASB	catheter-associated asymptomatic bacteriuria
CAUTI	catheter-associated urinary tract infection(s)
CFU	colony forming unit(s)
HAI	hospital acquired infection(s)
ICU	intensive care unit
IDSA	Infectious Diseases Society of America
RCT	randomize controlled trial
TMP	trimethoprim
TMP-SMX	trimethoprim-sulfamethoxazole
UTI	urinary tract infection(s)

B. De Simone (✉)
Department of Emergency and General Surgery, Azienda USL Reggio Emilia IRCSS, Reggio Emilia, Italy

M. Sartelli
Department of Surgery, Macerata Hospital, Macerata, Italy

L. Ansaloni
Department of Emergency and Trauma Surgery, University of Pavia, Pavia, Italy

F. Catena
Department of Emergency and Trauma Surgery, University Hospital of Parma, Parma, Italy

© Springer Nature Switzerland AG 2021
M. Sartelli et al. (eds.), *Infections in Surgery*, Hot Topics in Acute Care Surgery and Trauma, https://doi.org/10.1007/978-3-030-62116-2_8

8.1   Background

Urinary tract infections (UTI) are one of the most common hospital-acquired infections (HAI), representing up to 40% of all HAIs. Seventy–80% of these infections are attributable to an indwelling urethral catheter and as many as 95% of UTI in intensive care units (ICU) are associated with catheters [1–3]. In 2011, there were an estimated 93,000 cases of CAUTI in US acute care hospitals [3]. CAUTIs can lead to more serious complications such as sepsis and endocarditis, and it is estimated that over 13,000 deaths each year are associated with health-care-associated UTI [4].

The Centers for Disease Control and Prevention defines CAUTI as an UTI that develops in a patient who had an indwelling catheter in place at the time of infection onset or within 48 h before [5]. An indwelling catheter is specifically defined as a drainage tube inserted into the urinary bladder through the urethra, left in place, and connected to a closed collection system. As such, it excludes straight catheters, suprapubic catheters, nephrostomy tubes, and condom catheters. In addition to infection, catheter use is associated with nonbacterial urethral inflammation, urethral strictures, mechanical trauma, and mobility impairment. Genitourinary trauma events are reported to occur in 1.5% of catheter days [6].

The estimated rates of CAUTI vary by service: in an analysis of 15 hospitals in the Duke Infection Control Outreach Network, the rates were 1.83 per 1000 catheter days for patients in intensive care, compared with 1.55 per 1000 catheter days for other patients [7].

Specifically among surgical patients, rates of UTI range from 1.8% to 4.1% based on surgery type, and development of UTI has been associated with increased duration of hospital stay, increased incidence of surgical site infections, increased incidence of prosthetic infections, and increased mortality [8].

The risk of UTI with catheterization varies only slightly by catheter type but no study showed a statistically significant difference [9].

CAUTI are associated with increased morbidity, mortality, and costs. Hospital-associated bloodstream infection from a urinary source has a case fatality of 32.8%. Risk factors for developing hospital-acquired urinary tract–related bloodstream infection include neutropenia, renal disease, and male sex [10].

Each episode of CAUTI is estimated to cost $600; if associated with a bloodstream infection, costs increase to $2800. Nationally, CAUTIs result in an estimated $131 million annual excess medical costs in US [11].

An estimated 17% to 69% of CAUTI may be preventable with recommended infection control measures, which means that up to 380,000 infections and 9000 deaths related to CAUTI per year could be prevented and prevention has become a priority [11].

The most important risk factor for CAUTI is the prolonged use of the urinary catheter as summarized in Table 8.1. Reducing unnecessary catheter placement and minimizing the duration the catheter remains in situ are the primary strategies for CAUTI prevention (Table 8.2). Additional risk factors include female sex, older age, and not maintaining a closed drainage system.

Table 8.1 Simple main statements to prevent catheter-associated urinary tract infections

Simple main statements to prevent catheter-associated urinary tract infections
Sterile catheter insertion
Avoid unnecessary urinary catheters
Maintain urinary catheters based on recommended guidelines
Minimal duration of catheter placement

Table 8.2 Risk factors for catheter-associated urinary tract infections (CAUTI)

Risk factors for CAUTI modifiable	Risk factors for CAUTI non-modifiable
Duration of catheterization	Female sex
Non-aseptic catheter care	Aged>50
Lower professional training of inserter	Diabetes mellitus
Catheter insertion outside operating room	Serum creatinine >2 mg/dL
	Severe underlying disease

8.1.1 Key Points of the Problem

- Approximately 20% of patients have a urinary catheter placed at some time during their hospital stay, especially in ICUs, in long-term care facilities, and increasingly in home care settings [1].
- The daily risk of acquisition of bacteriuria varies from 3% to 10% when an indwelling urethral catheter remains in situ, approaching 100% after 30 days, which marks also the definition between short and long-term catheterization.
- Approximately 10–25% patients with bacteriuria progresses to symptomatic UTI and 1–4% develops urosepsis [12].
- Every single episode of catheterization in hospitalized patients represents a risk for CAUTI with high costs for health care systems.
- Inappropriate treatment of catheter-associated asymptomatic bacteriuria promotes antimicrobial resistance and Clostridium difficile infection in acute care facilities.

8.1.2 Definitions

UTIs are classified as:

- *Lower* that is UTI confined to the bladder;
- *Upper* that is pyelonephritis;
- *Uncomplicated* when UTI occurs in a normal host who has no structural or functional abnormalities, not pregnant, or who has not been instrumented (for example, with a catheter).
- *Complicated* is UTI that occurs in a host with predisposing conditions such as a catheter, regardless of the presenting clinical features or severity of illness. There is a wide spectrum of conditions represented in patients with complicated UTI,

including those with CAUTI, such as simple cystitis, pyelonephritis, pyelonephritis with abscess, prostatitis, and bacteremia [13].

8.2 Etiology, Microbiology, and Pathogenesis of CAUTIs

UTI develops from bacteriuria. In patients with indwelling urinary catheter or in patients with a recent history of urinary catheterization, the catheter represents the most common route of access for pathogens into the bladder [13].

The incidence of febrile UTI and bacteremia is relatively low since colonization of urethral catheters is caused mainly by less virulent organisms and a non-obstructed catheter effectively drains the infection [14].

The bacterial spectrum reflects the locally prevailing flora (e.g., community, hospital). Most microorganisms causing CAUTIs are from the endogenous microbiota of the perineum, that ascend the urethra along the external surface of the catheter. A smaller proportion of microorganisms (34%) come from the intraluminal contamination of the collection system from exogenous sources, such as frequently the health care personnel's hands [15].

Biofilm formation (that is a rapid process taking 1–3 days from contamination) is the first step for development of bacteriuria. Standard latex urinary catheters display a high propensity for biofilm formation owing to a favorable mix of hydrophobic and hydrophilic surface regions that allow for microorganisms' attachment. Biofilms are a dynamic collection of microbial organisms with continuing turnover that organize in a polysaccharide matrix on the extraluminal or intraluminal surface of the catheter. Patients continue to acquire new organisms at a rate of about 3–7% per day; up to 66% of extraluminal biofilms originate from the bacteria on the surrounding tissues in particular from gastrointestinal tract. Formation of biofilms on the intraluminal surface of the catheter occurs mainly through contamination of the closed-system urine collection bag, in fact pathogens identified on the intraluminal surface are often the same identified on the hands of health care personnel [16]. Over time, the urinary catheter becomes colonized with microorganisms living in a sessile state within the biofilm, rendering them resistant to antimicrobials and host defenses and virtually impossible to eradicate without removing the catheter [17].

The most frequent pathogens associated with CAUTI in hospitals reporting to National Healthcare Safety Network (NHSN) between 2006 and 2007 were *E. coli* (21.4%) and *Candida* spp. (21.0%), followed by *Enterococcus* spp. (14.9%), *P. aeruginosa* (10.0%), *K. pneumoniae* (7.7%), and *Enterobacter* spp. (4.1%), and *Acinetobacter baumannii* (1.2%). A smaller proportion was caused by other gram-negative bacteria and *Staphylococcus* spp. Moreover at one US tertiary care academic center, *Enterococcus* spp. (28.4%) and *Candida* spp. (19.7%) were reported to be the most common pathogens [18–20].

The persistence of *E. coli* in the urinary tract is related to the presence of Type 1 pili, an adhesin for uroepithelium as well as the Tamm–Horsfall protein [21]. *Enterococcus faecalis* and *Enterococcus faecium* are among the leading causes of hospital-acquired UTIs. Many enterococcal isolates can produce biofilms. Catheter implantation results in bladder inflammation and fibrinogen release and accumulation onto the catheter. *E. faecalis* takes advantage of the presence of fibrinogen and uses it as a resource through the production of proteases [22].

P. mirabilis is an organism of unique importance for CAUTIs. It is not typical in patients undergoing short-term catheterization, however the longer a catheter is in place the more likely *P. mirabilis* will be present. It was found in about 40% of urine samples collected from patients with chronic indwelling catheters. *P. mirabilis* has a strong biofilm forming activity compared to other uropathogens, and it is also a very potent urease producer. It hydrolyzes urea several times faster than other pathogens with urease activity. Organisms producing urease may cause a crystalline biofilm, which is similar to struvite stones, and it is associated with catheter encrustation and obstruction. Other urease producing species include *P. aeruginosa*, *K. pneumoniae*, *Morganella morganii*, other *Proteus* species, some *Providencia* spp. and some strains of *Staphylococcus aureus* and coagulase negative staphylococci [22–26].

Patients with urinary catheter also have an increased risk of UTI due to *Pseudomonas* spp. *that* is an opportunistic human pathogen, causing infections through biofilm formation on the surface of indwelling catheters. It uses a distinct mechanism to form biofilms, independent of exopolysaccharides during CAUTIs [27].

Another organism gram-negative bacillus involved in CAUTI is *Providencia stuartii* [25] and Acinetobacter Baumannii. Outbreaks of Acinetobacter urinary infections typically occur in healthcare settings treating very ill patients and rarely occur outside [22, 23].

Candiduria develops in 3–32% of patients with short-term catheterization. In case of long-term catheterization the reported incidence of candiduria was 17% [20].

Candida albicans with a growing incidence of *C glabrata* and *C tropicalis* readily causes a clinical UTI via the hematogenous route, but it can also cause ascending infection if an indwelling catheter is present, or after a long-term antibiotic therapy [18].

8.3 Clinical Features and Diagnosis of CAUTI

Patients presenting CAUTI can be symptomatic or bacteremic asymptomatic.

Diagnosis of symptomatic UTI requires both the presence of symptoms and positive urine culture that is obtained either while the indwelling catheter is in place or within 48 h of catheter removal [10, 15].

CAUTI is defined by the presence of symptoms or signs compatible with UTI, with no other identified source of infection, along with ~103 CFU/mL of ~1 bacterial species in a single catheter urine specimen or in a midstream voided urine specimen or a urine culture between 103 and 105 CFU/mL with a positive urinalysis (positive urinalysis includes the presence of nitrates, leukoesterases, pyuria, or microorganisms on gram stain) from a patient whose urethral, suprapubic, or condom catheter has been removed within the previous 48 h [28].

Symptoms considered signs of UTI are: fever, suprapubic tenderness, or costovertebral angle tenderness and systemic symptoms such as altered mentation, hypotension, or evidence of a systemic inflammatory response syndrome, when they are not attributable to another source. In patients with catheter removal in the previous 48 h, the presence of dysuria, urgency, and urinary frequency are considered clinical signs of UTI [12–18].

Diagnosis of asymptomatic catheter-associated bacteriuria and candiduria are defined as a urine culture of at least 108 colony forming units (CFU)/L and 106 CFU/L, respectively, of an identified microorganism(s) in the absence of signs and symptoms of UTI and a positive blood culture with at least one matching uropathogen to the urine culture [12–18].

Patients affected by pyelonephritis may complain nonspecific symptoms such as malaise, fever, flank pain, anorexia, altered mental status, and signs of sepsis [12–18].

Biochemical tests, such as urinary dipstick testing for nitrite and leukocyte esterase, can be performed quickly at the point-of-care with little cost. However, several factors affect the reliability and validity of these tests including the patient's intake of certain substances, urine color, the type of catheter materials used, and the strain of microorganism present in the urine [12–18].

Microbiological tests, such as quantitative urine culture, are considered to be the "gold standard" for determining significant bacteriuria. However, the diagnostic cutpoint for significant bacteriuria remains unclear and can vary between populations [12–18]. Culture specimens from the urine bag should not be obtained. It is recommended to obtain urine specimens through the catheter port using aseptic technique or, if a port is not present, puncturing the catheter tubing with a needle and syringe in patients with short-term catheterization. In long-term indwelling catheterization, the ideal method of obtaining urine for culture is to replace the catheter and collect the specimen from the freshly placed catheter. In a symptomatic patient, this should be done immediately prior to initiating antimicrobial therapy. Urine sample can be collected from suprapubic puncture also. Biofilm can be cultured directly from the catheter by a swab [12–18].

8.4   Management of CAUTIs

The aim of the antibiotic treatment in CAUTI is:

- The resolution of symptoms;
- The achievement of microbiological eradication;
- The prevention of microbiological relapse or reinfection.

The increasing antimicrobial resistance against different antimicrobials is an alarming problem with urinary pathogens. Chronic indwelling catheters are an important reservoir of different multiresistant gram-negative organisms, such as extended-spectrum beta-lactamase (ESBL) producing Enterobacteriaceae or carbapenem-resistant Enterobacteriaceae (CRE). As a consequence microorganisms may become almost impossible to eradicate and removing the catheter is the first step of treatment. While the catheter remains in situ, the spectrum of free-floating microorganisms and bacteria in the biofilms shows a dynamic turnover [29].

An early infection after short-term catheter placement (<1 month) is commonly asymptomatic and characterized by a monocolonization with the most frequently occurring bacteria such as *E. coli, Pseudomonas aeruginosa, Klebsiella pneumoniae, Proteus mirabilis, Staphylococcus epidermidis, Enterococcus* spp. and *Candida* spp.; it may be polymicrobial in up to 15% of case.

In long-term catheterized patients, polymicrobial bacteriuria occurs in up to 95% of the cases, with usually 3–5 isolated organisms: the commonest isolated bacteria is *E. coli*; associated with *Providencia stuartii, Pseudomonas, Proteus, Morganella* and *Acinetobacter, Enterococcus*, and *Candida* spp. [30–33].

In the annual summary of data reported to the National Healthcare Safety Network at the Centres for Disease Control and Prevention (2006–2007), 24.8% of *E. coli* isolates and 33.8% of *P. aeruginosa* isolates from CAUTIs were fluoroquinolone-resistant. Against ceftriaxone, resistance reported rate of *E. coli* and *K. pneumoniae* are 5.5% and 21.2%, respectively. Resistance reported rates for E.Coli, K. Pneumoniae, P. Aeruginosa and A.baumannii against Carbapenems are 4%, 10%, 25%, 25.6% respectively. Significant resistance was found against vancomycin (6.1%) and ampicillin (3.1%) in case of *E. faecalis* as well [17, 31].

The proportion of organisms that were multidrug-resistant, defined by nonsusceptibility to all agents in 4 classes, is 4% in *P. aeruginosa*, 9% in *K. pneumoniae*, and 21% in *Acinetobacter baumannii* [31].

The increasing incidence of resistant microorganisms is related to the increased antimicrobial exposure. Moreover the urinary catheter and bladder biofilm is a constantly evolving and dynamic environment with new organisms being continually incorporated in the biofilm [12].

Pyuria alone is not diagnostic of catheter-associated infection [33]. Pyuria and bacteriuria are common in catheterized patients and are not indicators for antibiotic treatment unless the patient is symptomatic. In the absence of symptoms, treatment of bacteriuria may contribute to inappropriate antimicrobial use and increased selection of antimicrobial-resistant uropathogens. Routine screening and treating catheterised patients with bacteriuria is not recommended in the absence of symptoms [33].

Treatment is only needed for symptomatic CAUTI. One exception is in pregnant women. RCTs involving non-catheterized women presenting with asymtomatic bacteriuria have shown that eradication of asymptomatic bacteriuria reduces the risk of pyelonephritis and the risk of low birth weight [34].

Another exception is in patients with cather-associated asymptomatic bacteriuria (CA-ASB) who undergo traumatic genitourinary procedures associated with mucosal bleeding, for whom studies have shown a high rate of post-procedure bacteremia and sepsis [30].

In clinical practice, consider removing or changing the catheter before treating the infection if it has been in place for more than 7 days. Catheters should be removed rather than changed when it is possible. An urine sample should be obtained from the sampling port of the catheter using an aseptic technique and sent for culture and susceptibility testing [35].

A meta-analysis was carried out to determine whether antibiotic prophylaxis at the time of removal of a urinary catheter reduces the risk of subsequent symptomatic UTI. Seven controlled studies (6 RCTs and 1 non-RC intervention study) had symptomatic UTI as endpoint were included in the analysis and authors reported that antibiotic prophylaxis was associated with benefit to the patient, with an absolute reduction in risk of UTI of 5.8% between intervention and control groups. The risk ratio was 0.45 (95% confidence interval 0.28 to 0.72). Nevertheless these outcomes, authors didn't recommend antibiotic prophylaxis for patients admitted to hospital who undergo short-term urinary catheterization at the time of removal of the urinary catheter because of the potential disadvantages of side effects and cost of antibiotics, and, above all, the development of antimicrobial resistance. They claimed the needing of identifying patients at risk for UTI who may benefit from this approach [31].

Women with CA-ASB after 48 h of a short-term catheter removal may be considered candidates for prophylactic treatment with trimethoprim/sulfamethoxazole. Methenamine salts may be used as prophylaxis in patients who require catheter placement for less than 1 week after gynecologic surgery [28].

8.4.1   Antimicrobial Selection for CAUTI

Antimicrobial agent selections for CAUTI depend on the gram stain and culture results. Routinely, 60–80% of CAUTIs have gram (−) origins, including *Escherichia coli*, *Klebsiella*, *Pseudomonas*, *Proteus*, and *Enterobacter* species. The other 20–40% are gram (+), with *Enterococcus* and *Staphylococcus* species being the most common.

Empirical antimicrobial treatment should be guided by considering factors that increase the risk of drug resistance, including the duration of hospital stay, prior antimicrobial treatments, residence at a long-term care facility, and local resistance patterns [36].

For acute uncomplicated cystitis, IDSA guidelines recommend treatment with trimethoprim-sulfamethoxazole (TMP-SMX) or trimethoprim (TMP) alone for 3 days as standard therapy. Other recommended treatments include a shorter course, such as a 3-day regimen of fluoroquinolones (e.g., ciprofloxacin, norfloxacin, and ofloxacin) that is reasonable for younger women under 65 years with mild CAUTI after catheter has been removed [28, 36] or a 7-day regimen of nitrofurantoin or a single-dose treatment with fosfomycin tromethamine. Nitrofurantoin has led to little resistance among *E. coli*, but it may have lower cure rates (85%), compared with those of other first-line agents (90–95%), and more side effects, especially acute and chronic pulmonary syndromes [30–36]. After a meta-analysis of 27 RCTs (fosfomycin versus other antibiotics), it was reported that fosfomycin may provide a valuable alternative option for the treatment of cystitis in non-pregnant and pregnant women and in elderly and pediatric patients. Fosfomycin is an old, broad-spectrum antibiotic with pharmacokinetic and pharmacodynamic aspects that favor its use for the treatment of UTIs. Specifically, after a single 3 g oral dose of fosfomycin tromethamine, the peak urine concentrations (above the minimal inhibitory concentrations of the common uropathogens) are achieved within 4 h and persist for 48 h [37]. Fluoroquinolones are not recommended as initial empirical therapy unless the prevalence of TMP-SMX or TMP resistance among local strains of *E. coli* exceeds 10–20% [30–36].

In patients suspected of having pyelonephritis, a urine culture and susceptibility test should always be performed, and initial empirical therapy should be tailored appropriately on the basis of the infecting uropathogen.

In treating pyelonephritis, a once-daily oral fluoroquinolone, including ciprofloxacin (1000 mg extended release or 500 mg twice daily, for 7 days) with or without an initial 400-mg dose of intravenous ciprofloxacin, or levofloxacin (750 mg for 5 days), is an appropriate choice for therapy in patients not requiring hospitalization where the prevalence of resistance of community uropathogens is not known to exceed 10% [30–36].

If the prevalence of fluoroquinolone resistance is thought to exceed 10%, an initial intravenous dose of a long-acting parenteral antimicrobial, such as 1 g of ceftriaxone or a consolidated 24-h dose of an aminoglycoside, is recommended [30–36].

Oral trimethoprim-sulfamethoxazole (160/800 mg [1 double-strength tablet] twice daily for 14 days) is an appropriate choice for therapy if the uropathogen is known to be susceptible. If trimethoprim-sulfamethoxazole is used when the susceptibility is not known, an initial intravenous dose of a long-acting parenteral antimicrobial, such as 1 g of ceftriaxone or a consolidated 24-h dose of an aminoglycoside, is recommended [30–36].

Oral β-lactam agents are less effective than other available agents for treatment of pyelonephritis. If an oral β-lactam agent is used, an initial intravenous dose of a long-acting parenteral antimicrobial, such as 1 g of ceftriaxone or a consolidated 24-h dose of an aminoglycoside, is recommended.

Recommended duration of therapy is 10–14 days for pyelonephritis with a β-lactam agent.

Women with pyelonephritis requiring hospitalization should be initially treated with an intravenous antimicrobial regimen, such as a fluoroquinolone; an aminoglycoside, with or without ampicillin; an extended-spectrum cephalosporin or extended-spectrum penicillin, with or without an aminoglycoside; or a carbapenem. The choice between these agents should be based on local resistance data, and the regimen should be tailored on the basis of susceptibility results [32].

In cases of CA-ASB with Candida, catheter removal should be a sufficient treatment. If symptomatic candiduria is identified, blood cultures should be drawn to assess for systemic infection. Rather than ascending from the kidneys, Candida often descends from a systemic blood infection. Systemic treatment with oral fluconazole 200 mg/day for 2 weeks is recommended for cystitis. For pyelonephritis, oral fluconazole 200 mg/day to 400 mg/day for 2 weeks may be administered for suscep-tible strains. Alternatives for resistant strains of Candida include flucytosine 25 mg/kg four times daily or amphotericin B 0.3 mg/kg/day to 0.7 mg/kg/day systemically [33].

Shorter duration of treatment is preferred in appropriate patients to limit devel-opment of resistance.

8.4.2 Practical Considerations for Treatment

- Nitrofurantoin is a key oral antibiotic stewardship program option in the treat-ment of acute uncomplicated cystitis due to multidrug-resistant gram (−) bacilli but is not is not recommended for people with an eGFR<45 ml/minute;
- Trimethoprim should only be prescribed if there is a lower risk of resistance. There is a higher risk of trimethoprim resistance with recent use and in older people in residential facilities.
- Amoxicillin is recommended only if culture results are available and bacteria are susceptible because resistance rates are high.
- Where nitrofurantoin, trimethoprim, or amoxicillin are not suitable, second choice oral antibiotics for people with no upper UTI symptoms are pivmecilli-nam or fosfomycin.
- For people with upper UTI symptoms, nitrofurantoin, trimethoprim, amoxicillin, pivmecillinam and fosfomycin are not appropriate and co-amoxiclav, ciprofloxa-cin or levofloxacin are recommended.
- In people unable to take oral antibiotics, co-amoxiclav or ciprofloxacin, ceftriax-one, gentamicin or amikacin in patients with severe infection or sepsis can be given intravenously.
- For pregnant women with CAUTI, cefalexin as the first-choice oral antibiotic for pregnant women who don't need intravenous antibiotics, and cefuroxime as the first-choice intravenous antibiotic are recommended [35].
- Regimens should be adjusted as appropriate depending on the culture and sus-ceptibility results and the clinical course.
- Treatment may need to be extended to 10–14 days if the patient's response to therapy is delayed; an abdominal computed tomography and a urologic evalua-tion may need to be performed if the patient does not have a prompt clinical response with defervescence by 72 h and presents signs of shock (Abnormal anatomy? Obstructive uropathy? Other causes of abdominal sepsis?).

8.4.3 Adverse Events Related to Antimicrobial Treatment

- Nitrofurantoin should be used with caution in those with renal impairment. It should be avoided at term in pregnancy because it may produce neonatal hemo-lysis. Adults (especially the elderly) and children on long-term therapy should be monitored for liver function and pulmonary symptoms;
- Trimethoprim has a teratogenic risk in the first trimester of pregnancy (folate antagonist), and the manufacturers advise avoidance during pregnancy;

- Quinolones are generally not recommended in children or young people who are still growing;
- Aminoglycosides doses are based on weight and renal function and whenever possible treatment should not exceed 7 days [28, 35].

8.5 Prevention of CAUTI

The clinical components of reducing CAUTI consist of three parts [35, 38–40]:

1. Avoid unnecessary urinary catheter.
2. Insert urinary catheter using aseptic technique.
3. Maintain urinary catheter based on recommended guidelines.
4. Review urinary catheter necessity daily and remove promptly: the duration of catheterization is the most important risk factor for development of infection.

Appropriate indications for indwelling urinary catheters are [38–40]:

- Acute urinary retention or obstruction.
- Urinary output monitoring in critically ill patients.
- Perioperative use in selected surgeries such as urologic surgery or surgery on contiguous structures of the genitourinary tract; prolonged surgery; large volume infusions or diuretics during surgery; intraoperative monitoring of urine output needed.
- Assistance with healing of stage III or IV perineal and sacral wounds in incontinent patients.
- Hospice/comfort/palliative care as an exception, at patient request to improve comfort (e.g., end-of-life care).
- Required immobilization for trauma or surgery.

Alternatives to indwelling catheters include [38–40]:

- External condom catheters for male patients without urinary retention or bladder outlet obstruction have lower risk of bacteriuria or symptomatic UTI.
- Intermittent catheterization several times per day may have the same or lower risk of infection, yet provide the patient with greater mobility and ensure an indwelling catheter is not left in place longer than necessary.

Inserting urinary catheters using aseptic technique requires trained personnel [38–40]. Both CDC and SHEA-IDSA note the following basic elements for insertion [35, 38]:

1. Utilize appropriate hand hygiene practice immediately before insertion of the catheter.
2. Insert an urinary catheter using aseptic technique and sterile equipment, specifically using:

- Gloves, a drape, and sponges; Standard precautions, include the use of gloves also during manipulation of the catheter site or apparatus.
- Sterile or antiseptic solution for cleaning the urethral meatus;
- Single-use packet of sterile lubricant jelly for insertion.
3. Use a small size catheter when it is possible, consistent with proper drainage, to minimize urethral trauma.

Catheter maintenance provides [38–40]:

- To maintain a sterile, continuously closed drainage system,
- To keep catheter properly secured to prevent movement and urethral traction,
- To keep collection bag below the level of the bladder at all times,
- To maintain unobstructed urine flow,
- To empty collection bag regularly, using a separate collecting container for each patient, and avoid allowing the draining spigot to touch the collecting container.

Practices to avoid during catheter maintenance include:

- Irrigating the catheter, except in cases of catheter obstruction;
- Disconnecting the catheter from the drainage tubing;
- Replacing catheter routinely (in the absence of obstruction or infection);
- If the collection system must replaced, use an aseptic technique.

Some approaches that should not be considered a routine part of CAUTI prevention, consequently [38–41]:

1. Do not routinely use antimicrobial/antiseptic-impregnated catheters.
2. Do not screen for asymptomatic bacteriuria in catheterized patients except in pregnant women and patients who undergo urologic procedures for which visible mucosal bleeding is anticipated.
3. Do not treat asymptomatic bacteriuria in catheterized patients except before invasive urologic procedures.
4. Avoid catheter irrigation: do not perform continuous irrigation of the bladder with antimicrobials as a routine infection prevention measure and if continuous irrigation is being used to prevent obstruction, maintain a closed system.
5. Do not use systemic antimicrobials routinely as prophylaxis.
6. Do not change the catheter routinely.

There are no clear clinical evidences about the use of antiseptic solution versus sterile saline for metal cleaning before catheter insertion, the use of urinary antiseptics (e.g., methenamine: the antimicrobial mechanism of methenamine is due to its hydrolysis in the body to form ammonia and formaldehyde that is bactericidal and

Table 8.3 Principles of a good management of catheter-associated urinary tract infections; CT: Computed Tomography

Principles of a good management of catheter-associated urinary tract infections
Consider removing (better) or changing the catheter before treating the infection if it has been in place for more than 7 days.
Obtain a urine sample from the sampling port of the catheter using an aseptic technique.
Take account of the severity of symptoms: If patient is hemodynamically stable, consider waiting until urine culture and susceptibility results are available before prescribing an antibiotic.
If patient presents signs of shock, offer an empiric antibiotic therapy to review according to susceptibility results, using narrow-spectrum antibiotics wherever possible.
Give oral antibiotics first-line if the person can take oral medicines, and the severity of their condition does not require intravenous antibiotics.
Review intravenous antibiotics by 48 h and consider stepping down to oral antibiotics where possible.
Ask for urological evaluation and CT scan if patient doesn't improve after 48–72 h of antibiotic therapy.
Optimal therapy duration is not well established but 7–14 days is reasonable in patients who had a satisfactory clinical response, including resolution of systemic manifestations.

broad spectrum; cranberry products: proanthocyanidins are the active ingredient in cranberries that acts as an antiadherent for bacteria within the urinary tract due to their tannin molecules containing irregular A-type linkages, which prevents adhesion of bacteria to the inner walls of the bladder) to prevent UTI, the use of catheters with valves (Table 8.3).

8.6   Conclusions (see below flowchart)

CAUTI represents a common hospital-acquired condition with potentially devastating clinical and economic consequences.

Urinary catheters should only be used for appropriate indications and should be removed as soon as they are no longer needed.

Antimicrobial resistance among urinary pathogens is an ever increasing problem. Inappropriate treatment of catheter-associated asymptomatic bacteriuria promotes antimicrobial resistance and *Clostridium difficile* infection in acute care facilities.

Antimicrobial treatment is only needed for symptomatic CAUTI. One exception is pregnant women and patients with catheter-associated asymptomatic bacteriuria who undergo traumatic genitourinary procedures associated with mucosal bleeding.

In the selection of antimicrobial agents consider the local epidemiology for antimicrobial resistance and the results of urine cultures.

If patient does not have a prompt clinical response or presents signs of shock, ask for an abdominal computed tomography and urologic evaluation.

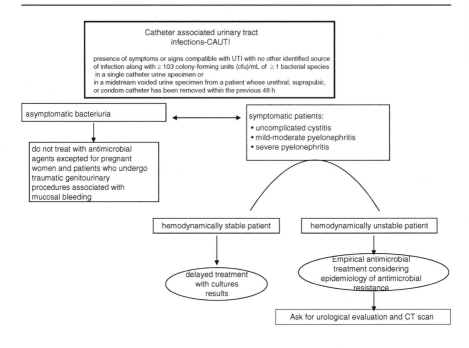

References

1. Burton D, Edwards J, Srinivasan A, et al. Trends in catheter-associated urinary tract infection in adult intensive care units-United States, 1990–2007. Infect Control Hosp Epidemiol. 2011;32:748–56.
2. Cairns S, Reilly J, Stewart S, Tolson D, Godwin J, Knight P. The prevalence of health care-associated infection in older people in acute care hospitals. Infect Control Hosp Epidemiol. 2011;32(8):763–7. https://doi.org/10.1086/660871.
3. Magill SS, Edwards JR, Bamberg W, et al. Multistate point-prevalence survey of health care–associated infections. N Engl J Med. 2014;370:1198–208. https://doi.org/10.1056/NEJMoa1306801.
4. Klevens RM, Edwards JR, Richards CL, et al. Estimating health care-associated infections and deaths in U.S. hospitals, 2002. Public Health Rep. 2007;122:160–6. https://doi.org/10.1177/003335490712200205.
5. Gould CV, Umscheid CA, Agarwal RK, et al. Guideline for prevention of catheter-associated urinary tract infections. 2009. https://www.cdc.gov/infectioncontrol/guidelines/cauti/
6. Lo E, Nicolle LE, Coffin SE, et al. Strategies to prevent catheter-associated urinary tract infections in acute care hospitals: 2014 update. Infect Control Hosp Epidemiol. 2014;35:S32–47. https://doi.org/10.1017/S0899823X00193845.
7. Lewis SS, Knelson LP, Moehring RW, Chen LF, Sexton DJ, Anderson DJ. Comparison of non-intensive care unit (ICU) versus ICU rates of catheter-associated urinary tract infection in community hospitals. Infect Control Hosp Epidemiol. 2013;34(7):744–7. https://doi.org/10.1086/671000.

8. Weber DJ, Sickbert-Bennett EE, Gould CV, Brown VM, Huslage K, Rutala WA. Incidence of catheter-associated and non-catheter-associated urinary tract infections in a healthcare system. Infect Control Hosp Epidemiol. 2011;32(8):822–3. https://doi.org/10.1086/661107.
9. Trickey AW, Crosby ME, Vasaly F, et al. Using NSQIP to investigate SCIP deficiencies in surgical patients with a high risk of developing hospital-associated urinary tract infections. Am J Med Qual. 2014;29:381–7.
10. Pickard R, Lam T, Maclennan G, et al. Types of urethral catheter for reducing symptomatic urinary tract infections in hospitalised adults requiring short-term catheterisation: multicentre randomised controlled trial and economic evaluation of antimicrobial- and antiseptic-impregnated urethral catheters (the CATHETER trial). Health Technol Assess. 2012;16:1–197.
11. Foxman B. Urinary tract infection syndromes: occurrence, recurrence, bacteriology, risk factors, and disease burden. Infect Dis Clin N Am. 2014;28(1):1–13. https://doi.org/10.1016/j.idc.2013.09.003. Epub 2013 Dec 8
12. Zimlichman E, Henderson D, Tamir O, Franz C, Song P, Yamin CK, Bates DW. Health careassociated infections: a meta-analysis of costs and financial impact on the US health care system. JAMA Intern Med. 2013; https://doi.org/10.1001/jamainternmed.2013.9763.
13. Ramanathan R, Duane TM. Urinary tract infections in surgical patients. Surg Clin North Am. 2014;94(6):1351–68. https://doi.org/10.1016/j.suc.2014.08.007. Epub 2014 Oct 3
14. Johnson JR. Definitions of complicated urinary tract infection and pyelonephritis. Clin Infect Dis. 64(3):390. https://doi.org/10.1093/cid/ciw712.
15. Blodgett TJ, Gardner SE, Blodgett NP, Peterson LV, Pietraszak M. A tool to assess the signs and symptoms of catheter-associated urinary tract infection: development and reliability. Clin Nurs Res. 2015;24(4):341–56. https://doi.org/10.1177/1054773814550506.
16. Chenoweth CE, Saint S. Urinary tract infections. Infect Dis Clin N Am. 2011;25(1):103–15. https://doi.org/10.1016/j.idc.2010.11.005. Epub 2010 Dec 18
17. Tambyah PA, Halvorson KT, Maki DG. A prospective study of pathogenesis of catheter-associated urinary tract infections. Mayo Clin Proc. 1999;74:131–6.
18. Köves B, Magyar A, Tenke P. Spectrum and antibiotic resistance of catheter-associated urinary tract infections. GMS Infect Dis. 2017;5:Doc06. Published 2017 Nov 22. https://doi.org/10.3205/id000032.
19. [https://www.intechopen.com/books/microbiology-of-urinary-tract-infections-microbial-agents-and-predisposing-factors/microbiology-of-catheter-associated-urinary-tract-infection].
20. Hidron AI, Edwards JR, Patel J, Horan TC, Sievert DM, Pollock DA, Fridkin SK. National Healthcare Safety Network team; participating National Healthcare Safety Network facilities. NHSN annual update: antimicrobial-resistant pathogens associated with healthcare-associated infections: annual summary of data reported to the National Healthcare Safety Network at the Centers for Disease Control and Prevention, 2006–2007. Infect Control Hosp Epidemiol. 2008;29(11):996–1011. https://doi.org/10.1086/591861.
21. Chang R, Greene MT, Chenoweth CE, Kuhn L, Shuman E, Rogers MA, Saint S. Epidemiology of hospital-acquired urinary tract-related bloodstream infection at a university hospital. Infect Control Hosp Epidemiol. 2011;32(11):1127–9. https://doi.org/10.1086/662378.
22. Ikäheimo R, Siitonen A, Kärkkäinen U, Mäkelä PH. Virulence characteristics of Escherichia coli in nosocomial urinary tract infection. Clin Infect Dis. 1993;16(6):785–91. https://doi.org/10.1093/clind/16.6.785.
23. Guiton PS, Hannan TJ, Ford B, Caparon MG, Hultgren SJ. Enterococcus faecalis overcomes foreign body-mediated inflammation to establish urinary tract infections. Infect Immun. 2013;81(1):329–39. https://doi.org/10.1128/IAI.00856-12.
24. Matsukawa M, Kunishima Y, Takahashi S, Takeyama K, Tsukamoto T. Bacterial colonization on intraluminal surface of urethral catheter. Urology. 2005;65(3):440–4. https://doi.org/10.1016/j.urology.2004.10.065.

25. Warren JW, Tenney JH, Hoopes JM, Muncie HL, Anthony WC. A prospective microbiologic study of bacteriuria in patients with chronic indwelling urethral catheters. J Infect Dis. 1982;146(6):719–23. https://doi.org/10.1093/infdis/146.6.719.

26. Jones BD, Mobley HL. Genetic and biochemical diversity of ureases of Proteus, Providencia, and Morganella species isolated from urinary tract infection. Infect Immun. 1987;55(9):2198–203.

27. Cole SJ, Records AR, Orr MW, Linden SB, Lee VT. Catheter-associated urinary tract infection by Pseudomonas aeruginosa is mediated by exopolysaccharide-independent biofilms. Infect Immun. 2014;82(5):2048–58. https://doi.org/10.1128/IAI.01652-14.

28. Hooton TM, Bradley SF, Cardenas DD, Colgan R, Geerlings SE, Rice JC, Saint S, Schaeffer AJ, Tambayh PA, Tenke P, Nicolle LE. Diagnosis, prevention, and treatment of catheter-associated urinary tract infection in adults: 2009 international clinical practice guidelines from the Infectious Diseases Society of America. Clin Infect Dis. 2010;50(5):625–63. https://doi.org/10.1086/650482.

29. Brennan BM, Coyle JR, Marchaim D, Pogue JM, Boehme M, Finks J, Malani AN, VerLee KE, Buckley BO, Mollon N, Sundin DR, Washer LL, Kaye KS. Statewide surveillance of carbapenem-resistant enterobacteriaceae in Michigan. Infect Control Hosp Epidemiol. 2014;35(4):342–9. https://doi.org/10.1086/675611.

30. Nicolle LE, Gupta K, Bradley SF, Colgan R, DeMuri GP, Drekonja D, Eckert LO, Geerlings SE, Köves B, Hooton TM, Juthani-Mehta M, Knight SL, Saint S, Schaeffer AJ, Trautner B, Wullt B, Siemieniuk R. Clinical practice guideline for the Management of Asymptomatic Bacteriuria: 2019 update by the Infectious Diseases Society of America. Clin Infect Dis. 2019;68(10):e83–e110. https://doi.org/10.1093/cid/ciy1121.

31. Marschall J, Carpenter CR, Fowler S, Trautner BW. CDC prevention epicenters program. Antibiotic prophylaxis for urinary tract infections after removal of urinary catheter: meta-analysis [published correction appears in BMJ. 2013;347:f5325]. BMJ. 2013;346:f3147. Published 2013 June 11. https://doi.org/10.1136/bmj.f3147.

32. Gupta K, Hooton TM, Naber KG, Wullt B, Colgan R, Miller LG, Moran GJ, Nicolle LE, Raz R, Schaeffer AJ, Soper DE. International clinical practice guidelines for the treatment of acute uncomplicated cystitis and pyelonephritis in women: a 2010 update by the Infectious Diseases Society of America and the European Society for Microbiology and Infectious Diseases. Clin Infect Dis. 2011;52(5):e103–20. https://doi.org/10.1093/cid/ciq257.

33. Trautner BW. Management of catheter-associated urinary tract infection. Curr Opin Infect Dis. 2010;23(1):76–82. https://doi.org/10.1097/QCO.0b013e328334dda8.

34. Smaill FM, Vazquez JC. Antibiotics for asymptomatic bacteriuria in pregnancy. Cochrane Database Syst Rev. 2015;(8):CD000490. https://doi.org/10.1002/14651858.CD000490.pub3.

35. https://www.nice.org.uk/guidance/ng109/chapter/Recommendations#choice-of-antibiotic; https://www.nice.org.uk/guidance/ng111/chapter/Recommendations

36. Wagenlehner FME, Pilatz A, Naber KG, et al. Anti-infective treatment of bacterial urinary tract infections. Curr Med Chem. 2008;15:1412–27.

37. Falagas ME, Vouloumanou EK, Togias AG, Karadima M, Kapaskelis AM, Rafailidis PI, Athanasiou S. Fosfomycin versus other antibiotics for the treatment of cystitis: a meta-analysis of randomized controlled trials. J Antimicrob Chemother. 2010;65(9):1862–77. https://doi.org/10.1093/jac/dkq237.

38. http://www.icpsne.org/SHEA%202014%20Updated%20CAUTI%20Prevention%20Guidelines%20(1).pdf

39. https://www.ahrq.gov/sites/default/files/publications/files/implementation-guide_0.pdf

40. https://www.urotoday.com/images/catheters/pdf/IHIHowtoGuidePreventCAUTI.pdf

41. Cortese YJ, Wagner VE, Tierney M, Devine D, Fogarty A. Review of catheter-associated urinary tract infections and in vitro urinary tract models. J Healthc Eng. 2018;2018:2986742. Published 2018 Oct 14. https://doi.org/10.1155/2018/2986742.

How to Prevent and Treat Catheter-Related Bloodstream Infections

9

Cristian Tranà

9.1   Introduction

Central venous catheters (CVCs) are integral to the modern clinical practices and are inserted for the administration of fluids, blood products, medication, nutritional solutions, hemodialysis, and for hemodynamic monitoring [1]. They are the main source of bacteremia in hospitalized patients and therefore should be used only if they are really necessary.

About half of nosocomial bloodstream infections occur in intensive care units, and the majority of them are associated with intravascular device. Central-venous-catheter-related bloodstream infections (CRBSIs) are an important cause of healthcare-associated infections [1].

The 2010 United States National Health-care Safety Network (NHSN) report that covered 2473 hospitals reported nearly 11,000 cases of laboratory-confirmed CRBSI, with estimated CRBSI rates of up to 3.5% [2]. A study involving four European countries (France, Germany, Italy and the UK) estimated there were between 8400 to 14,400 episodes of CRBSI per year in these countries, with associated annual costs of between EUR 35.9 and EUR 163.9 million [3].

In the setting of CRBSIs, prevention is a cornerstone and the clinician must well know risk factors to develop a CRBSI.

9.2   Risk Factors

Risk factors for CRBSI include patient-, catheter-, and operator-related factors [4–9]:

C. Tranà (✉)
Department of Oncologic and General Surgery, Macerata Hospital, Macerata, Italy

© Springer Nature Switzerland AG 2021   89
M. Sartelli et al. (eds.), *Infections in Surgery*, Hot Topics in Acute Care Surgery
and Trauma, https://doi.org/10.1007/978-3-030-62116-2_9

- Prolonged hospitalization before catheterization.
- Prolonged duration of catheterization.
- Heavy microbial colonization at the insertion site.
- Heavy microbial colonization of the catheter hub.
- Internal jugular catheterization.
- Femoral catheterization in adults.
- Neutropenia.
- Prematurity (i.e., early gestational age).
- Reduced nurse-to-patient ratio in the ICU [10, 11].
- Total parenteral nutrition.
- Substandard catheter care (e.g., excessive manipulation of the catheter).
- Transfusion of blood products (in children).

The catheter itself can be involved in 4 different pathogenic pathways [1]:

- Colonization of the catheter by microorganisms from the patient's skin and occasionally the hands of healthcare workers,
- Intraluminal or hub contamination,
- Secondary seeding from a bloodstream infection, and, rarely,
- Administration of contaminated infusate or additives.

9.3   Strategies to Prevent CRBSIs

Shea/IDSA recommendations divide strategies to prevent CRBSIs into several categories [12, 13].

Before Insertion
The use of a clear and evidence-based list of indications for CVC use to minimize unnecessary CVC placement is useful. Is also mandatory to require education of healthcare personnel involved in insertion, care, and maintenance of CVCs with periodic re-training also using simulation programs and with a credentialing process. Preoperative bathing with chlorhexidine preparation seems to reduce CRBSIs in ICU patients over 2 months of age. In children under 2 months chlorhexidine gluconate based topical antiseptic products can be used with care because they may cause irritation or chemical burns. There is also a risk of systemic absorption. Alternative agents, such as povidone-iodine or alcohol, can be used in this age group. Do not administer systemic antimicrobial prophylaxis routinely before insertion or during use of an intravascular catheter to prevent catheter colonization or CRBSI.

At Insertion
It is mandatory to have in the hospital a written guideline with a checklist for CVC insertion in ICU and non-ICU settings with a special effort to the use of aseptic technique. There must be a strict observation of these recommendations. The

performing of hand hygiene with alcohol-based waterless product or antiseptic soap and water is very important. Remember that use of gloves does not obviate hand hygiene.

Another important item is the choose of the right insertion site. Avoid the use of femoral vein for central venous access especially in obese adult patients when the catheter is placed under planned and controlled conditions. Only in emergency settings is allowed the use of femoral vein. In children, the femoral site has not been associated with an increased risk of infection. Do not use peripherally inserted CVCs (PICCs) as a strategy to reduce the risk of CRBSIs: they present the same risk of internal jugular or subclavian CVCs.

The use of ultrasound guidance for internal jugular catheter insertion and maximum sterile barrier precautions during CVC insertion (such as mask, cap, sterile gown, and a sterile drape over the patient) with the use an alcoholic chlorhexidine antiseptic for skin preparation can minimize the risk of CRBSIs.

After Insertion

It is important to maintain the appropriate nurse-to-patient ratio (at least 1 to 2), to reduce the incidence of CRBSIs in ICU. Catheter hubs, needleless connectors, and injection ports before accessing the catheter must be disinfected with vigorously apply mechanical friction for no less than 5 sec with an alcoholic chlorhexidine preparation, 70% alcohol, or povidone-iodine. Alcoholic chlorhexidine may have additional residual activity compared with alcohol for this purpose.

Non-essential catheter, also without signs of infections must be removed. The dressing of CVC insertion site has to be transparent. Insertion site care must to be performed with a chlorhexidine-based antiseptic every 5–7 days or immediately if the dressing is soiled, loose, or damp; change gauze dressings every 2 days or earlier if the dressing is soiled, loose, or damp. If there is drainage from the catheter exit site, use gauze dressings instead of transparent dressings until drainage resolves.

Antimicrobial ointments can be used for hemodialysis catheter-insertion sites. Polysporin "triple" (where available) or povidone-iodine ointment should be applied to hemodialysis catheter insertion if compatible with the catheter material. Avoid mupirocin ointment the risks of facilitating mupirocin resistance and the potential damage to polyurethane catheters.

Last but not least the surveillance for CRBSIs: Measure the unit-specific incidence of CRBSIs (CRBSIs per 1000 catheter-days) and report the data on a regular basis to the units, physician and nursing leadership, and hospital administrators overseeing the units; Compare these data with historical for individual units and with national rates and perform audit with multidisciplinary involvement.

A special issue: catheter impregnation, coating, or bonding for reducing central venous catheter-related infections in adults [14].

Currently, modifications of the CVC itself, in the form of antimicrobial impregnation, coating, or bonding, have also been used to prevent CRBSI. two major types of antimicrobial agents are used as CVC coatings: antiseptics and antibiotics. 'Antiseptic' refers to an agent that destroys or inhibits the growth of a range of microorganisms that are present in or on living tissues (e.g., hand washes or surgical scrubs), while 'antibiotic' refers to an agent that acts in similar fashion to an antiseptic, but targets selected micro-organisms, especially bacteria, and works generally in low concentrations [15]. Various forms of antiseptic and antibiotic catheter impregnation have been introduced since the late 1980s, including chlorhexidine-silver sulphadiazine (C-SS) and minocycline-rifampicin (MR) impregnation, which are the most commonly used and studied [16, 17]. Impregnation was only applied at the external surface of the first C-SS-impregnated catheters, but MR impregnation is applied to both external and luminal surfaces. More recently, second generation C-SS-impregnated catheters have been introduced, with both the external and luminal surfaces of the catheters impregnated [18]. Several other compounds that have demonstrated antibacterial activities in vitro, like silver, platinum, carbon and heparin have also been evaluated as CVC-impregnation materials in clinical studies [19–21]. Silver and platinum were found to inhibit bacterial cell growth and division [22, 23], while heparin was thought to reduce bacterial growth via a prevention of fibrin deposition and thrombus formation in the catheters [19]. Carbon nanotubes were seen to cause cell wall damage to bacteria that were in direct contact with them [24], and combining these with platinum and silver enhanced their overall antibacterial properties [25].

About this topic a Cochrane Systematic Review [14] demonstrate that there is significant benefits with impregnated CVCs for catheter-related outcomes, such as catheter colonization, in trials conducted in intensive care units (ICUs) only. There is also a high-quality, but smaller body of evidence that shows no significant benefit of these catheters in reducing mortality, and moderate-quality evidence shows no difference in clinically diagnosed sepsis. Therefore, there remains uncertainty about the value of these modified catheters in improving overall patient mortality and morbidity.

9.4   CRBSIs Diagnosis

The diagnosis of CRBSI is often suspected clinically in a patient using a CVC who presents with fever or chills, unexplained hypotension, and no other localizing signs [1]. Diagnosis of CRBSI requires establishing the presence of bloodstream infection and demonstrating that the infection is related to the catheter. Blood cultures should not be drawn solely from the catheter port as these are frequently colonized with skin contaminants, thereby increasing the likelihood of a false-positive blood culture.

According to IDSA guidelines [26] a definitive diagnosis of CRBSI requires culture of the same organism from both the catheter tip and at least one percutaneous blood culture. Alternatively, culture of the same organism from at least two blood samples (one from a catheter hub and the other from a peripheral vein or second lumen) meeting criteria for quantitative blood cultures or differential time to positivity. Most laboratories do not perform quantitative blood cultures, but many laboratories are able to determine differential time to positivity. Quantitative blood cultures demonstrating a colony count from the catheter hub sample $\geq$ three-fold higher than the colony count from the peripheral vein sample (or a second lumen) supports a diagnosis of CRBSI. Differential time to positivity (DTP) refers to growth detected from the catheter hub sample at least two hours before growth detected from the peripheral vein sample.

Quantitative blood cultures and/or DTP should be done before initiation of antimicrobial therapy and with the same volume of blood per bottle. Evidence is insufficient to recommend that blood cultures be routinely obtained after discontinuation of antimicrobial therapy for CRBSI.

In Fig. 9.1 you can see a proposed algorithm for diagnosis of CRBSIs.

9.5   CRBSIs Therapy

The CVC and arterial catheter, if present, should be removed and cultured if the patient has unexplained sepsis or erythema overlying the catheter-insertion site or purulence at the catheter-insertion site.

Antibiotic therapy for catheter-related infection is often initiated empirically. The initial choice of antibiotics will depend on the severity of the patient's clinical disease, the risk factors for infection, and the likely pathogens associated with the specific intravascular device. Resistance to antibiotic therapy due to biofilm formation also has an important role in the management of bacteremia. In fact the nature of biofilm structure makes microorganisms difficult to eradicate and confer an inherent resistance to antibiotics.

As soon as possible, a target therapy is mandatory based upon the microbiological data. Nowadays there is the possibility from a blood sample to know after few hours if the patient has gram positive or gram negative bacteria with the precise identification of the pathogen. There is also the possibility to detect the main mechanisms of antimicrobial resistance. So we can give the right antibiotic to the right patient in the right time to fight CRBSIs.

Prophylactic antimicrobial or antiseptic lock solution should be considered for the following: Patients with long-term hemodialysis catheters, Patients with limited venous access and a history of recurrent CLABSI and Pediatric cancer patients with long-term catheters [27].

Figure 9.2 shows a therapeutical algorithm for short-term CVC related infections or arterial catheter-related infections.

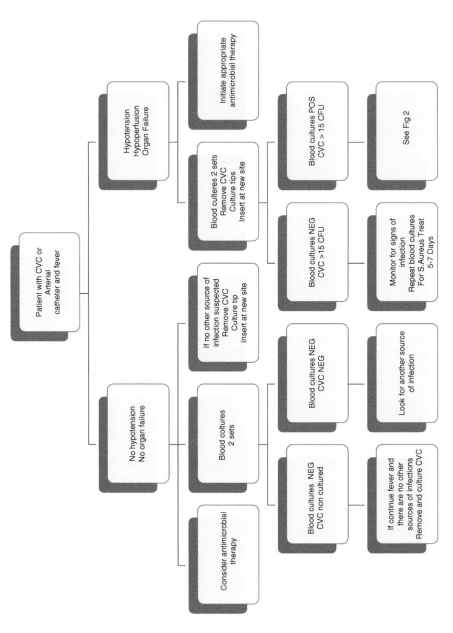

Fig. 9.1 Algorithm for the diagnosis [26]

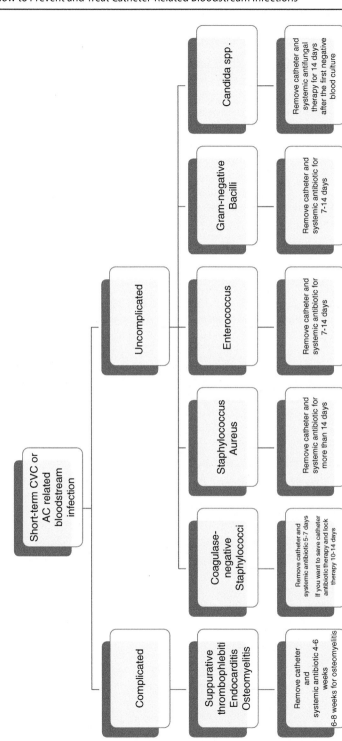

Fig. 9.2 Approach to the management of patients with short-term CVC related or arterial (AC)-related bloodstream infections [26]

9.6   Lock Therapy

Antibiotic lock therapy, a method for sterilizing the catheter lumen, involves instilling high concentrations of antibiotics into the catheter lumen for extended periods of time. Results from in vitro studies demonstrate stability of antibiotics while maintaining high concentrations for prolonged periods of time. In vivo studies show antibiotic lock technique as an effective and safe option for both prevention and treatment of CRBSIs [28].

However, removal of an infected catheter in combination with antimicrobial therapy is the most reliable method of eradicating infection. Retention of the CVC may result in failure to clear the organism from the catheter with subsequent relapse of infection. In some cases it may nevertheless be desirable to consider catheter salvage, for example:

- High risk of replacing catheter e.g., coagulopathy.
- Alternative vascular access sites limited or not available.

While a decision to salvage a catheter requires careful consideration of the risks and benefits, in general catheter salvage should not be attempted in the following circumstances [29]:

- Organisms known to be difficult to eradicate e.g., *Staphylococcus aureus*, fungi including *Candida* spp., *P. aeruginosa*, mycobacteria, environmental non-fermenting gram-negative bacilli e.g., *Stenotrophomonas maltophilia*.
- Severe sepsis and hemodynamic instability resulting from the CVC-associated infection.
- Bacteremia persisting despite 72 h of antimicrobial therapy.
- Metastatic complications e.g., infective endocarditis, osteomyelitis.
- Relapse of infection following a previous course of antimicrobial therapy.

Indications for lock therapy [28].

- Antibiotic lock is indicated for patients with catheter-related bloodstream infections involving long-term catheters with no signs of exit site or tunnel infection for whom catheter salvage is the goal.
- For CRBSI, antibiotic lock therapy should not be used as monotherapy; It should be used in conjunction with systemic antimicrobial therapy.

- Dwell times for an antibiotic lock solution should not exceed 48 h before reinstallation of lock solution; preferably reinstallation should take place every 12–24 h.
- Catheter removal is generally recommended for CRBSI due to *S.aureus* and *Candida* species instead of treatment with antibiotic lock and catheter retention.

The evidence base to support the use of antibiotic line locks is poor [29]. The majority of the trials are open-label or observational case studies with unclear participant allocation to the control and intervention groups. The trials lacked statistical power and the confidence intervals were too large to allow reliable conclusions to be drawn.

In most of the randomized controlled trials the method of blinding was unclear and none of the trials were done with an intention to treat analysis, increasing the likelihood of 'chance' findings. The definitions of a CRBSI varied between trials and some trials did not perform peripheral blood cultures to confirm a CRBSI. The primary outcome in some trials was a blood stream infection rather than a CRBSI, this may have overestimated the response rate with antibiotic line locks. Most of the randomized controlled trials looked at prevention rather than treatment of a CRBSI. Furthermore, some trials used antibiotic flush solutions rather than antibiotic line locks.

Two controlled trials showed successful treatment with antibiotic line locks in comparison to the control groups, however they lack statistical power. Recurrent bacteremia was more likely if the catheter wasn't removed.

All trials used different types of antibiotics at different concentrations. However, the majority of the trials used vancomycin antibiotic line locks. One trial reported immediate precipitation of Ciprofloxacin with heparin and significant absorbance changes with heparin and the following: Ceftazidime and Gentamicin.

Short-term and long-term adverse effects of antibiotic line locks were not assessed and are unknown. Furthermore, an increase in antibiotic resistance is a concern. None of the trials that used Vancomycin as an antibiotic line lock, showed an increase in vancomycin-resistant enterococci.

The Infectious Diseases Society of America (IDSA) recommends the use of antibiotic lock therapy in uncomplicated CRBSI with the use of systemic antibiotics, where catheter salvage is considered the best option for the patient [26].

In Fig. 9.3 you can see a proposal algorithm for treatment of long-term CVC infections or port-related infections.

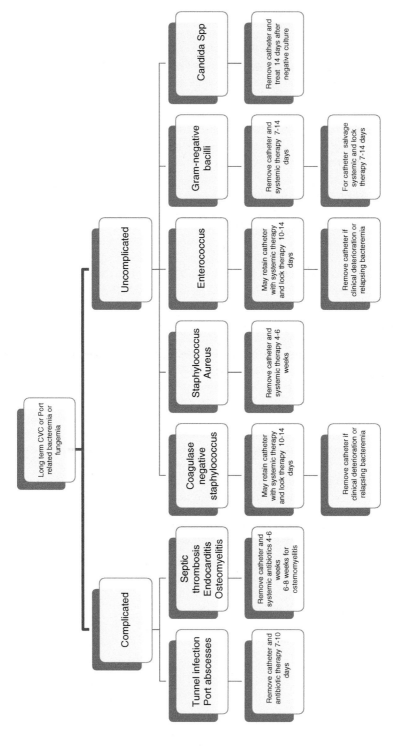

Fig. 9.3 Approach to the treatment of a patient with a long-term CVC or a port-related bloodstream infection [26]

References

1. Sartelli M. Central-venous-catheter-related bloodstream infections. In: Global Alliance for Infections in Surgery. http://www.infectionsinsurgery.org
2. Dudeck M, Horan T, Peterson K, Allen-Bridson K, Morrell G, Pollock D, et al. National Healthcare Safety Network (NHSN) report, Data Summary for 2010, Device-associated Module. National Healthcare Safety Network (NHSN) annual reports 7 July 2011.
3. Tacconelli E, Smith G, Hieke K, Lafuma A, Bastide P. Epidemiology, medical outcomes and costs of catheter-related bloodstream infections in intensive care units of four European countries: literature- and registry-based estimates. J Hosp Infect. 2009;72(2):97–103.
4. Mermel LA. Infections caused by intravascular devices. In: Pfeiffer JA, editor. APIC text of infection control and epidemiology. 2nd ed. St. Louis: Mosby; 2000. p. 30–8.
5. Almuneef MA, Memish ZA, Balkhy HH, Hijazi O, Cunningham G, Francis C. Rate, risk factors and outcomes of catheter-related bloodstream infection in a paediatric intensive care unit in Saudi Arabia. J Hosp Infect. 2006;62(2):207–13.
6. Alonso-Echanove J, Edwards JR, Richards MJ, et al. Effect of nurse staffing and antimicrobial-impregnated central venous catheters on the risk for bloodstream infections in intensive care units. Infect Control Hosp Epidemiol. 2003;24(12):916–25.
7. Lorente L, Henry C, Martin MM, Jimenez A, Mora ML. Central venous catheter–related infection in a prospective and observational study of 2,595 catheters. Crit Care. 2005;9(6):R631–5.
8. Rey C, Alvarez F, De-La-Rua V, et al. Intervention to reduce catheter-related bloodstream infections in a pediatric intensive care unit. Intensive Care Med. 2011;37(4):678–85.
9. Lorente L, Jimenez A, Naranjo C, et al. Higher incidence of catheter-related bacteremia in jugular site with tracheostomy than in femoral site. Infect Control Hosp Epidemiol. 2010;31(3):311–3.
10. Fridkin SK, Pear SM, Williamson TH, Galgiani JN, Jarvis WR. The role of understaffing in central venous catheter–associated bloodstream infections. Infect Control Hosp Epidemiol. 1996;17(3):150–8.
11. Cimiotti JP, Haas J, Saiman L, Larson EL. Impact of staffing on bloodstream infections in the neonatal intensive care unit. Arch Pediatr Adolesc Med. 2006;160:832–6.
12. Marschall J, Mermel LA, Fakih M, et al. Strategies to prevent central line–associated bloodstream infections in acute care hospitals: 2014 update. Infect Control Hosp Epidemiol. 2014;35(7):753–71. Cambridge University Press on behalf of The Society for Healthcare Epidemiology of America
13. O'Grady NP, Alexander M, Burns LA, et al. Guidelines for the prevention of intravascular catheter-related infections. Clin Infect Dis. 2011;52(9):e162–93.
14. Lai NM, Chaiyakunapruk N, Lai NA, O'Riordan E, Pau WSC, Saint S. Catheter impregnation, coating or bonding for reducing central venous catheter-related infections in adults. Cochrane Database Syst Rev. 2016;(3):CD007878. https://doi.org/10.1002/14651858.CD007878.pub3.
15. McDonnell G, Russell AD. Antiseptics and disinfectants: activity, action, and resistance. Clin Microbiol Rev. 1999;12(1):147–79. [PUBMED: 9880479]
16. Falagas ME, Fragoulis K, Bliziotis IA, Chatzinikolaou I. Rifampicin-impregnated central venous catheters: a meta-analysis of randomized controlled trials. J Antimicrob Chemother. 2007;59:359–69. [PUBMED: 17255143]
17. Mermel LA. New technologies to prevent intravascular catheter-related bloodstream infections. Emerg Infect Dis. 2001;7:197–9. [PUBMED: 11294705]
18. Ramritu P, Halton K, Collignon P, Cook D, Fraenkel D, Battistutta D, et al. A systematic review comparing the relative effectiveness of antimicrobial-coated catheters in intensive care units. Am J Infect Control. 2008;36:104–17. [PUBMED: 18313512]
19. Abdelkefi A, Achour W, Ben Othman T, Ladeb S, Torjman L, Lakhal A, et al. Use of heparin-coated central venous lines to prevent catheter-related bloodstream infection. J Support Oncol. 2007;5(6):273–8. [PUBMED: 17624052]

20. Hanna H, Bahna P, Reitzel R, Dvorak T, Chaiban G, Hachem R, et al. Comparative in vitro efficacies and antimicrobial durabilities of novel antimicrobial central venous catheters. Antimicrob Agents Chemother. 2006;50(10):3283–8. [PUBMED: 17005806]
21. Khare MD, Bukhari SS, Swann A, Spiers P, McLaren I, Myers J. Reduction of catheter-related colonization by the use of a silver zeolite-impregnated central vascular catheter in adult critical care. J Infect. 2007;54(2):146–50. [PUBMED: 16678904]
22. Jung WK, Koo HC, Kim KW, Shin S, Kim SH, Park YH. Antibacterial activity and mechanism of action of the silver ion in Staphylococcus aureus and Escherichia coli. Appl Environ Microbiol. 2008;74(7):2171–8. [PUBMED: 18245232]
23. Rosenberg B, Van Camp L, Grimley EB, Thomson AJ. The inhibition of growth or cell division in Escherichia coli by different ionic species of platinum (IV) complexes. J Biol Chem. 1967;242(6):1347–52. [PUBMED: 5337590]
24. Kang S, Pinault M, Pfefferle LD, Elimelech M. Single-walled carbon nanotubes exhibit strong antimicrobial activity. Langmuir. 2007;23(17):8670–3. [PUBMED: 17658863]
25. Narayan R, Abernathy H, Riester L, Berry C, Brigmon R. Antimicrobial properties of diamond-like carbon-silver-platinum nanocomposite thin films. J Mater Eng Perform. 2005;14:435–40. https://doi.org/10.1361/105994905X56197.
26. Mermel LA, Allon M, Bouza E, et al. Clinical practice guidelines for the diagnosis and management of intravascular catheter-related infection: 2009 update by the Infectious Diseases Society of America. Clin Infect Dis. Jul 1 2009;49(1):1–45.
27. Ling, et al. APSIC guide for prevention of Central Line Associated Bloodstream Infections (CLABSI). Antimicrob Resist Infect Control. 2016;5:16. https://doi.org/10.1186/s13756-016-0116-5.
28. Mui E. Antibiotic lock therapy guideline. Stanford Hospital and Clinics Pharmacy Department Policies and Procedures. Issue Date: 06/2011.
29. Nottingham Antimicrobial Guidelines Committee. Antibiotic line lock guideline. Nottingham University Hospital. October 2017.

Clostridium difficile Infection in Surgical Patients

10

John Woods, Nikita Bhatt, and Raul Coimbra

10.1   Introduction

A marked increase in the incidence and severity of *Clostridium difficile* infection (CDI) has been observed in the last 30 years. CDI is the most common cause of diarrhea in hospitalized patients.

Age, comorbidities, drug-induced immunosuppression, immunosuppressive diseases, hypoproteinemia, inflammatory bowel disease, and previous use of antibiotics in the hospital setting all constitute known risk factors for the development of the disease [1–3]. Additionally, surgical procedures not only predispose patients to CDI but it can also be used as a treatment modality in cases of very severe CDI (toxic megacolon).

In this chapter we will review the etiology, pathophysiology, clinical manifestations, and the most modern treatment options for different stages of CDI.

J. Woods
University of California Riverside, Riverside, CA, USA

Riverside University Health System Medical Center, Moreno Valley, CA, USA

N. Bhatt
Riverside University Health System Medical Center, Moreno Valley, CA, USA

R. Coimbra (✉)
Riverside University Health System Medical Center, Moreno Valley, CA, USA

Loma Linda University, Loma Linda, CA, USA
e-mail: r.coimbra@ruhealth.org

© Springer Nature Switzerland AG 2021
M. Sartelli et al. (eds.), *Infections in Surgery*, Hot Topics in Acute Care Surgery and Trauma, https://doi.org/10.1007/978-3-030-62116-2_10

10.2 Etiology

Clostridioides difficile, formerly known as *Clostridium difficile*, is a gram-positive, obligate anaerobe capable of producing spores which allow it to survive in aerobic conditions then contributing to transmission in healthcare settings [4]. Although historically *C. difficile* has not been found to be a normal commensal organism of the human gastrointestinal tract, it now colonizes 4–15% of the adult population [5]. Colonization typically occurs via the fecal-oral route and the disruption of microbial ecosystem with antibiotics leads to clinical disease. Awareness and prevention of risk factors for infection is of paramount importance as *C. difficile* is one of the most common causes of hospital-acquired infections with half a million annual cases and more than 29,000 deaths occurring annually in the United States [6].

The organism is spread among humans by the fecal-oral route, and when transformed to its spore state, it is difficult to eradicate with alcohol-based and other traditional surface cleaners. The spores, which can be shed by both symptomatic and asymptomatic patients, can remain on contaminated surfaces for up to 5 months [7]. This puts patients at risk for infection from contact with the healthcare environment or healthcare workers' hands. Implementation of infection control measures such as the use of personal protective equipment, hand washing with soap and water, use of sporicidal agents for cleaning surfaces, and isolation of patients are key in preventing hospital-acquired infections caused by *C. difficile*.

10.3 Pathophysiology

Disease severity can range from mild diarrhea to pseudomembranous colitis which was identified as caused by *C. difficile* over 40 years ago [8]. Both host factors (age >65 years, previous CDI episode, and immunocompromised status) and environmental risk factors (antibiotic and proton pump inhibitor exposure) play a role in the development of *C. difficile*-associated diarrhea (CDAD).

Upon transmission via the fecal-oral route, the vegetative cells are killed by the acidic environment of the stomach while the acid-resistant spores are able to pass to the small bowel where they are converted to the vegetative form under favorable conditions leading to toxin production. It is important to note that only toxin-producing strains cause clinical disease. The prime conditions for infection with *C. difficile* occur when the commensal bacterial population of the colon has been altered and exposure to *C. difficile* toxins alters the gut epithelium invoking an immune response which is responsible for CDAD symptoms [9].

There are two main toxins responsible for the disease course, Toxin A (TcdA) and Toxin B (TcdB). Both toxins work synergistically to promote recruitment of macrophages, and monocytes which in turn promote release of inflammatory markers resulting in neutrophil recruitment. When the colonic lining becomes inflamed with infiltration of macrophages and neutrophils, frequent watery diarrhea results [10]. The manifestations of the disease can vary from mild diarrhea to pseudomembranous colitis based on age, immune response, and virulence of the strain of *C. difficile* to which a host is exposed.

Some *C. difficile* strains, particularly BI/NAP1/027, may produce a binary toxin called *C. difficile* transferase (CDT). This hypervirulent strain causes more toxin production, higher rates of recurrence, and higher mortality rates than other strains and is a result of resistance acquired in *C. difficile* due to increase in use of fluoroquinolones. Given that certain antibiotics can select for resistance in *C. difficile* it is even more important to focus on antimicrobial stewardship strategies as a way to slow down the *C. difficile* epidemic.

10.4   Clinical Manifestations

The spectrum of disease produced by toxic strains of *C. difficile* is variable, ranging from asymptomatic infection or mild diarrhea to severe disease that may result in toxic megacolon, multisystem organ failure, and death. Up to 30% of patients may develop recurrent CDI [6, 11–13]. Symptoms of CDI can present after the first day of antibiotic use or up to six weeks after completion of an antibiotic course. Most commonly, symptoms develop within the first 5 to 10 days after exposure to antibiotics. Though diarrhea is the hallmark symptom of CDI, it may not be present initially. This can be secondary to colonic dysmotility from previous underlying pathology or from the disease process itself. This is especially important in surgical patients who may have a concomitant ileus. Thus, in surgical patients it is critical to have a high index of suspicion for the diagnosis of CDI.

Mild disease is defined as diarrhea without any systemic symptoms, such as fever, renal failure, or hemodynamic instability. Diarrhea can be accompanied by mild abdominal pain and cramps. If symptoms are prolonged, this can result in electrolyte imbalance and volume depletion. If this occurs in patients with multiple or severe comorbidities, particularly after surgery, non-severe CDI can lead to increased morbidity.

Moderate disease can result in profuse diarrhea, abdominal distension, abdominal pain, fever, tachycardia, and/or oliguria. This readily responds to fluid resuscitation. It is important to recognize that *C. difficile* colitis can present without diarrhea; usually severe leukocytosis and abdominal distension will be present.

Severe or fulminant disease may result in occult bleeding, renal failure with oliguria, hemodynamic instability requiring vasopressor support, and/or cardiopulmonary failure requiring mechanical ventilation. Severe CDI is relatively infrequent and only develops in 1 to 3% of cases [14–18]. Severe CDI can lead to ileus, toxic megacolon, intestinal perforation, multisystem organ failure, and death. The first warning sign can be diminishing diarrhea due to decreased colonic muscle tone. Other signs that can lead to the diagnosis include fever without obvious cause, severe leukocytosis, abdominal distension with or without tenderness, recent or current antibiotic use, and obtundation of the patient. The clinician must maintain a high level of suspicion for diagnosing CDI in the at-risk population. Important predictors of severe CDI are; WBC $>15 \times 10^3$cells/mL, increase in serum creatinine level >1.5 times the baseline level, temperature >38.5 °C, and albumin <2.5 g/dL [14–19].

Mortality in this group of patients remains high due to the development of toxic megacolon with colonic perforation, peritonitis, and septic shock with subsequent multisystem organ failure. Systemic symptoms arise from toxin induced inflammatory mediators released locally in the colon as well as toxins being released into the bloodstream.

There has been a significant rise in the number of cases of severe CDI associated with multisystem organ failure and increased mortality in the last several years. This has been associated with the hypervirulent 027 strain of *C. difficile* [14, 20, 21]. Early diagnosis and treatment are important in reducing the mortality associated with severe CDI. Patients who present with organ failure including increased serum lactate or vasopressor requirements, should be assessed immediately with regard to early operative intervention.

Recurrence of symptoms after initial treatment for CDI develops in 10–30% of patients. For patients with 1–2 previous episodes of CDI, the risk of recurrence can be as high as 40–65% [6, 12–15]. Recurrence of CDI (RCDI) is associated with an impaired immune response to the *C. difficile* toxins and/or alterations of the colonic flora. RCDI is a result of germinating resident spores that remain after treatment with antibiotics, or due to reinfection from an environmental source. Distinction between recurrence and reinfection can only be achieved if the strain of *C. difficile* is identified using molecular techniques. Recurrent episodes are less severe compared to the first episode.

Patients who develop CDI have increased hospital length of stay, increased medical costs, increased readmission rates, as well as higher morbidity and mortality rates. The same is true of surgical patients with CDI [6, 22, 23].

10.5 Diagnosis

The diagnosis of CDI should be based on clinical signs in conjunction with laboratory testing. Stool testing should only be performed on diarrheal stools from at-risk patients that have >3 loose stools in a 24-h period and no alternative reason for signs and symptoms, such as stool softener use or enteral nutrition. This is especially relevant in patients with known risk factors, like recent antibiotic use, hospitalization, and advanced age. In patients with ileus who are unable to produce a stool specimen, performing polymerase chain reaction testing of perirectal swabs provides an acceptable alternative [14].

C. difficile strains with hypervirulent traits, have been described in the last decade. Particularly, *C. difficile* strain 027, has been associated with increased disease severity, recurrence, and high mortality rates [20–26].

In order to effectively manage CDI, it is important to have a prompt and precise diagnosis to initiate treatment in a timely manner. Identifying CDI as early as possible allows for earlier treatment and improved outcomes. Rapid isolation of infected patients is key in controlling the potential transmission of CDI in the hospital setting.

C. difficile has been shown to colonize the intestinal tract of healthy individuals. Therefore, diagnostic testing for CDI should only be performed on diarrheal stools of patients presenting with symptoms concerning for CDI. The testing of formed stools can result in false positive tests, which can result in unnecessary antibiotic treatment.

Radiographs of the abdomen in CDI may be normal, or they may show ileus, colonic dilation, thumb printing, or haustral thickening. CT imaging is suggested for patients with clinical manifestations of severe CDI. However, due to the low sensitivity of CT it is not recommended for screening purposes alone. CT imaging can assist with an early diagnosis and can help determine the severity of the disease in patients with CDI. CT findings of CDI include colonic wall thickening (pancolitis), dilation of the colon, pericolonic stranding, "accordion sign" (high-attenuation oral contrast in the colonic lumen alternating with low-attenuation inflamed mucosa), "target sign" (IV contrast displaying varying degrees of attenuation caused by submucosal inflammation), and ascites. The most common finding on CT, colonic wall thickening, is non-specific and can be found in other etiologies of colitis. CT diagnosis of CDI has a sensitivity of 52%, specificity of 93%, and positive and negative predictive values of 88% and 67%, respectively [14, 27, 28].

CDI can also be detected endoscopically by the presence of ulcers, plaques, and pseudomembranes. These lesions will be present in 90% of fulminant colitis cases versus 23% in mild cases. The pathognomonic lesion in CDI is the pseudomembrane, which is characteristically raised, yellowish, with skipped areas of normal appearing mucosa. Endoscopy can be hazardous in the setting of fulminant colitis, as there is an increased risk of colonic perforation. For this reason, endoscopy should be used sparingly, as the diagnosis can be made readily via laboratory testing.

10.6   Medical Management

Metronidazole and oral vancomycin have been the mainstay of CDI for the past 30 years with vancomycin being reserved for severe infections. However, recent evidence and the availability of newer agents has brought a shift in the management of CDI.

Several randomized controlled trials [29, 30] have shown that oral vancomycin is superior to metronidazole, even in mild to moderate disease. Given the recent evidence, metronidazole has fallen out of favor in the updated 2017 Infectious Diseases Society of America (IDSA)/Society of Healthcare Epidemiology of America (SHEA) guidelines and is no longer recommended as first-line treatment.

Treatment should be guided by whether the episode is initial or recurrent, as well as by the severity of the infection (Table 10.1).

The first step in approaching treatment is to discontinue unnecessary antibiotics whenever possible as this may influence the risk of recurrent CDI. Supportive measures include correcting electrolyte disturbances, discontinuation of unnecessary proton pump inhibitors as these have been associated with the development of CDIs, and the use of antiperistalic agents. Probiotics have been used to recolonize the GI

Table 10.1 Management of adult patients with *C. difficile* infection

Episode type and disease severity	Clinical parameters	Treatment	Considerations
Initial episode, non-severe	Leukocytosis with a white blood cell count of ≤15,000 cells/mL and a serum creatinine level <1.5 mg/dL	VAN 125 mg PO 4 times daily × 10 days, OR FDX 200mg PO twice daily × 10 days. If above agents are unavailable, metronidazole 500mg PO three times a day × 10 days	Treatment may be extended up to 14 days in patients who have delayed resolution of symptoms, or those are treated with metronidazole
Initial episode, severe	Leukocytosis with a white blood cell count of >15,000 cells/mL or a serum creatinine level >1.5 mg/dL	VAN 125 mg PO 4 times daily × 10 days, OR FDX 200mg PO twice daily × 10 days	Treatment may be extended up to 14 days in patients who have delayed resolution of symptoms
Initial episode, fulminant	Hypotension or shock, ileus, megacolon	VAN 500 mg 4 times per day orally or by nasogastric tube. For ileus: • Consider rectal instillation of VAN • Add intravenous metronidazole 500 mg every 8 h to oral or rectal VAN	Consider early surgical consultation, and consult ID or GI
First recurrence		VAN 125 mg PO 4 times daily × 10 days if metronidazole was used for the initial episode, OR Vancomycin in a taper and pulsed-dose regimen if a standard VAN regimen was used for the initial episode: 125 mg PO 4 times/ day × 10–14 days, then 125 mg PO 2 times/ day × 1 week, then 125 mg PO daily for 1 wk, then 125 mg PO every 2 or 3 days for 2–8 weeks, OR FDX 200 mg PO 2 times a day × 10 days if VAN was used for the initial episode	Consider ID or GI consult

Table 10.1 (continued)

Episode type and disease severity	Clinical parameters	Treatment	Considerations
Second or subsequent recurrence		Vancomycin in a taper and pulsed-dose regimen, OR VAN 125 mg PO 4 times a day × 10 days followed by rifaximin 400 mg PO 3 times a day for 20 days, OR FDX 200 mg PO 2 times/ day for 10 day, OR Fecal microbiota transplantation (generally reserved for >2 recurrent episodes [i.e., >3 CDI episodes])	Consider ID or GI consult

Van Vancomycin, *FDX* Fidaxomicin, *PO* Orally, *ID* Infectious diseases, *GI* Gastrointestinal

tract, but the data is limited by size and quality of studies along with inconsistency in the type of formulations that have been used leading to a lack of consensus in recommending their use.

10.7   Treatment of Initial Episode of CDI

Either oral vancomycin 125 mg four times daily, or fidaxomicin 200 mg oral twice daily is recommended over metronidazole for an initial episode of CDI in adults, regardless of severity (Table 10.1). Cost and availability may limit fidaxomicin use. Oral metronidazole is recommended only if vancomycin or fidaxomicin are unavailable or contraindicated.

Typical treatment duration is 10 days, but may be extended up to 14 days in patients who have not had resolution of symptoms by 10 days [31].

There has been variability in the factors that determine severity of disease, but the IDSA/SHEA guidelines recommend using leukocyte count of >15,000 cells/mL or a serum creatinine level >1.5 mg/dL as indicators of severe disease. The recommended dosage of vancomycin is 125 mg given 4 times daily regardless of disease severity because this dose achieves adequate bactericidal concentration in the intestinal lumen and a higher dose does not confer any additional benefit. When comparing vancomycin to fidaxomicin the clinical cure rate with fidaxomicin is non-inferior to vancomycin, but the rate of recurrence is significantly lower with fidaxomicin use thus fidaxomicin may be reserved in patients at an increased risk of CDI recurrence.

10.8 Fulminant CDI

Fulminant CDI may be characterized by hypotension or shock, ileus, or megacolon. Treatment is higher dose vancomycin 500 mg orally four times daily for 10 days. If ileus is present, rectal instillation of vancomycin 500 mg in 100 mL normal saline every 6 h as a retention enema can be considered (Table 10.1). Intravenous metronidazole 500 mg every 8 h is recommended as an addition to oral or rectal vancomycin if ileus is suspected since ileus may interfere with the distribution of orally administered vancomycin in the gut lumen. In patients with an inadequate response to vancomycin and metronidazole, tigecycline or intravenous immunoglobulins may be used, but studies have provided limited evidence [31]. Studies have shown that a rising WBC count (>25,000 cells/mL) or rising lactate level (>5 mmol/L) is associated with higher mortality and early surgical intervention is key for survival, hence expert surgical consultation must be sought earlier in the course of fulminant CDI with ileus [21].

10.9 Treatment of Recurrent CDI

Approximately 25% of patients will experience recurrent CDI. Risk factors for recurrent CDI are administration of antibiotics during or after treatment of previous CDI, increased severity of underlying disease, advanced age, and immune compromise. Recurrent CDI can result from the same strain (relapse) or a different *C. difficile* strain (new infection), but the management of this infection is the same regardless of etiology.

Treatment of the first recurrent episode varies based on the agent used to treat the initial episode of CDI (Table 10.1). Patients who received metronidazole for their initial episode must be treated with a standard 10-day course of oral vancomycin 125 mg four times daily. Patients who received a standard course of oral vancomycin as initial treatment must be treated with a tapered, pulse-dose regimen of vancomycin, or a 10-day course of fidaxomicin. Metronidazole is not recommended for recurrent CDI. Patients with multiple recurrent CDIs may receive an extended course of oral vancomycin (tapered or pulse regimen), or oral vancomycin followed by rifaximin, or fidaxomicin. There is no additional benefit in extending the treatment duration.

Fecal microbiota transplantation (FMT) has been used successfully to correct the antibiotic-related dysbiosis in the gut microbiome which contributes to the development of CDIs. Reported FMT success rates have been higher in non-randomized trials than randomized controlled trials. Success rates are high regardless of route of installation of feces and range from 77% to 94% with the highest success rates with colonic instillation [32–37]. Data in severe, refractory CDI is limited. There is no consensus on the number of antibiotic treatment courses for recurrent CDI before using FMT, but IDSA/SHEA recommends appropriate antibiotic treatment of at least 2 recurrences, or a total of 3 CDI episodes, before initiating FMT. Complications of FMT are limited and may be related to infectious complications or physical complications from instillation, long-term consequences are unknown at this time.

Bezlotoxumab, a Toxin B binding monoclonal antibody, was approved in 2016 to reduce the risk of recurrence in adult patients concomitantly receiving antibiotics for CDI treatment and shows significant promise.

10.10   Consultation

Gastroenterology or infectious diseases consultation must be considered in patients with an inadequate response or recurrent infection. Surgery must be consulted in patients with a rising WBC count and lactate levels or with fulminant CDI associated with ileus.

10.11   Surgical Management

Patients with fulminant colitis (FC) who progress to systemic toxicity require surgical intervention. Predictive clinical and laboratory findings included: age (>70 years), prior CDI, profound leukocytosis (>18,000/mm^3), hemodynamic instability, use of anti-peristaltic medications, and clinical findings of increasing abdominal pain, distension, diarrhea, and change in mental status [6, 12–14]. Patients with severe CDI who progress to systemic toxicity are likely to have multiple comorbidities. Delaying surgery in this group leads to an increased likelihood of poor outcomes. There is some evidence that shows a short period of medical optimization can improve outcomes before colectomy [38].

There is no reliable clinical or laboratory findings that can predict those patients who will respond to medical management and those who will require surgery. In the setting of severe CDI emergency colectomy provides a survival benefit compared to continuing antibiotics [16–18]. Patients presenting with organ failure (acute renal failure, cardiopulmonary compromise, or change in mental status) also need prompt intervention since the timing of surgical intervention is crucial for survival of these patients. There is a decrease in mortality associated with surgery performed before the onset of cardio/pulmonary failure or vasopressor requirements, especially in patients <65 years of age. Mortality rates rise when surgical exploration is performed after the development of respiratory failure and the use of vasopressors. Optimal timing for surgery remains controversial in CDI, but most studies support surgical intervention 3–5 days after diagnosis in patients who are worsening or not clinically improving. It is strongly recommended that patients with severe CDI undergo early surgery prior to developing shock and requiring vasopressors [1, 14, 19, 39–43].

Resection of the entire colon with end ileostomy should be considered to treat patients with fulminant colitis. Diverting loop ileostomy with antegrade colonic lavage is a potential useful alternative to resection of the entire colon [44, 45]. The most commonly performed operation for the treatment of fulminant colitis is total colectomy with end ileostomy. When deciding for colonic resection, if total colectomy is not performed, reoperation to resect further bowel is usually required. Once a decision has been made to operate for FC a total abdominal colectomy should be performed. The surgeon should not be deterred by the external appearance of the colon, as it may appear relatively benign. Almost universally, the colon will be extremely edematous and boggy, containing liters of fluid. Pericolic inflammation and sterile inflammatory ascites is commonly encountered as well. Sometimes, especially if surgery has been delayed, the colonic wall may be necrotic with or without perforation.

Given the severity of illness in these patients, surgery should be performed in an expeditious manner. The operation should be performed open, ligating the mesenteric vessels before they branch, to facilitate a quick resection. The intraperitoneal portion of the colon should be removed and the rectum divided at or near the peritoneal reflection.

A diverting loop ileostomy with antegrade colonic lavage can be a colon preserving alternative to total colectomy. Patients with FC are managed by a loop ileostomy, intraoperative colonic lavage with warmed polyethylene glycol 3350/electrolyte solution via the ileostomy and postoperative antegrade instillation of vancomycin flushes via the ileostomy. The operation can be performed laparoscopically in the hemodynamically stable patient. Pre-procedure predictors of mortality for colonic lavage include age, elevated serum lactate levels, timing of operation, vasopressor use, and presence of acute renal failure [44, 45].

10.12 Outcomes

The outcomes of patients with fulminant colitis due to *C. difficile* are dependent on their selection and the timing of surgical intervention. Patients with age >65 years, cardiopulmonary failure, vasopressor requirements, renal failure, and severe leukocytosis have a mortality rate that exceeds 50%. When these predictors are not present the majority of patients survive with good recovery.

Physiologic support including invasive monitoring in an intensive care unit and aggressive resuscitation is often necessary in fulminant colitis. The diarrhea from CDI results in significant volume depletion and electrolyte abnormalities; therefore, fluid and electrolyte imbalances should be corrected. Early detection of shock and aggressive management of underlying organ dysfunction are essential for improved outcomes in patients with fulminant colitis. Supportive measures, such as intravenous fluid resuscitation, albumin supplementation and electrolyte replacement, should be provided to all patients with severe *C. difficile* infection.

References

1. Lessa FC, Gould CV, McDonald LC. Current status of *Clostridium difficile* infection epidemiology. Clin Infect Dis. 2012;55:65–70.
2. Gourarzi M, Seyedjacadi SS, Goudarzi H, Mehdizadeh Aghdam E, Nazeri S. *Clostridium difficile* infection: epidemiology, pathogenesis risk factors and therapeutic options. Scientifica. 2014;2014:916826.
3. To KB, Napolitano LM. *Clostridium difficile* infection: update on diagnosis, epidemiology, and treatment strategies. Surg Infect (Larchmt). 2014;15:490–502.

4. Abt MC, McKenney PT, Pamer EG. *Clostridium difficile* colitis: pathogenesis and host defence. Nat Rev Microbiol. 2016;14(10):609–20. https://doi.org/10.1038/nrmicro.2016.108.
5. Furuya-Kanamori L, Marquess J, Yakob L, et al. Asymptomatic *Clostridium difficile* colonization: epidemiology and clinical implications. BMC Infect Dis. 2015;15:516. https://doi.org/10.1186/s12879-015-1258-4.
6. Lessa FC, Mu Y, Bamberg WM, et al. Burden of *Clostridium difficile* infection in the United States. N Engl J Med. 2015;372:825–34.
7. Fekety R, Kim KH, Brown D, Batts DH, Cudmore M, Silva J Jr. Epidemiology of antibiotic-associated colitis; isolation of *Clostridium difficile* from the hospital environment. Am J Med. 1981;70(4):906–8.
8. George RH, Symonds JM, Dimock F, et al. Identification of *Clostridium difficile* as a cause of pseudomembranous colitis. Br Med J. 1978;1(6114):695. https://doi.org/10.1136/bmj.1.6114.695.
9. Yacyshyn B. Pathophysiology of *Clostridium difficile*-associated diarrhea. Gastroenterol Hepatol (N Y). 2016;12(9):558–60.
10. Poxton IR, McCoubrey J, Blair G. The pathogenicity of *Clostridium difficile*. Clin Microbiol Infect. 2001;7(8):421–4.
11. Kent KC, Rubin MS, Wroblewski L, Hanff PA, Silen W. The impact of *Clostridium difficile* on a surgical service: a prospective study of 374 patients. Ann Surg. 1998;227:296–301.
12. Rodrigues MA, Brady RR, Rodrigues J, Graham C, Gibb AP. *Clostridium difficile* infection in general surgery patients; identification of high-risk populations. Int J Surg. 2010;8:368–72.
13. Kim MJ, Kim BS, Kwon JW, Ahn SE, Lee SS, Park HC, Lee BH. Risk factors for the development of *Clostridium difficile* colitis in a surgical ward. J Korean Surg Soc. 2012;83:14–20.
14. Sartelli M, Di Bella S, McFarland LV, et al. 2019 update of the WSES guidelines for management of *Clostridium difficile* infection in surgical patients. World J Emerg Surg. 2019;14:8. https://doi.org/10.1186/s13017-019-0228-3.
15. Bagdasarian N, Rao K, Malani PN. Diagnosis and treatment of *Clostridium difficile* in adults: a systematic review. JAMA. 2015;313:398–408.
16. Kim PK, Zhao P, Teperman S. Evolving treatment strategies for severe *Clostridium difficile* colitis: defining the therapeutic window. In: Sartelli M, Bassetti M, Martin-Loeches I, editors. Abdominal sepsis. Hot topics in acute care surgery and trauma. Springer; 2018.
17. Girotra M, Kumar V, Khan JM, Damisse P, Abraham RR, Aggarwal V, Dutta SK. Clinical predictors of fulminant colitis in patients with *Clostridium difficile* infection. Saudi J Gastroenterol. 2012;18:133–9.
18. Kaiser AM, Hogen R, Bordeianou L, Alavi K, Wise PE, Sudan R. CME committee of the SSAT. *Clostridium difficile* infection from a surgical perspective. J Gastrointest Surg. 2015;19:1363–77.
19. Carchman EH, Peitzman AB, Simmons RL, Zuckerbraun BS. The role of acute care surgery in the treatment of severe, complicated *Clostridium difficile*-associated disease. J Trauma Acute Care Surg. 2012;73:789–800.
20. Warny M, Pepin J, Fang A, Killgore G, Thompson A, Brazier J, Frost E, McDonald LC. Toxin production by an emerging strain of *Clostridium difficile* associated with outbreaks of severe disease in North America and Europe. Lancet. 2005;366:1079–84.
21. Lamontagne F, Labb AC, Haeck O, et al. Impact of emergency colectomy on survival of patients with fulminant *Clostridium difficile* colitis during an epidemic caused by a hypervirulent strain. Ann Surg. 2007;245:267–72.
22. Miller AT, Tabrizian P, Greenstein AJ, et al. Long-term follow-up of patients with fulminant *Clostridium difficile* colitis. J Gastrointest Surg. 2009;13(5):956–9.
23. Halabi WJ, Nguyen VQ, Carmichael JC, Pigazzi A, Stamos MJ, Mills S. *Clostridium difficile* colitis in the United States: a decade of trends, outcomes, risk factors for colectomy, and mortality after colectomy. J Am Coll Surg. 2013;217:802–12.
24. Sailhamer EA, Carson K, Chang Y, et al. Fulminant *Clostridium difficile* colitis; patterns of care and predictors of mortality. Arch Surg. 2009;144(5):433–9.

25. Surawicz CM, Brandt LJ, Binion DG, Ananthakrishnan AN, Curry SR, Gilligan PH, McFarland LV, Mellow M, Zuckerbraun BS. Guidelines for diagnosis, treatment, and prevention of Clostridium difficile infections. Am J Gastroenterol. 2013;108:478–98.
26. Guyatt G, Gutterman D, Baumann MH, Addrizzo-Harris D, Hylek EM, Phillips B, Raskob G, Lewis SZ, Schunemann H. Grading strength of recommendations and quality of evidence in clinical guidelines: report from an American College of Chest Physicians task force. Chest. 2006;129:174–81.
27. Lee DY, Chung EL, Guend H, Whelan RL, Wedderburn RV, Rose KM. Predictors of mortality after emergency colectomy for Clostridium difficile colitis: an analysis of ACS-NSQIP. Ann Surg. 2014;259:148–56.
28. Boland GW, Lee MJ, Cats AM, Gaa JA, Saini S, Mueller PR. Antibiotic-induced diarrhea: specificity of abdominal CT for the diagnosis of Clostridium difficile disease. Radiology. 1994;191:103–6.
29. Johnson S, Louie TJ, Gerding DN, et al. Polymer alternative for CDI treatment (PACT) investigators. vancomycin, metronidazole, or tolevamer for Clostridium difficile infection: results from two multinational, randomized, controlled trials. Clin Infect Dis. 2014;59:345–54.
30. Zar FA, Bakkanagari SR, Moorthi KM, Davis MB. A comparison of vancomycin and metronidazole for the treatment of Clostridium difficile-associated diarrhea, stratified by disease severity. Clin Infect Dis. 2007;45:302–7.
31. McDonald LC, Gerding DN, Johnson S, Bakken JS, Carroll KC, Coffin SE, et al. Clinical practice guidelines for Clostridium difficile infection in adults and children: 2017 update by the Infectious Diseases Society of America (IDSA) and Society for Healthcare Epidemiology of America (SHEA). Clin Infect Dis. 2018;66:e1–e48.
32. Gough E, Shaikh H, Manges AR. Systematic review of intestinal microbiota transplantation (fecal bacteriotherapy) for recurrent Clostridium difficile infection. Clin Infect Dis. 2011;53:994–1002.
33. MacConnachie AA, Fox R, Kennedy DR, Seaton RA. Faecal transplant for recurrent Clostridium difficile-associated diarrhoea: a UK case series. QJM. 2009;102:781–4.
34. Brandt LJ, Aroniadis OC, Mellow M, et al. Long-term follow-up of colonoscopic fecal microbiota transplant for recurrent Clostridium difficile infection. Am J Gastroenterol. 2012;107:1079–87.
35. Hamilton MJ, Weingarden AR, Sadowsky MJ, Khoruts A. Standardized frozen preparation for transplantation of fecal microbiota for recurrent Clostridium difficile infection. Am J Gastroenterol. 2012;107:761–7.
36. Jorup-Rönström C, Håkanson A, Sandell S, et al. Fecal transplant against relapsing Clostridium difficile-associated diarrhea in 32 patients. Scand J Gastroenterol. 2012;47:548–52.
37. Mattila E, Uusitalo-Seppälä R, Wuorela M, et al. Fecal transplantation, through colonoscopy, is effective therapy for recurrent Clostridium difficile infection. Gastroenterology. 2012;142:490–6.
38. Clanton J, Fawley R, Haller N, Daley T, Porter J, Paranjape C, Bonilla H. Patience is a virtue: an argument for delayed surgical intervention in fulminant Clostridium difficile colitis. Am Surg. 2014;80:614–9.
39. Stewart DB, Hollenbeak CS, Wilson MZ. Is colectomy for fulminant Clostridium difficile colitis life saving? A systematic review. Colorectal Dis. 2013;15:798–804.
40. Chan S, Kelly M, Helme S, Gossage J, Modarai B, Forshaw M. Outcomes following colectomy for Clostridium difficile colitis. Int J Surg. 2009;7:78–81.
41. Seder CW, Villalba MR Jr, Robbins J, Ivascu FA, Carpenter CF, Dietrich M, Villalba MR Sr. Early colectomy may be associated with improved survival in fulminant Clostridium difficile colitis: an 8-year experience. Am J Surg. 2009;197:302–7.
42. Ferrada P, Velopulos CG, Sultan S, Haut ER, Johnson E, Praba-Egge A, Enniss T, Dorion H, Martin ND, Bosarge P, Rushing A, Duane TM. Timing and type of surgical treatment of Clostridium difficile-associated disease: a practice management guideline from the Eastern Association for the Surgery of Trauma. J Trauma Acute Care Surg. 2014;76:1484–93.

43. Lee DY, Chung EL, Guend H, Whelan RL, Wedderburn RV, Rose KM. Predictors of mortality after emergency colectomy for *Clostridium difficile* colitis: an analysis of ACS-NSQIP. Ann Surg. 2014;259:148–56.

44. Neal MD, Alverdy JC, Hall DE, Simmons RL, Zuckerbraun BS. Diverting loop ileostomy and colonic lavage: an alternative to total abdominal colectomy for the treatment of severe, complicated *Clostridium difficile* associated disease. Ann Surg. 2011;254:423–37.

45. Ferrada P, Callcut R, Zielinski MD, Bruns B, Yeh DD, Zakrison TL, et al. EAST Multi-Institutional Trials Committee. Loop ileostomy versus total colectomy as surgical treatment for *Clostridium difficile*-associated disease: an Eastern Association for the Surgery of Trauma multicenter trial. J Trauma Acute Care Surg. 2017;83:36–40.

Source Control in Intra-Abdominal Infections

11

Joshua D. Jaramillo, Joseph D. Forrester, and David A. Spain

11.1   Definitions

Source control in surgery is the act of eliminating or reducing foci of infection contributing to physiologic derangement of the human host, allowing the host defenses to control the remainder of the infection. In combination with appropriate and targeted antibiotic therapy, source control is one of the two pillars of care of the patients with intra-abdominal infections. Such intra-abdominal infections (IAI) include appendicitis, cholecystitis, diverticulitis, gastroduodenal perforations, necrotizing pancreatitis, salmonella, tuberculosis, trauma, urinary tract pathology, gynecologic pathology, and iatrogenic injury, among others [1]. Terms including IAI, peritonitis, and abdominal sepsis are often used interchangeably in vernacular conversation, but should be used to define similar but distinct clinical states.

The distinction between an uncomplicated and a complicated IAI has fluctuated over time. Historically, infections limited to, and contained within, a hollow viscus were considered uncomplicated. When infections breached their native anatomic boundaries and entered normally sterile areas of the abdomen, they were termed complicated IAI [2–4]. Functionally, to satisfy regulatory bodies such as the FDA, complicated IAI have been defined as those that have required source control interventions [2]. Yet there are clearly conditions that are contained to a lumen that require source control, fulminant *Clostridioides* (*Clostridium*) *difficile* infection being but one. The 2017 Surgical Infection Society/Infectious Disease Society of America Revised Guidelines on the Management of Intra-Abdominal Infection updated the definition of complicated IAI to reflect the range of pathology— "Patients with complicated IAI may be characterized as manifesting secondary or tertiary peritonitis, single or multiple intra-abdominal abscesses, or an intra-abdominal phlegmon" [2].

J. D. Jaramillo · J. D. Forrester · D. A. Spain (✉)
Division of General Surgery, School of Medicine, Stanford University, Stanford, CA, USA
e-mail: joshjara@stanford.edu; jdf1@stanford.edu; dspain@stanford.edu

© Springer Nature Switzerland AG 2021
M. Sartelli et al. (eds.), *Infections in Surgery*, Hot Topics in Acute Care Surgery and Trauma, https://doi.org/10.1007/978-3-030-62116-2_11

Fig. 11.1 Natural history of three clinical outcomes that can occur with intra-abdominal infections. (Adapted from Cheadle et al. In: Cheadle WG, Spain DA. The continuing challenge of intra-abdominal infection. Am J Surg. 2003;186(5A):15S–22S: 16S; Figure 2)

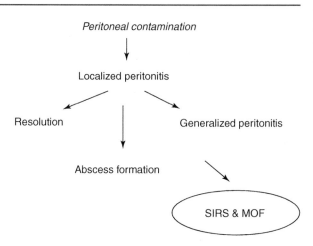

Localized peritonitis is peritoneal inflammation resulting from loss of integrity of the gastrointestinal tract or from infected viscera, at the site of infection. When a patient develops localized peritonitis, there are three potential outcomes (Fig. 11.1). In the first outcome, the patient's host response can clear the infection. In these cases, it is possible the patient may never even seek care. In the second outcome, the body is able to contain, but not clear the infection. Mechanisms for controlling more widespread spillage include migration of inflammatory cells including neutrophils and macrophages, local fibrin production by fibroblasts, complement activation, and walling off sites of inflammation with omentum or small bowel [5]. In the third outcome, rapid or persistent contamination, an expanding localized infection, or free rupture of a hollow viscus can overwhelm intrinsic localizing mechanisms. In such cases, widespread bacterial contamination results in generalized peritonitis.

Traditionally, peritonitis has been divided into primary, secondary, and tertiary peritonitis [5, 6]. Primary peritonitis includes infection of the peritoneal cavity that occur without breakdown of normal anatomic barriers to infection, as in the case of spontaneous bacterial peritonitis in patients with cirrhosis, or among patients undergoing peritoneal dialysis [6]. Offending pathogens tend to be isolated to a single species, with the main pathogens in adults being coliform bacteria [5]. Secondary peritonitis occurs as a result of infections arising from alimentary tract microbes contaminating an otherwise sterile peritoneal cavity [6, 7]. This definition clearly has overlap with historic definitions of complicated IAI. These infections are more commonly multi-species, and involve coliform bacteria [5]. Finally tertiary peritonitis refers to patients who require more than one operation for IAI, or who develop treatment failure after initial source control attempts [6, 7]. However, the terms secondary and tertiary peritonitis lack specificity or consistency, and do not contain specifics of chronicity or extent [2]. Given these constraints, the more functional localized or generalized, acute or chronic, complicated, or uncomplicated terminology has been used in this chapter.

11.2   Epidemiology

Acute abdominal pain is one of the most common indications for surgical consultation in the emergency department (ED) and hospital, and intra-abdominal infections are a common cause of acute abdominal pain. Acute abdominal pain is responsible for 10% of emergency department visits annually in the US, and approximately 10% of these cases have abdominal pathology requiring surgical intervention [8–10]. Sepsis frequently accompanies intra-abdominal infection. Among patients presenting with sepsis worldwide, 15–43% had intra-abdominal sources and among patients who develop sepsis in-hospital, more than 60% were the result of an invasive procedure [11, 12].

In the early 1900s, mortality of an intra-abdominal infection was near 90% [5]. By the 1950s mortality rates had been reduced to 50% and by the 1970s mortality rates were less than 30–40% [5]. Modern understanding of physiology, a wide range of antibiotics, intensive care, and improved diagnostic capability have reduced the mortality rates associated with intra-abdominal infections to <30% [5]. A recent international multicenter observational study among high-, middle- and low-income countries, conducted in 132 centers over 4 month period enrolled 4553 patients with complex intra-abdominal infections and observed an overall 9.2% (416/4533) mortality rate [13]. This mortality rate is similar to 30-day mortality rate (8%) and operative mortality rate (6%) observed among patients undergoing emergency general surgery for abdominal pathology in the US, England, and Australia [14].

Patients with sepsis as a result of an intra-abdominal infection may be at particularly high risk of an untoward outcome. The overzealous immune response seen in sepsis can lead to shock, multiple organ system failure, and death. Patients with severe sepsis secondary to complicated intra-abdominal infection have reported mortality rates ranging from 20–60% [15–18]. In the US, a postoperative diagnosis of septic shock was associated with 30% and 40% mortality rate for elective and emergency general surgery patients, respectively [19]. Addressing both the underlying intra-abdominal infection and the subsequent sepsis are critical to increase chances of a positive outcome.

11.3   Initial Resuscitation

Once an IAI is suspected, antibiotic administration, appropriate volume resuscitation, and restoration of normal physiology should be the goal prior to performing an operation. Resuscitation priorities have been eloquently depicted in the Surviving Sepsis Campaign bundle [20]. Among patients with sepsis and septic shock, blood cultures should be obtained, broad-spectrum antibiotics should be administered, lactate levels should be measured, a 30 ml/kg crystalloid bolus should be given for patients with hypotension or a lactate ≥4 mmol/L, and vasopressors should be started if a patient is hypotensive during or after fluid bolus administration with a goal to maintain a mean arterial pressure ≥65 mmHg [20]. Initial empiric antibiotic therapy should be broad but account for likely sources of infection and the host risk factors [2]. Ideally blood cultures should be obtained prior to initiating antibiotic therapy as sterilization of cultures can occur within minutes of appropriate antibiotic therapy [21, 22]. But obtaining blood cultures should not delay starting antibiotic therapy; delays in antibiotic therapy lead to an increase in mortality [23, 24].

If a patient does not respond to these initial resuscitative interventions, an operation should not be postponed. Clinical worsening could signal progression of intra-abdominal sepsis. In these situations, operative intervention should be pursued as expeditiously and aggressively as possible. Delays in obtaining source control lead to worse outcomes [25–27].

11.4 Diagnosis

Localizing the offending source may help guide operative exposure and technique. Yet little has changed since Sir Zachary Cope first published *Early Diagnosis of the Acute Abdomen* [28]. "The necessity of making a thorough physical examination in every acute abdominal case should not need much emphasis. Radiologic or ultrasonic examinations, CT, and the vast array of laboratory tests available to all of us today will not compensate for a poor or incomplete history and physical" [29]. Physical exam may provide early identification of an intra-abdominal infection and obviate the need for additional imaging, particularly for patients *in extremis* or with generalized peritonitis (Fig. 11.2).

In cases of diagnostic uncertainty, additional imaging may provide information that can target intervention. Upright, plain radiograph (X-ray) may be useful in identifying free air under the diaphragm or pneumatosis of the biliary tree or bowel. While portable and quick, these plain films are neither sensitive nor specific for a wide range of abdominal pathology. However, for patients with free air and a concerning exam, no further imaging may be needed. Ultrasound is an important diagnostic tool; it can be performed in the ED or ICU, is low-cost, repeatable, and lacks radiation exposure. Patients with acute abdominal pain who experienced surgeon-performed ultrasound in the ED were 1.6 times more likely to proceed directly to the OR from the ED ($P < 0.001$) [30].

Among patients who initially respond to resuscitative efforts, computed tomography (CT) may provide more detailed information about specific intra-abdominal organs, vasculature, muscle, other soft tissue and bones. CT scans can be performed rapidly, and many surgeons are facile with interpreting this imaging modality. An abdominal CT scan with oral and intravenous contrast is the imaging modality of choice [7, 31]. Contrast administration must be judicious. Intravenous contrast may not be appropriate for patients with contrast allergy or renal impairment, and oral contrast may not be appropriate for patients at risk of aspiration. Magnetic resonance imaging (MRI) is an alternative for cross-sectional abdominal imaging. However, MRI is time-consuming and costly, and is not appropriate for a patient *in extremis*. For those patients who can tolerate the study however, MRI remains an important diagnostic adjunct. Magnetic resonance cholangiopancreatography in

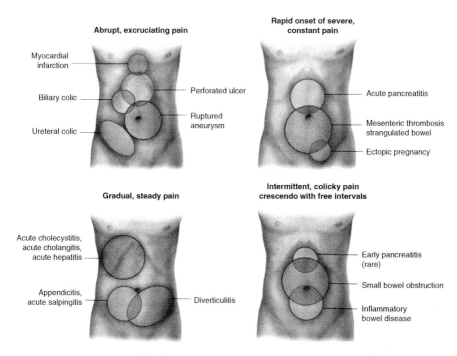

Fig. 11.2 The differential diagnosis of the acute abdomen with signs and symptoms elicited during physical exam. (Adapted from Britt, LD, ed Acute Care Surgery. In: Britt LD, Peitzman AB, Barie PS, Jurkovich GJ. Acute Care Surgery. 2nd Edition. Philadelphia: Lippincott Williams & Wilkins; 2019:534; Figure 41.1)

particular may be useful for assessing the integrity and patency of the bile and pancreatic ducts.

Ultimately, imaging should not delay operative intervention, particularly among patients with clear physical exam or who remain hemodynamically compromised despite initial attempts at resuscitation [25–27]. In these cases, a "cut-scan" is the safest method of definitively diagnosing the underlying pathology.

11.5 Treatment

Techniques for obtaining source control vary widely depending on the site of infection, acuity of infection, and physiologic state of the host (Table 11.1). In cases of IAI where the intrinsic mechanisms of infection containment are successful, delayed operative therapy temporized with percutaneous drainage may be appropriate [32]. Examples of such situations where such tactics may be acceptable include infected pancreatic necrosis, hepatic abscess, perforated appendicitis with abscess, acalculous cholecystitis, and diverticular abscess, among others. In these situations, percutaneous drainage can be viewed as temporary source control. Pathology such as

Table 11.1 Common intra-abdominal infections and source control options

Abdominal pathology	Source control options	Guideline recommendations
Perforated peptic ulcer (PPU) (<2 cm) [71]	Simple closure +/− omental patch	• Operative treatment of any PPU with pneumoperitoneum and signs of peritonitis • Nonoperative management may be appropriate in stable, non-peritonitic, not severely septic patients without significant pneumoperitoneum • Laparoscopic repair offers postoperative recovery advantages and superior visualization of peritoneal cavity in stable patients in presence of appropriate laparoscopic skills • Primary repair in cases of PPU >5 mm and <2 cm protected with omental patch • Open surgery is recommended in presence of bleeding peptic ulcers
Perforated peptic ulcer (PPU) (>2 cm) [71]	Resectional gastroduodenal surgery	• Resectional surgery in cases of PPU defect >2 cm, presence of malignant ulcers, significant bleeding or obstructing ulcers • Diversion techniques including Roux en-Y or pyloric exclusion to protect large duodenal repairs • Consider external bile drainage (via trans-cystic tube) if large duodenal ulcer • Duodenostomy in presence of large ulcers with severe tissue inflammation
Acute, non-perforated appendicitis [72, 73]	Appendectomy or ileocolonic resection	• Timely appendectomy for non-perforated appendicitis is preferred source control method rather than nonoperative management with antibiotics • Both open and laparoscopic approaches to appendectomy are appropriate based on surgeon preference and equipment availability • Nonoperative management with antibiotics is a viable option for certain patients in cases of non-complicated appendicitis understanding treatment failure rates, recurrence rates, and rare malignancy in setting of available outpatient antibiotics and follow up [74–78]
Perforated appendicitis [72, 73]	Appendectomy or ileocolonic resection	• Emergency appendectomy is required in cases of free perforation with diffuse peritonitis in patients who are septic and hemodynamically unstable • Rescue appendectomy may be required in cases of failed nonoperative management with antibiotics with or without percutaneous drainage • Operative technique is similar to non-perforated appendicitis except in severe infections with free perforation or generalized peritonitis where ileocolonic resection instead of appendectomy would be required for source control. In these cases, a lower midline incision is preferable • Copious irrigation has failed to demonstrate benefit [46, 47] • Peritoneal drains are not necessary after perforated appendicitis [79] • Short course of antibiotics (4 days) recommended after appendectomy for perforated appendicitis [50]

Peri-appendiceal abscess [72, 73, 80–82]	Appendectomy or percutaneous drainage +/− interval appendectomy	• Consider immediate appendectomy in cases of perforated appendicitis with abscess when no evidence of phlegmon • Percutaneous abscess drainage can provide source control and decrease complications, especially in cases with phlegmon and significant inflammation which would require extended bowel resection • Interval appendectomy after nonoperative management of perforated appendicitis suggested to exclude appendiceal neoplasm
Small bowel ischemia [83]	Resection	• When diagnosis of acute bowel ischemia is made the following should be initiated immediately: resuscitation, nasogastric decompression, broad-spectrum antibiotics • Prompt laparotomy with bowel resection to obtain source control • Damage control surgery for patients in shock with planned re-laparotomy • Be aware of underlying cause as may require anticoagulation for venous thrombosis, endovascular vs open repair for thrombotic injury to improve mesenteric perfusion • Massive intestinal necrosis requires understanding and judgment related to patient's comorbidities and advance directives to direct appropriate treatment
Small bowel perforation	Primary repair or resection	• Diagnosis of small bowel perforation should prompt resuscitative measures, nasogastric decompression, broad-spectrum antibiotics, and urgent surgical intervention • Operative repair technique depends on severity of injury • Primary repair appropriate for injuries that involve <50% of wall circumference imbricating the mucosal edges • Resection required for larger defects or where surround tissue not viable for closure
Colonic diverticulitis (<4 cm abscess) [84, 85]	Antibiotics alone	• Nonoperative treatment includes oral or intravenous antibiotics depending on severity of infection in hemodynamically stable patients without drainable collection • After resolution of acute episode, colon should be endoscopically evaluated to confirm diagnosis • Individualized surgical plan for elective colectomy after uncomplicated based on patient preferences and comorbidities
Colonic diverticulitis (>4 cm abscess) [84, 85]	Percutaneous drainage followed by elective colectomy	• Image guided percutaneous drainage in hemodynamically stable patients with drainable diverticular abscess • Elective colectomy, open vs laparoscopic based on surgeon expertise, recommended after complicated diverticulitis (free perforation, abscess, fistula, bowel obstruction, or stricture) • Elective resection should include entire involved colon with margins of healthy colon and rectum • All left sided colectomies for diverticulitis should be taken distally to the upper rectum

(continued)

Table 11.1 (continued)

Abdominal pathology	Source control options	Guideline recommendations
Colonic diverticulitis with peritonitis or failure of conservative therapy [84, 85]	Colectomy	• Urgent colectomy required for patients with diffuse peritonitis, hemodynamic instability, or failure of nonoperative management of acute diverticulitis • Operative therapy without resection is not an appropriate alternative to colectomy • Source control involves resection of the involved colon with Hartmann procedure • Restoration of bowel continuity after resection must incorporate comorbidities and surgeon preference
Large bowel ischemia [86]	Resection +/− diversion	• When diagnosis of acute colonic ischemia is made the following should be initiated immediately: resuscitation, bowel rest, and broad-spectrum antibiotics • In cases of colonic ischemia with severe features (hypotension, tachycardia, peritonitis, or radiographic evidence of gangrene) patient should undergo prompt laparotomy and segmental resection as indicated • Damage control surgery for patients in septic shock with planned re-laparotomy • Be aware of underlying cause as may require anticoagulation for venous thrombosis, endovascular vs open repair for thrombotic injury to improve colonic perfusion • Significant colonic necrosis requires understanding and judgment related to patient's comorbidities and advance directives to direct appropriate treatment
Large bowel perforation	Resection +/− diversion	• Diagnosis of large bowel perforation should prompt resuscitative measures, nasogastric decompression, broad-spectrum antibiotics and urgent surgical intervention • Operative repair depends on severity of injury • Primary repair appropriate for injuries that involve <50% of wall circumference imbricating the mucosal edges • Resection required for larger defects or where surround tissue not viable for closure
Rectal perforation [87, 88]	Primary repair/resection + diversion	• Operative repair depends on severity of injury related to primary repair vs resection as described above • Primary anastomosis preferred over diverting colostomy in hemodynamically stable patients • Damage control surgery methods should be employed in hemodynamically unstable patients with planned re-laparotomy

Condition	Procedure	Details
Acute cholecystitis [89, 90]	Cholecystectomy	• Early cholecystectomy is recommended for source control of patients with acute cholecystitis (<7 days) • In patients with pain >7–10 days, immediate antibiotics and delayed cholecystectomy is preferred unless there is peritonitis or sepsis where emergency surgery would be required • Laparoscopic cholecystectomy, when feasible, is preferred though open is valid option for "difficult gallbladder" • Intraoperative cholangiogram is appropriate when there is clinical suspicion of choledocholithiasis
Gangrenous cholecystitis [89–91]	Cholecystectomy or cholecystostomy	• Laparoscopic approach should be attempted except in case of septic shock • Subtotal cholecystectomy is valid option for advanced inflammation or gangrenous gallbladder or where anatomy is difficult to recognize • Percutaneous cholecystostomy drainage should be considered as possible surgical alternative in subset of patients unfit for emergency surgery due to severe comorbidities
Acute cholangitis [89–91]	ERCP, PTBD, or surgical decompression	• Upon diagnosis, resuscitate, and initiate antimicrobial treatment. If septic, should follow Surviving Sepsis guidelines and consider ICU admission • Perform early biliary track drainage via ERCP (preferred) or PTBD. Surgical common bile duct exploration may be necessary as third line alternative. If there is lack of facilities or personnel, consider transferring the patient • Cholecystectomy should be performed for cholelithiasis after acute cholangitis has resolved
Pancreatic necrosis [33, 34, 92–94]	Step-up approach of pancreatic debridement	• Pancreatic debridement is indicated in patients with pancreatic necrosis and associated sepsis secondary to severe pancreatitis • Late debridement is preferred, ideally 4 weeks after onset of acute pancreatitis • Patients who require pancreatic debridement should be treated in a tertiary referral center where surgical, endoscopic, and radiologic expertise are available • Minimally invasive approaches to debridement include CT guided catheter drainage and endoscopic debridement Surgical approaches include open debridement with internal vs external drainage, open packing, laparoscopic debridement
Hepatic abscess [95–97]	Drainage and antibiotic therapy	• Drainage should be attempted when feasible • Drainage techniques include: image guided percutaneous drainage, drainage by ERCP, laparoscopic drainage, open drainage • Multiple loculated abscesses may require surgical drainage

(continued)

Table 11.1 (continued)

Abdominal pathology	Source control options	Guideline recommendations
Echinococcal cyst [98]	Antihelminthic therapy ± drainage	• Treatment depends on WHO classification severity and treatment options include various combinations of antihelminthic therapy, PAIR (puncture, aspiration, injection, reaspiration), and surgery
Splenic abscess [99, 100]	Drainage, resection or splenectomy	• Standard of care is splenectomy
Fulminant C. *difficile* colitis [101–103]	Subtotal colectomy	• Surgery for C. *difficile* colitis should be reserved for patients with severe colitis that fail medical management, have peritonitis or colonic perforation • Subtotal colectomy with ileostomy is the operative procedure of choice • Diverting loop ileostomy with colonic lavage may be an alternative to colectomy for patients with severe C. *difficile* colitis
Postoperative abscess [32, 104]	Percutaneous drainage	• In stable patients with contained abscess <3 cm antimicrobial therapy may be sufficient • In stable patients with contained abscess >3 cm, percutaneous drainage is ideal • Patients with abscess and peritonitis or septic shock should be surgically explored • In cases of unstable patients with phlegmon where drainage is not safe, proximal diversion should be considered
Postoperative leak [104]	Reoperation	• In cases of free intraperitoneal anastomotic leak, the patient should be taken for surgical management if <7 days from initial procedure
Esophageal perforation [105, 106]	Operation at GE junction, stenting	• Upon diagnosis, resuscitate, make NPO, and initiate broad-spectrum antibiotics • Thorough knowledge of esophageal anatomy and surrounding structures is essential for operative planning and approach (cervical vs thoracic vs abdominal perforations) • Devitalized tissue at the perforation site should be debrided • Primary repair by first exposing the extent of mucosal injury followed by layered closure • Esophageal endoscopic covered stents can be used in selected patients to manage perforation
Mesenteric ischemia [83]	Operation	• When diagnosis of acute mesenteric ischemia is made the following should be initiated immediately: resuscitation, nasogastric decompression, broad-spectrum antibiotics • Prompt laparotomy with bowel resection to obtain source control • Damage control surgery for patients in septic shock with planned re-laparotomy • Be aware of underlying cause as may require anticoagulation for venous thrombosis, endovascular vs open repair for thrombotic injury to improve mesenteric perfusion • Massive intestinal necrosis requires understanding and judgment related to patient's comorbidities and advance directives to direct appropriate treatment

infected pancreatic necrosis or a hepatic abscess may be sufficiently addressed by percutaneous drainage alone [33–35]. For those patients with an appendiceal or diverticular abscess or acalculous cholecystitis, definitive source control can be performed at a later date when the patient has returned to a more favorable physiologic state. In some cases, subjecting the patient to an operation to resect the offending organ may no longer be required.

Uncontrolled sepsis can also be driven by infected fluid collections not amenable to percutaneous drainage due to the organ infected (such as a splenic abscess) or being inaccessible given proximity to surrounding structures, as in the case of an inter-mesenteric abscess. In these cases, surgery should focus on removing devitalized or infected tissue, irrigation of the abdomen, and achieving copasetic physiology.

Among patients who are physiologically robust in the immediate preoperative period, and remain so intraoperatively, restoration of gastrointestinal continuity can, and should, occur. In patients with profound physiologic derangement as a result of the initial septic insult, damage control surgery is warranted. While there are no definitive cut-offs for when damage control surgery should be performed, hypothermia (temperature <35 °C), pH < 7.2, base deficit of 8 or more, and evidence of coagulopathy, either alone or in combination, are reasonable thresholds [36, 37]. Source control should be obtained expeditiously with a combination of resection of devitalized or infected tissue and wide drainage. Restoration of intestinal continuity may not be warranted given anticipated need for continued resuscitation and anticipated bowel wall edema, questionably viable tissue, and guarded physiologic status [36]. In these cases the patient will need to be left with an open abdomen, and should receive temporary coverage rather than definitive abdominal closure. Among a mixed surgical and trauma population negative pressure therapy (NPT) systems were associated with higher rates of primary fascial closure and are recommended [36, 38, 39]. However, few prospective randomized trials of high-quality exist, and if NPT is not available, other options are likely adequate [36, 39]. The critical decision is not the type of device used to cover the abdomen, but the decision to leave the abdomen open due to the patient being physiologically deranged [36, 37].

The patient should be taken to the ICU, warmed, and resuscitated. Once the patient's physiology has been restored, they can be returned to the operating room for definitive repair and abdominal closure [36]. In these cases, planned or repeat laparotomy should be performed ideally within 24 h pending improvement in a given patient's physiology. Working toward abdominal closure as expeditiously as the patient's condition allows is critical to optimize chances of primary fascial closure [36]. While the data are scant among patients with an intra-abdominal infection, each hour delay in returning to the operating room (24 h after initial laparotomy) was associated with 1.1% decrease in achieving primary fascial closure for trauma patients [40]. Early closure may avoid the potentially severe side effects of an open abdomen, and will improve resource utilization [36]. Fascia should only be closed after source control is assured.

Peritoneal lavage is widely practiced during source control procedures in the setting of complex intra-abdominal infections, yet its benefits are not clear [41, 42].

Proponents of peritoneal lavage claim that irrigating the abdomen dilutes the bacterial load decreasing risk of postoperative infectious complications. Hence the surgical dictum "the solution to pollution is dilution." However, randomized controlled trails as well as meta-analysis have failed to show benefit of lavage in patients with peritonitis [43–48]. The frequency and choice of lavage varies widely and includes saline, aqueous betadine, water, and antibiotic fluid. Lavage solutions may reduce antimicrobial burden through dilution, direct antimicrobial affects from dissolved antimicrobial drugs, or pathogen lysis from osmotic gradients. Most surgeons practice lavage with warm saline until the fluid is clear using 500–1000 mL [49]. There is no robust data to suggest that antibiotic-containing irrigant or irrigant with iodine or chlorhexidine reduces risk of infection [45, 49]. In light of risking antimicrobial resistance and healthcare costs, these tactics should not be encouraged. Using water or other hypotonic irrigant solutions may increase lysis of microbial pathogens, but may negatively affect host cells. Given these considerations, warmed sterile isotonic crystalloid solution is the most appropriate irrigant solution. Careful consideration should be given to aggressive irrigation when the infection is localized, as lavage may further spread bacteria and other pathogens in an otherwise unperturbed abdomen.

Source control is but one of two pillars of effective therapy for intra-abdominal infections. Targeted antimicrobial therapy is also required for patients with complicated intra-abdominal infections. For uncomplicated infections like acute cholecystitis or non-perforated appendicitis, perioperative antibiotics are sufficient. But for patients with complicated intra-abdominal infections, four to five days of antibiotic therapy are sufficient after source control, as demonstrated in the STOP-IT trial [50]. Readers are directed to the chapter discussing antibiotic therapy for an in-depth review of antibiotic options and recommended durations of therapy.

To help tailor therapy, peritoneal cultures should be obtained to allow for pathogen-directed antimicrobial therapy when sensitivities result [2]. Treatment failure in some cases may be secondary to resistant pathogens [51, 52]. Studies show that patients with intra-abdominal infections with antimicrobial resistant organisms are at risk of adverse outcomes [52–55]. Furthermore, there is an increasing proportion of multidrug-resistant organisms in intra-abdominal infections [51, 56, 57]. Prompt identification of an antimicrobial resistant infection is essential for the surgeon, as it should inform clinical management.

Utility of prophylactic drain placement after abdominal operations has long been the subject of debate. Amongst a wide range of procedures, drains paradoxically increase the risk of developing an surgical site infection even among contaminated (class III) wounds; among dirty (class IV) wounds this effect is not as pronounced [58]. Among patients undergoing colorectal operations drains are not routinely recommended, unless a technically challenging low-pelvic anastomosis is performed [59, 60]. Similarly, drains are not recommended after complicated acute appendectomies or cholecystectomies and may increase hospital cost and length of stay [61–63]. Even among patients who undergo hepatic or major upper gastrointestinal resections, no benefit is observed with routine drainage [64, 65]. Pancreatic resections may benefit from short-term drainage in some cases, but meta-analysis do not support routine drain use [66]. Despite the overwhelming body of evidence that suggests no benefit to drainage (and potential harm), drain placement after source control operations is disconcertingly common. Drains should not be routinely left after source control operations.

Treatment failure after initial attempts at source control may occur in up to 20% of patients [2, 36]. Patients should be assessed for source control failure if there is progressive organ dysfunction within the first 12–48 h after initial source control [2]. In these situations, abdominal re-exploration should strongly be considered. After 72 h, use of CT to identify fluid collections amenable to percutaneous drainage may become more useful [2]. The traditional teaching that the sensitivity and specificity of an abdominal CT scan to distinguish between failures of source control and normal postoperative fluid improves the further the duration of time from surgery to CT scan has been debated [67–69]. However, we and others have found it beneficial to hold off on obtaining a CT scan to assess for failure of source control until day 5 or greater to maximize the chances of detecting pathology that is likely to be successfully addressed through percutaneous intervention [2, 70].

11.6   Conclusion

Source control is an old concept in surgery, but one that remains essential to the management of patients with intra-abdominal infections. Patients with peritonitis secondary to an intra-abdominal infection require aggressive and timely intervention. Imaging may be useful, but should not delay operative intervention in clear cases. Damage control tactics, with delayed restoration of normal anatomy, may be desirable when the patient is profoundly physiologically unstable. Targeted antibiotic therapy is an important adjunct after source control has been achieved in complicated infections. While cautious optimism may be tempting after source control procedure, high suspicion for missed injury, ongoing infection or inadequate source control is prudent and preferable. When treatment failure is detected, an early return to the operating room is a sign of good judgment and a humble surgeon.

References

1. Sartelli M. A focus on intra-abdominal infections. World J Emerg Surg. 2010;5:9.
2. Mazuski JE, Tessier JM, May AK, et al. The surgical infection society revised guidelines on the management of intra-abdominal infection. Surg Infect (Larchmt). 2017;18(1):1–76.
3. Solomkin JS, Mazuski JE, Bradley JS, et al. Diagnosis and management of complicated intra-abdominal infection in adults and children: guidelines by the Surgical Infection Society and the Infectious Diseases Society of America. Clin Infect Dis Off Publ Infect Dis Soc Am. 2010;50(2):133–64.
4. Blot S, De Waele JJ. Critical issues in the clinical management of complicated intra-abdominal infections. Drugs. 2005;65(12):1611–20.
5. Ordoñez CA, Puyana JC. Management of peritonitis in the critically ill patient. Surg Clin North Am. 2006;86(6):1323–49.

6. Cheadle WG, Spain DA. The continuing challenge of intra-abdominal infection. Am J Surg. 2003;186(5A):15S–22S.
7. Sartelli M, Viale P, Koike K, et al. WSES consensus conference: guidelines for first-line management of intra-abdominal infections. World J Emerg Surg W. 2011;6:2.
8. Cervellin G, Mora R, Ticinesi A, et al. Epidemiology and outcomes of acute abdominal pain in a large urban Emergency Department: retrospective analysis of 5,340 cases. Ann Transl Med. 2016;4(19):362.
9. Hastings RS, Powers RD. Abdominal pain in the ED: a 35 year retrospective. Am J Emerg Med. 2011;29(7):711–6.
10. Mazzei MA, Guerrini S, Cioffi Squitieri N, et al. The role of US examination in the management of acute abdomen. Crit Ultrasound J. 2013;5(Suppl 1):S6.
11. Rhodes A, Phillips G, Beale R, et al. The Surviving Sepsis Campaign bundles and outcome: results from the International Multicentre Prevalence Study on Sepsis (the IMPreSS study). Intensive Care Med. 2015;41(9):1620–8.
12. NCEPOD – Sepsis: Just Say Sepsis! 2015. https://www.ncepod.org.uk/2015sepsis.html. Accessed 21 Aug 2019.
13. Sartelli M, Abu-Zidan FM, Catena F, et al. Global validation of the WSES Sepsis Severity Score for patients with complicated intra-abdominal infections: a prospective multicentre study (WISS Study). World J Emerg Surg. 2015;10(1):61.
14. Chana P, Joy M, Casey N, et al. Cohort analysis of outcomes in 69 490 emergency general surgical admissions across an international benchmarking collaborative. BMJ Open. 2017;7(3):e014484.
15. Angus DC, Linde-Zwirble WT, Lidicker J, Clermont G, Carcillo J, Pinsky MR. Epidemiology of severe sepsis in the United States: analysis of incidence, outcome, and associated costs of care. Crit Care Med. 2001;29(7):1303–10.
16. Pacelli F, Doglietto GB, Alfieri S, et al. Prognosis in intra-abdominal infections. Multivariate analysis on 604 patients. Arch Surg. 1996;131(6):641–5.
17. Wacha H, Hau T, Dittmer R, Ohmann C. Risk factors associated with intraabdominal infections: a prospective multicenter study. Peritonitis Study Group. Langenbecks Arch Surg. 1999;384(1):24–32.
18. Mulier S, Penninckx F, Verwaest C, et al. Factors affecting mortality in generalized postoperative peritonitis: multivariate analysis in 96 patients. World J Surg. 2003;27(4):379–84.
19. Moore LJ, Moore FA, Todd SR, Jones SL, Turner KL, Bass BL. Sepsis in general surgery: the 2005–2007 national surgical quality improvement program perspective. Arch Surg Chic Ill 1960. 2010;145(7):695–700.
20. Levy MM, Evans LE, Rhodes A. The Surviving Sepsis Campaign bundle: 2018 update. Intensive Care Med. 2018;44(6):925–8.
21. Zadroga R, Williams DN, Gottschall R, et al. Comparison of 2 blood culture media shows significant differences in bacterial recovery for patients on antimicrobial therapy. Clin Infect Dis Off Publ Infect Dis Soc Am. 2013;56(6):790–7.
22. Kanegaye JT, Soliemanzadeh P, Bradley JS. Lumbar puncture in pediatric bacterial meningitis: defining the time interval for recovery of cerebrospinal fluid pathogens after parenteral antibiotic pretreatment. Pediatrics. 2001;108(5):1169–74.
23. Ferrer R, Martin-Loeches I, Phillips G, et al. Empiric antibiotic treatment reduces mortality in severe sepsis and septic shock from the first hour: results from a guideline-based performance improvement program. Crit Care Med. 2014;42(8):1749–55.
24. Kumar A, Roberts D, Wood KE, et al. Duration of hypotension before initiation of effective antimicrobial therapy is the critical determinant of survival in human septic shock. Crit Care Med. 2006;34(6):1589–96.
25. Sartelli M, Catena F, Ansaloni L, et al. Complicated intra-abdominal infections in Europe: a comprehensive review of the CIAO study. World J Emerg Surg. 2012;7(1):36.
26. Soop M, Carlson GL. Recent developments in the surgical management of complex intra-abdominal infection. Br J Surg. 2017;104(2):e65–74.

27. Azuhata T, Kinoshita K, Kawano D, et al. Time from admission to initiation of surgery for source control is a critical determinant of survival in patients with gastrointestinal perforation with associated septic shock. Crit Care. 2014;18(3):R87.

28. Cope SZ. The early diagnosis of the acute abdomen. Oxford: H. Frowde; Hodder & Stoughton; 1921.

29. Silen W, Cope SZ. Cope's early diagnosis of the acute abdomen. 22nd ed. Oxford: Oxford University Press; 2010.

30. Lindelius A, Törngren S, Pettersson H, Adami J. Role of surgeon-performed ultrasound on further management of patients with acute abdominal pain: a randomized controlled clinical trial. Emerg Med J. 2009;26(8):561–6.

31. Foinant M, Lipiecka E, Buc E, et al. Impact of computed tomography on patient's care in nontraumatic acute abdomen: 90 patients. J Radiol. 2007;88(4):559–66.

32. Cinat ME, Wilson SE, Din AM. Determinants for successful percutaneous image-guided drainage of intra-abdominal abscess. Arch Surg. 2002;137(7):845–9.

33. Mowery NT, Bruns BR, MacNew HG, et al. Surgical management of pancreatic necrosis: a practice management guideline from the Eastern Association for the Surgery of Trauma. J Trauma Acute Care Surg. 2017;83(2):316–27.

34. Leppäniemi A, Tolonen M, Tarasconi A, et al. 2019 WSES guidelines for the management of severe acute pancreatitis. World J Emerg Surg. 2019;14:27.

35. Cai Y-L, Xiong X-Z, Lu J, et al. Percutaneous needle aspiration versus catheter drainage in the management of liver abscess: a systematic review and meta-analysis. HPB. 2015;17(3):195–201.

36. Waibel BH, Rotondo MF. Damage control for intra-abdominal sepsis. Surg Clin North Am. 2012;92(2):243–57.

37. Coccolini F, Montori G, Ceresoli M, et al. The role of open abdomen in non-trauma patient: WSES consensus paper. World J Emerg Surg. 2017;12:39.

38. Cheatham ML, Demetriades D, Fabian TC, et al. Prospective study examining clinical outcomes associated with a negative pressure wound therapy system and Barker's vacuum packing technique. World J Surg. 2013;37(9):2018–30.

39. Cirocchi R, Birindelli A, Biffl WL, et al. What is the effectiveness of the negative pressure wound therapy (NPWT) in patients treated with open abdomen technique? A systematic review and meta-analysis. J Trauma Acute Care Surg. 2016;81(3):575–84.

40. Pommerening MJ, DuBose JJ, Zielinski MD, et al. Time to first take-back operation predicts successful primary fascial closure in patients undergoing damage control laparotomy. Surgery. 2014;156(2):431–8.

41. Parcells JP, Mileski JP, Gnagy FT, Haragan AF, Mileski WJ. Using antimicrobial solution for irrigation in appendicitis to lower surgical site infection rates. Am J Surg. 2009;198(6):875–80.

42. Roth RM, Gleckman RA, Gantz NM, Kelly N. Antibiotic irrigations. A plea for controlled clinical trials. Pharmacotherapy. 1985;5(4):222–7.

43. Gammeri E, Petrinic T, Bond-Smith G, Gordon-Weeks A. Meta-analysis of peritoneal lavage in appendicectomy. BJS Open. 2019;3(1):24–30.

44. Hunt JL. Generalized peritonitis. To irrigate or not to irrigate the abdominal cavity. Arch Surg. 1982;117(2):209–12.

45. Schein M, Gecelter G, Freinkel W, Gerding H, Becker PJ. Peritoneal lavage in abdominal sepsis. A controlled clinical study. Arch Surg. 1990;125(9):1132–5.

46. St Peter SD, Adibe OO, Iqbal CW, et al. Irrigation versus suction alone during laparoscopic appendectomy for perforated appendicitis: a prospective randomized trial. Ann Surg. 2012;256(4):581–5.

47. Moore CB, Smith RS, Herbertson R, Toevs C. Does use of intraoperative irrigation with open or laparoscopic appendectomy reduce post-operative intra-abdominal abscess? Am Surg. 2011;77(1):78–80.

48. Penna M, Markar SR, Mackenzie H, Hompes R, Cunningham C. Laparoscopic lavage versus primary resection for acute perforated diverticulitis: review and meta-analysis. Ann Surg. 2018;267(2):252–8.

49. Whiteside OJH, Tytherleigh MG, Thrush S, Farouk R, Galland RB. Intra-operative peritoneal lavage—who does it and why? Ann R Coll Surg Engl. 2005;87(4):255–8.
50. Sawyer RG, Claridge JA, Nathens AB, et al. Trial of short-course antimicrobial therapy for intraabdominal infection. N Engl J Med. 2015;372(21):1996–2005.
51. Labricciosa FM, Sartelli M, Abbo LM, et al. Epidemiology and risk factors for isolation of multi-drug-resistant organisms in patients with complicated intra-abdominal infections. Surg Infect (Larchmt). 2018;19(3):264–72.
52. Christou NV, Turgeon P, Wassef R, Rotstein O, Bohnen J, Potvin M. Management of intra-abdominal infections. The case for intraoperative cultures and comprehensive broad-spectrum antibiotic coverage. The Canadian Intra-abdominal Infection Study Group. Arch Surg. 1996;131(11):1193–201.
53. Hopkins JA, Lee JC, Wilson SE. Susceptibility of intra-abdominal isolates at operation: a predictor of postoperative infection. Am Surg. 1993;59(12):791–6.
54. Montravers P, Martin-Loeches I. Source control and intra-abdominal infections: still many questions and only limited answers. J Crit Care. 2019;52:265–6.
55. Sotto A, Lefrant JY, Fabbro-Peray P, et al. Evaluation of antimicrobial therapy management of 120 consecutive patients with secondary peritonitis. J Antimicrob Chemother. 2002;50(4):569–76.
56. Seguin P, Laviolle B, Chanavaz C, et al. Factors associated with multidrug-resistant bacteria in secondary peritonitis: impact on antibiotic therapy. Clin Microbiol Infect. 2006;12(10):980–5.
57. Seguin P, Fédun Y, Laviolle B, Nesseler N, Donnio P-Y, Mallédant Y. Risk factors for multidrug-resistant bacteria in patients with post-operative peritonitis requiring intensive care. J Antimicrob Chemother. 2010;65(2):342–6.
58. Mujagic E, Zeindler J, Coslovsky M, et al. The association of surgical drains with surgical site infections – a prospective observational study. Am J Surg. 2019;217(1):17–23.
59. Puleo FJ, Mishra N, Hall JF. Use of intra-abdominal drains. Clin Colon Rectal Surg. 2013;26(3):174–7.
60. Jesus EC, Karliczek A, Matos D, Castro AA, Atallah AN. Prophylactic anastomotic drainage for colorectal surgery. Cochrane Database Syst Rev. 2004;(4):CD002100.
61. Gurusamy KS, Koti R, Davidson BR. Routine abdominal drainage versus no abdominal drainage for uncomplicated laparoscopic cholecystectomy. Cochrane Database Syst Rev. 2013;(9):CD006004.
62. Cheng Y, Zhou S, Zhou R, et al. Abdominal drainage to prevent intra-peritoneal abscess after open appendectomy for complicated appendicitis. Cochrane Database Syst Rev. 2015;(2):CD010168.
63. Chilton CP, Mann CV. Drainage after cholecystectomy. Ann R Coll Surg Engl. 1980;62(1):60–5.
64. Shrikhande SV, Barreto SG, Shetty G, et al. Post-operative abdominal drainage following major upper gastrointestinal surgery: single drain versus two drains. J Cancer Res Ther. 2013;9(2):267–71.
65. Messager M, Sabbagh C, Denost Q, et al. Is there still a need for prophylactic intra-abdominal drainage in elective major gastro-intestinal surgery? J Visc Surg. 2015;152(5):305–13.
66. Zhang W, He S, Cheng Y, et al. Prophylactic abdominal drainage for pancreatic surgery. Cochrane Database Syst Rev. 2018;(6):CD010583.
67. Antevil JL, Egan JC, Woodbury RO, Rivera L, Oreilly EB, Brown CVR. Abdominal computed tomography for postoperative abscess: is it useful during the first week? J Gastrointest Surg. 2006;10(6):901–5.
68. Norwood SH, Civetta JM. Abdominal CT scanning in critically ill surgical patients. Ann Surg. 1985;202(2):166–75.
69. Nielsen JW, Kurtovic KJ, Kenney BD, Diefenbach KA. Postoperative timing of computed tomography scans for abscess in pediatric appendicitis. J Surg Res. 2016;200(1):1–7.
70. Okita Y, Mohri Y, Kobayashi M, et al. Factors influencing the outcome of image-guided percutaneous drainage of intra-abdominal abscess after gastrointestinal surgery. Surg Today. 2013;43(10):1095–102.

71. Di Saverio S, Bassi M, Smerieri N, et al. Diagnosis and treatment of perforated or bleeding peptic ulcers: 2013 WSES position paper. World J Emerg Surg. 2014;9(1):45.
72. Di Saverio S, Birindelli A, Kelly MD, et al. WSES Jerusalem guidelines for diagnosis and treatment of acute appendicitis. World J Emerg Surg. 2016;11:34.
73. Rushing A, Bugaev N, Jones C, et al. Management of acute appendicitis in adults: a practice management guideline from the Eastern Association for the Surgery of Trauma. J Trauma Acute Care Surg. 2019;87(1):214–24.
74. Vons C, Barry C, Maitre S, et al. Amoxicillin plus clavulanic acid versus appendicectomy for treatment of acute uncomplicated appendicitis: an open-label, non-inferiority, randomised controlled trial. Lancet Lond Engl. 2011;377(9777):1573–9.
75. Hansson J, Körner U, Khorram-Manesh A, Solberg A, Lundholm K. Randomized clinical trial of antibiotic therapy versus appendicectomy as primary treatment of acute appendicitis in unselected patients. Br J Surg. 2009;96(5):473–81.
76. Eriksson S, Granström L. Randomized controlled trial of appendicectomy versus antibiotic therapy for acute appendicitis. Br J Surg. 1995;82(2):166–9.
77. Styrud J, Eriksson S, Nilsson I, et al. Appendectomy versus antibiotic treatment in acute appendicitis. A prospective multicenter randomized controlled trial. World J Surg. 2006;30(6):1033–7.
78. Salminen P, Paajanen H, Rautio T, et al. Antibiotic therapy vs appendectomy for treatment of uncomplicated acute appendicitis: the APPAC randomized clinical trial. JAMA. 2015;313(23):2340–8.
79. Petrowsky H, Demartines N, Rousson V, Clavien P-A. Evidence-based value of prophylactic drainage in gastrointestinal surgery: a systematic review and meta-analyses. Ann Surg. 2004;240(6):1074–84.
80. Brown CVR, Abrishami M, Muller M, Velmahos GC. Appendiceal abscess: immediate operation or percutaneous drainage? Am Surg. 2003;69(10):829–32.
81. Oliak D, Yamini D, Udani VM, et al. Initial nonoperative management for periappendiceal abscess. Dis Colon Rectum. 2001;44(7):936–41.
82. Mällinen J, Rautio T, Grönroos J, et al. Risk of appendiceal neoplasm in periappendicular abscess in patients treated with interval appendectomy vs follow-up with magnetic resonance imaging: 1-year outcomes of the peri-appendicitis acuta randomized clinical trial. JAMA Surg. 2019;154(3):200–7.
83. Bala M, Kashuk J, Moore EE, et al. Acute mesenteric ischemia: guidelines of the World Society of Emergency Surgery. World J Emerg Surg. 2017;12:38.
84. Feingold D, Steele SR, Lee S, et al. Practice parameters for the treatment of sigmoid diverticulitis. Dis Colon Rectum. 2014;57(3):284–94.
85. Moore FA, Catena F, Moore EE, Leppaniemi A, Peitzmann AB. Position paper: management of perforated sigmoid diverticulitis. World J Emerg Surg. 2013;8(1):55.
86. Brandt LJ, Feuerstadt P, Longstreth GF, Boley SJ. American College of Gastroenterology. ACG clinical guideline: epidemiology, risk factors, patterns of presentation, diagnosis, and management of colon ischemia (CI). Am J Gastroenterol. 2015;110(1):18–44.
87. Herr MW, Gagliano RA. Historical perspective and current management of colonic and intraperitoneal rectal trauma. Curr Surg. 2005;62(2):187–92.
88. Demetriades D, Murray JA, Chan L, et al. Penetrating colon injuries requiring resection: diversion or primary anastomosis? An AAST prospective multicenter study. J Trauma. 2001;50(5):765–75.
89. Mayumi T, Okamoto K, Takada T, et al. Tokyo guidelines 2018: management bundles for acute cholangitis and cholecystitis. J Hepato-Biliary-Pancreat Sci. 2018;25(1):96–100.
90. Ansaloni L, Pisano M, Coccolini F, et al. 2016 WSES guidelines on acute calculous cholecystitis. World J Emerg Surg. 2016;11:25.
91. Mori Y, Itoi T, Baron TH, et al. Tokyo guidelines 2018: management strategies for gallbladder drainage in patients with acute cholecystitis (with videos). J Hepato-Biliary-Pancreat Sci. 2018;25(1):87–95.

92. Besselink MGH, van Santvoort HC, Nieuwenhuijs VB, et al. Minimally invasive "step-up approach" versus maximal necrosectomy in patients with acute necrotising pancreatitis (PANTER trial): design and rationale of a randomised controlled multicenter trial [ISRCTN13975868]. BMC Surg. 2006;6:6.

93. van Santvoort HC, Besselink MG, Bakker OJ, et al. A step-up approach or open necrosectomy for necrotizing pancreatitis. N Engl J Med. 2010;362(16):1491–502.

94. van Brunschot S, van Grinsven J, van Santvoort HC, et al. Endoscopic or surgical step-up approach for infected necrotising pancreatitis: a multicentre randomised trial. Lancet. 2018;391(10115):51–8.

95. Rajak CL, Gupta S, Jain S, Chawla Y, Gulati M, Suri S. Percutaneous treatment of liver abscesses: needle aspiration versus catheter drainage. AJR Am J Roentgenol. 1998;170(4):1035–9.

96. Yu SCH, Ho SSM, Lau WY, et al. Treatment of pyogenic liver abscess: prospective randomized comparison of catheter drainage and needle aspiration. Hepatology. 2004;39(4):932–8.

97. Mohsen AH, Green ST, Read RC, McKendrick MW. Liver abscess in adults: ten years experience in a UK centre. QJM Mon J Assoc Physicians. 2002;95(12):797–802.

98. Brunetti E, Kern P, Vuitton DA. Writing Panel for the WHO-IWGE. Expert consensus for the diagnosis and treatment of cystic and alveolar echinococcosis in humans. Acta Trop. 2010;114(1):1–16.

99. Robinson SL, Saxe JM, Lucas CE, Arbulu A, Ledgerwood AM, Lucas WF. Splenic abscess associated with endocarditis. Surgery. 1992;112(4):781–6.

100. Ting W, Silverman NA, Arzouman DA, Levitsky S. Splenic septic emboli in endocarditis. Circulation. 1990;82(5 Suppl):IV105–9.

101. Steele SR, McCormick J, Melton GB, et al. Practice parameters for the management of *Clostridium difficile* infection. Dis Colon Rectum. 2015;58(1):10–24.

102. Sartelli M, Di Bella S, McFarland LV, et al. 2019 update of the WSES guidelines for management of Clostridioides (Clostridium) difficile infection in surgical patients. World J Emerg Surg. 2019;14:8.

103. Neal MD, Alverdy JC, Hall DE, Simmons RL, Zuckerbraun BS. Diverting loop ileostomy and colonic lavage: an alternative to total abdominal colectomy for the treatment of severe, complicated *Clostridium difficile* associated disease. Ann Surg. 2011;254(3):423–7.

104. Phitayakorn R, Delaney CP, Reynolds HL, et al. Standardized algorithms for management of anastomotic leaks and related abdominal and pelvic abscesses after colorectal surgery. World J Surg. 2008;32(6):1147–56.

105. de Schipper JP, Pull ter Gunne AF, HJM O, van Laarhoven CJHM. Spontaneous rupture of the oesophagus: Boerhaave's syndrome in 2008. Literature review and treatment algorithm. Dig Surg. 2009;26(1):1–6.

106. Fischer A, Thomusch O, Benz S, von Dobschuetz E, Baier P, Hopt UT. Nonoperative treatment of 15 benign esophageal perforations with self-expandable covered metal stents. Ann Thorac Surg. 2006;81(2):467–72.

Ongoing Peritonitis (Tertiary Peritonotis)

12

Vittoria Pattonieri, Gennaro Perrone, Antonio Tarasconi, Hariscine K. Abongwa, and Fausto Catena

12.1 Definition

Recurrent intra-abdominal infections remain a formidable challenge to the surgeon. The associated severe inflammatory response originating from the peritoneal damage causes a high percentage of septic course. Depending on the underlying pathology, infectious peritonitis in classified into primary peritonitis (spontaneous bacterial peritonitis, arises in the absence of an identifiable anatomical derangement), secondary peritonitis, which is the most frequent entity and is defined as an infection of the peritoneal cavity resulting from loss of integrity of the gastrointestinal tract, and tertiary peritonitis. TP is less common and is defined as a severe recurrent or persistent intra-abdominal infection occurring 48–72 h following apparently successful and adequate surgical control of SP [1]. Whereas antibiotics are the mainstay of therapy of primary peritonitis, source control in the form of surgical or percutaneous drainage or removal of a colonized device is needed to resolve SP. These measures, combined with adequate physiologic support, result in cure of the infectious process in most patients. It has been recognized that appropriate surgical and antimicrobial therapy does not result in full resolution of all cases of peritonitis, particularly in the most gravely ill patients. Rather, a clinical syndrome evolves characterized by a prolonged systemic inflammation, organ dysfunction leading to a high rate of SIRS and severe sepsis or septic shock, in associations with recurrent peritoneal infection with organism of low intrinsic pathogenicity. In these critically ill patient, with impaired immune defense and a considerable number of subsequent surgical interventions, infectious complications as well as a mortality double as high ranging between 30 and 63% [2–6]. The microbial flora encountered in TP is different from SP and displays mostly opportunistic and nosocomial facultative pathogenic bacteria and fungi (e.g., *Enterococci, Enterobacter,*

V. Pattonieri · G. Perrone · A. Tarasconi · H. K. Abongwa · F. Catena (✉)
Department of Emergency Surgery, Maggiore Hospital, Parma, Italy

© Springer Nature Switzerland AG 2021
M. Sartelli et al. (eds.), *Infections in Surgery*, Hot Topics in Acute Care Surgery and Trauma, https://doi.org/10.1007/978-3-030-62116-2_12

Candida). Due to broad-spectrum antibiotic therapy, a significant proportion of microbes develop multiresistance to antibiotics.

It is often difficult to differentiate between SP and TP since there is a continuum between both clinical situations and the exact time point when SP turns into TP is often missed [3]. Although TP may be diagnosed during relaparotomy as a simple discrete point in the illness, in reality, it evolves gradually over several hours or days.

Tertiary peritonitis poses a significant problem for clinicians, not only due to its treatment-resistant course, but also because of lack of consensus over the precise definition of the syndrome. Several authors define it as a diffuse, therapy resistant peritonitis with fungi or low-grade pathogenic bacteria in the absence of well-defined infective focus after apparently adequate therapy [4, 6–8]. Other author postulated that TP occurred when the initial peritoneal infection continued because surgical treatment was not successful [9, 10]. Clinical and laboratory parameters may remain pathologic or slowly decreasing 48 h after source control, so that reliable recognition of TP may be difficult. On the other hand, a time period of 7 days might miss adequate therapy strategy for TP.

The latest ICU consensus conference guidelines provide a precise definition of TP as intra-abdominal infection that persists or recurs $\geq$48 h following successful and adequate surgical source control. This definition contains two essential conditions, which have to be met: the time period ($\geq$48 h) and successful surgical source control [11].

Unfortunately, by the time most patients develop the clinical signs of tertiary peritonitis, the window for meaningful intervention may have passed [7].

12.2 Diagnosis

The value of clinical and laboratory parameters and scoring systems for sufficient diagnosis and monitoring of TP is still discussed controversially. It is often difficult to differentiate between SP and TP since they are in continuum between both clinical situation and the exact time point when SP turns into TP is often missed. A subset of patients that received a surgical source control for SP will however develop clinical signs of recurrent or persistent intra-abdominal infection in spite of apparently successful source control, which often results in reoperation. During subsequent laparotomies, recurrent or persistent peritonitis is encountered in spite of adequate surgical source control during the initial operation. This form of peritonitis is referred to TP. The diagnosis of TP can only be made in the absence of an obvious anatomical defect or disruption of the gastrointestinal hollow viscera; otherwise, the peritonitis has to be classified as ongoing SP (primary failure of surgical source control). The most frequent way to diagnose TP is a planned or on demand relaparotomy, performed in the interval after initial operation [12]. However, the ICU consensus conference provided three categories for the diagnostic certainty of TP: "microbiologically confirmed," "probable," and "possible".

It is desirable to identify patients at risk for developing TP as early as possible or at least during the first days after initial operation for SP. In order to assess the severity of intra-abdominal infection, multiple scales for evaluation of critically ill patients with peritonitis admitted to ICU have been described. Mannheim Peritonitis Index (MPI), APACHE II score, SAPS II score, C-reactive protein (CRP), and procalcitonin (PCT) are early and easily accessible parameters which may be utilized for identification of patients who might develop TP.

The Mannheim Peritonitis Index (MPI) represents a scoring system that estimates the severity and prognosis of SP at the onset of this clinical condition. It is applied under routine conditions during initial surgery for SP in the operating room. Since 1987, it has been developed and validated in several studies for SP [13, 14]. The MPI includes information about age, sex, organ failure, cancer and duration of peritonitis, involvement of colon, extent of spread, and the character of peritoneal fluid.

The Acute Physiology and Chronic Health Evaluation (APACHE) II score predicts mortality and multi-organ failure (MOF) throughout the documentation of permanent changes in labor and ICU parameters. It measures biochemical parameters, blood pressure, pulse and temperature (acute physiology score) alongside age (age points), and chronic organ insufficiency assessment including liver, kidney, and cardiovascular, respiratory, and immune system (chronic health points). The APACHE II score has been shown to have limitations in patients with TP or severe sepsis/septic shock. In this patient population resuscitation frequently occurs in places other than ICU, including the operating room, emergency room and transferring institution. As a result, the patients may be relatively stable at the time of ICU admission, and the APACHE II score may not reflect the initial magnitude of physiologic derangement [6].

The Simplified Acute Physiology Score II (SAPS II) was initially designed to predict mortality and disease severity of critically ill patients on surgical intensive care units [15].

C-reactive protein constitutes a routine parameter in patients with abdominal infections. The main problem of CRP is the lack of specificity for abdominal infections, and a rise of CRP during the postoperative period may simply be the result of the operative trauma [9, 10]. CRP and PCT have also rarely been evaluated in the diagnosis of TP. Concentration of CRP have been used to follow septic patients, but is unable to predict the outcome of disease or severity. During the postoperative period sepsis can be difficult to distinguish from the noninfectious situations, such as postoperative systemic inflammatory response syndrome (SIRS), related to surgical trauma. SIRS can be self-limiting or may progress to severe sepsis or septic shock [16]. Major surgical trauma may induce a non-septic SIRS which can be difficult to distinguish from early postoperative septic complications. PCT could helpful in the early diagnosis of postoperative infection after major surgery. PCT is known to be an early marker of severe sepsis, but it is correlated with the severity of SIRS after severe trauma [17, 18] and so may be distorted by major surgery. PCT was identified as a better discriminator then CRP in characterizing the degree of inflammation related to infection. PCT was more specific for sepsis-induced inflammation than CRP, but no better than CRP at identifying infection uncomplicated by sepsis or organ failure [19]. PCT measurements may be useful for early diagnosis of septic postoperative complications. Early diagnosis and treatment of septic patients may greatly improve outcome [20].

In response to infection or surgical trauma, the peritoneal environment produces cytokines. Proinflammatory cytokines recruit inflammatory cells to combat pathogens, stimulate wound repair and clear damaged tissue. To protect the host from damage by this inflammatory response, anti-inflammatory cytokines are also produced. Homeostasis is restored when the infection is controlled by a balanced immune response. Initially, a predominant proinflammatory reaction causes septic shock with organ dysfunction. If peritonitis persists and TP develops after a series of interventions, the anti-inflammatory cascade prevails, causing suppression of the immune system. Because of this, peritoneal inflammation is lacking, and there is no tendency toward the healing of wound or organ recovery. The immune system can be considered as one failing organ in the syndrome of multiple organ failure. Predisposing factors for immune paralysis include patient-related factors, such as genetic immune deficiencies, malnutrition and age, iatrogenic factors as surgery, immunosuppressive drugs and blood transfusions, and underlying diseases, as malignancy and neutropenia [4, 21, 22]. Immune paralysis can be defined by the critical level of deactivated monocytes with less than 30% HLA-DR expression [23]. This decreased cellular immunity is associated with high infection rates and mortality [24].

Beside these clinical and laboratory parameters, Mokart et al. have recently shown that IL-6 is a good independent early marker of postoperative sepsis, severe sepsis or septic shock after major surgery [25]. The pattern of change of IL-6 is similar to that of PCT (postoperatively increased levels in septic patients, early marker of postoperative infections following major surgery), contrariwise is not yet available for routine diagnosis.

However, the value of clinical (MPI, SAPS II, APACHE II) and laboratory parameters (CRP, PCT) for sufficient diagnosis is limited, even if the MPI could be significantly higher in patients that later on developed TP compared to SP. MPI is an early marker for TP [3].

It would be desirable to have diagnostic markers that could predict at the onset of peritonitis—during the initial operation or the first postoperative days after— whether the individual patient will develop TP or not.

12.3   Risk Factors and Microbial Flora

Age of patients, underlying etiology of peritonitis, malnutrition, endocrine dysfunction, and presence of multidrug-resistant microorganisms are some of the important epidemiologic and clinical risk factors which may predispose toward TP.

Comorbidities of patients with SP and TP do not significantly differ from each other. Nevertheless, cardiopulmonary and malignant comorbidities are associated with higher mortality. Less than a half of patients with SP die compared to those suffering from TP [8]. Advanced age is a significant factor associated with TP as confirmed in literature [10, 26]. Higher age is a predictive factor for development of persisting peritonitis and organ failure, according to Barie et al.

Endocrine pathways play an important role in the body's physiological response to peritonitis: in response to infectious insult the hypothalamic-pituitary-adrenal axis in activated, resulting in increased serum cortisol concentrations. The role of corticosteroids is essential to restore homeostasis. In persistent stress, such as complicated or persistent peritonitis, the adrenocortical response can be deranged and a phenomenon called relative adrenal insufficiency could develop. The etiology is not fully clear, but is thought to be caused by depletion of the adrenal cortex and glucocorticoid receptor resistance. Substitution of corticosteroids in patients with relative adrenal insufficiency can reverse the septic-shock state drastically [27]. Prolonged critical illness is characterized catabolism of whole-body protein stores, resulting in muscle wasting and negative nitrogen balance, associated with increased morbidity and mortality [28].

Many authors have shown that there is a microbial shift in TP toward *Enterococcus, Enterobacter, Pseudomonas, Candida albicans*, and other opportunistic bacteria and fungi, cultured from the peritoneal cavity during operation [6, 8]. Indeed, pathogens frequently cultured from the peritoneal cavity in TP include multiresistant gram-negative organisms, endogenous organisms of low intrinsic pathogenicity [29]. This shift may reflect antibiotic pressure, as these organisms are resistant to most first-line antibiotics used in the surgical ICU. The main source of these pathogens in thought to be the patient's gastrointestinal tract. In critical illness intestinal hypoperfusion, intestinal starvation, and elimination of normal gut flora by antimicrobial agents cause mucosal atrophy with subsequent loss of gut barrier function and microbial translocation [30, 31]. Moreover, manipulation during surgery may damage the bowel, promoting translocation of pathogens. Microbes and toxins moving from the gut lumen into the bloodstream and the peritoneal cavity activate the host's immune inflammatory defense mechanisms, thus the immune response will be both uncontrolled and unbalanced, leading to tissue destruction and multiple organ failure. Finally, the superinfection of TP may arise as a result of the translocation of the infecting species from the adjacent gastrointestinal tract. The characteristic flora of TP includes the same organisms that have been shown to overgrow the proximal gastrointestinal tract of the critically ill patients, and there is a strong correlation between gut colonization and the development of peritoneal infection with the same species [32]. After appropriate surgical management, the combination of intact host defenses and appropriate antimicrobial therapy results in complete resolution of most cases of SP; TP develops when the interaction of therapeutic intervention and host defenses fails. There is evidence in literature that adequate perfusion and enteral feeding are important for preservation and restoration of the gastrointestinal tract and maintenance of barrier function. Moreover, mucosal immunity, originating in GALT (gut associate lymphoid tissue) appears to be preserving by enteral feeding. There is substantial evidence in both critically ill and high-risk surgical patients that enteral feeding leads to significantly fewer infectious complications [33, 34].

Patients suffering from TP have a significantly higher number of different infecting organisms than those with SP. Microbiological specimen in immune-suppressed patients with TP are different from those with SP. The number of opportunistic bacterial organism, mostly colonizing gastrointestinal tract, and fungi such as *Candida* increase, and organism become aggressive due to the immune weakness and prolonged peritoneal infection. The flora of TP is often identical to that predominating in nosocomial ICU-acquired infections [29]. Moreover, although we could not commonly demonstrate bacteremia in association with episode of TP, all of the predominant organisms—*Candida, Enterobacter,* coagulase-negative staphylococci, and enterococci—are common causes of bacteremia in ICU.

The microbial resistograms of these microbes revealed two- to threefold higher resistance rates compared with those in secondary peritonitis leading to a challenge in the initiation of an adequate and specific antibiotic treatment.

12.4 Therapy

Antimicrobial treatment in TP remains a matter of debate. Early goal-directed therapy provides benefits in outcome of patients with severe sepsis [6]. Initial antibiotic therapy for intra-abdominal infections is typically empirical in nature because a patient with abdominal sepsis/PS needs immediate treatment and microbiological data resulting from culture and swabs can require 24–48 h before they are available. In the context of intra-abdominal sepsis the major pathogens involved are community-acquired microbes. TP are instead commonly caused by more resistant flora and complex multidrug regimen may be necessary for first-line, empiric therapy. TP is a life-threatening intra-abdominal infection with high rates of mortality due to high rate of multidrug-resistant infections and invasive candidiasis. In these critically ill patients antimicrobial therapy should be started as soon as possible; moreover, clinicians should always consider, especially in these patients, the physiopathological status of the patient as well as the pharmacokinetic properties of the employed antibiotics to ensure timely and effective administration of antibiotics [35]. Treatment of choice in patients with TP is conservative management. As these patients have no perforations or leaks, early enteral nutrition in advisable. It prevents atrophy of the gastrointestinal mucosa, maintains immunocompetence and preserves normal gut flora. Major septic complications are reduced as presented in a meta-analysis of prospective randomized trials [36].

For all these reasons, in TP the surgical strategy does not appear to be the pivotal factor and reoperations for severe abdominal infections are correlated to considerable deterioration and fatal outcome [37]. Proinflammatory mediator levels such as IL-6 raise after surgical treatment, resulting in aggravated peritoneal permeability and at least septic shock and MOF. The predominant finding noted at relaparotomies in patients with TP in the presence of poorly localized collections of fluid, rather than discrete abscesses [6]. Mechanosurgical solutions are likely to have reached their limit once TP has developed. Indeed, repeated interventions may play a fundamental role in causing a further deterioration of the local immune response.

Furthermore, manipulation of the viscera may endanger the integrity of the intestine and thereby promote translocation.

12.5 Conclusions

Tertiary peritonitis represent the current limit of the surgical approach to sever intra-abdominal infection. Specific pathogens are cultured from the peritoneal cavity, although these appear more a symptom then the cause of critical illness. Elevated prognostic scores, advanced age, endocrine dysfunction, and fungal infections are associated with high mortality and tertiary peritonitis. Patients with more than one infecting organism suffer more frequently from TP and fatal outcome is correlated with cardiovascular and malignant comorbidities. Due to high mortality and often delayed diagnosis, it is crucial to identify patients at risk for developing TP as early as possible: at the initial operation and during the first postoperative days. Lack of peritoneal inflammation with systemic energy suggests immune paralysis and this state can have both endogenous or exogenous origins. Moreover, the endocrine stress response is essential for metabolic, cardiovascular and immunological homeostasis.

Organ failure is the main cause of death and is significantly high in patients with TP.

Early detection of nosocomial infections and increased rate of an adequately initiated antibiotic treatment in the patients with a high infectious risk are the pillars of TP management: definitive recognition of TP and optimal treatment in the first critical days provide maximal benefit in terms of outcome.

References

1. Calandra T, Cohen J. The international sepsis forum consensus conference on definition of infection in the intensive care unit. Crit Care Med. 2005;33:1538–48.
2. Weiss G, Steffanie W, Lippet H. Peritonitis: main reason of severe sepsis in surgical intensive care. Zentralbl Chir. 2007;132:130–7.
3. Chromik AM, Meiser A, Hölling J, Sülberg D, Daigeler A, Meurer K, et al. Identification of patients at risk for development of tertiary peritonitis on a surgical intensive care unit. J Gastrointest Surg. 2009;13:1358–67.
4. Buijk SE, Bruining HA. Future directions in the management of tertiary peritonitis. Intensive Care Med. 2002;28:1024–9.
5. Marshall JC, Innes M. Intensive care unit management of intraabdominal infection. Crit Care Med. 2003;31:2228–37.
6. Nathens AB, Rotstein O, Marshall JC. Tertiary peritonitis: clinical features of a complex nosocomial infection. World J Surg. 1998;22:158–63.
7. Evans HL, Raymond DP, Pelletier SJ, et al. Tertiary peritonitis (recurrent diffuse or localized disease) is not an independent predictor of mortality in surgical patients with intraabdominal infection. Surg Infect. 2001;2:255–63.
8. Pahnofer P, Iazy B, Riedl M, Ferenc V, Ploder M, Jakesz R, et al. Age microbiology and prognostic scores help to differentiate between secondary and tertiary peritonitis. Langebecks Arch Surg. 2009;394:265–71.

9. Evans HL, Raymond DP, Pelletier SJ, et al. Diagnosis of intra-abdominal infections in the critically ill patient. Curr Opin Crit Care. 2001;7:117–21.
10. Malangoni MA. Evaluation and management of tertiary peritonitis. Am Surg. 2000;66:157–61.
11. Mishra SP, Tiwary SK, Mishra M, Gupta SK. An introduction on tertiary peritonitis. J Emerg Trauma Shock. 2014;7:121–3.
12. Koperna T. Surgical management of severe secondary peritonitis. Br J Surg. 2000;87:378.
13. Billing A, Fröhlich D. Prediction of outcome using the Mannheim peritonitis index in 2003 patients. Br J Surg. 1994;81:209–13.
14. Linder MM, Wacha H, Feldmann U, Wesch G, Streifensand RA, Gundlach E. The Mannheim Peritonitis Index. An instrument for the intraoperative prognosis of peritonitis. Chirurg. 1987;58:84–92.
15. Weiss G, Meyer F, Lippert H. Infectiological diagnostic problems in tertiary peritonitis. Langenbeck's Arch Surg. 2006;391:473–82.
16. Rangel-Fausto MS, Pittet D, et al. The natural history of the systemic inflammatory response syndrome (SIRS). A prospective study. JAMA. 1995;273:117–23.
17. Hensel M, Volk T, Docke WD, et al. Hyperprocalcitoninemia in patients with noninfectious SIRS and pulmonary dysfunction associated with cardiopulmonary bypass. Anesthesiology. 1998;89:93–104.
18. Mimoz O, Benoist JF, et al. Procalcitonin ad C-reactive protein during the early posttraumatic systemic inflammatory response syndrome. Intensive Care Med. 1998;24:185–8.
19. Ugarte H, Silva E, Mercan D, De Mendoca A, Vincent JL. Procalcitonin used as a marker of infection in the intensive care unit. Crit Care Med. 1999;27:498–504.
20. Rivers E, Nguyen B, Havstad S, et al. Early goal-directed therapy in the treatment of severe sepsis and septic shock. N Engl J Med. 2001;345:1368–77.
21. Heiss MM, Fraunberger P, Delanoff C, Stets R, Allgayer H, et al. Modulation of immune response by blood transfusion: evidence for a differential effect of allogeneic and autologous blood in colorectal cancer surgery. Shock. 1997;8:402–8.
22. Lundy J, Ford CM. Surgery, trauma and immune suppression. Evolving the mechanism. Ann Surg. 1983;197:434–8.
23. Asadullah K, Woiciechowsky C, Docke WD, et al. Very low monocytic HLA-DR expression indicates high risk of infection-immunomonitoring for patients after neurosurgery and patients during high dose steroid therapy. Eur J Emerg Med. 1995;2:184–90.
24. Cheadle WG, Mercer-Jones M, Heinzelmann M, Polk HC Jr. Sepsis and septic complications in the surgical patient: who in at risk? Shock. 1996;6:S6–9.
25. Mokart D, Merlin M, et al. Procalcitonin, interleukin 6 and systemic inflammatory response syndrome (SIRS): early markers of postoperative sepsis after major surgery. Br J Anaesth. 2005;94:767–73.
26. Bohen J, Mustard RA, Oxholm SE, Schouten D. APACHE II score and abdominal infection. Arch Surg. 1988;123:225.229.
27. Briegel J, Forst H, Haller M, Schelling G, Kilger E, Kuprat G, Hemmer B, Hummel T, Lenhart A, Heyduck M, Stoll C, Peter K. Stress doses of hydrocortisone reverse hyperdynamic sepsis shock: a prospective, randomized, double-blind, single-center study. Crit Care Med. 1999;27:723–32.
28. Douglas RG, Shaw JH. Metabolic response to sepsis and trauma. Br J Surg. 1989;76:115–22.
29. Nathens AB, Chu PT, Marshall JC. Nosocomial infection in the surgical intensive care unit. Infect Dis Clin N Am. 1992;6:657–75.
30. Swank GM, Deitch EA. Role of the gut in multiple organ failure: bacterial translocation and permeability changes. World J Surg. 1996;20:411–7.
31. Carrico CJ, Maekins JL, Marshall JC, Fry D, Maier RV. Multiple-organ-failure syndrome. Arch Surg. 1986;121:196–208.
32. Marshall JC, Christou NV, Meakins JL. The gastrointestinal tract: the "undrained abscess" of multiple organ failure. Ann Surg. 1993;218:111.
33. Minard G, Kudsk KA. Is early feeding beneficial? New Horiz. 1994;2:156–63.

34. Kudsk KA, Li J, Renegar KB. Loss of upper respiratory tract immunity with parenteral feeding. Ann Surg. 1996;223:629–35.
35. Sartelli M, Chichom-Mefire A, Labricciosa FM, Hardcastle T, Abu-Zidan FM, Adesunkanmi AK, et al. The management of intra-abdominal infections from a global perspective: 2017 WSES guidelines for management of intra-abdominal infections. World J Emerg Surg. 2017;12:29.
36. Moore FA, Feliciano DV, Andrassy RJ, McArdle AH, Booth FV, Morgenstein-Wagner TB, Kellum JM, Welling RE, Moore EE. Early enteral feeding, compared with parenteral, reduces postoperative septic complications. The results of a meta-analysis. Ann Surg. 1992;216:172–83.
37. Sautner T, Götzinger P, Redl-Wenzl EM, Dittrich K, Felfernig M, Sporn P, Roth E, Függer R. Does reoperation for abdominal sepsis enhance the inflammatory host response? Arch Surg. 1997;123:250–5.

The Challenge of Postoperative Peritonitis Due to Anastomotic Leakage

13

J. J. M. Claessen, F. F. van den Berg, and M. A. Boermeester

Anastomotic leakage is a common cause for postoperative peritonitis and associated with high mortality and morbidity. Management of secondary peritonitis remains challenging and requires a multidisciplinary approach, adequate ICU support and 24/7 decision-making. Contrast-enhanced CT imaging is required before relaparotomy. Current evidence points towards on-demand strategy as the preferable strategy for ongoing or recurrent peritonitis with primary abdominal closure following emergency surgery. Temporary closure techniques using mesh-mediated negative pressure treatment devices can be used to promote abdominal closure and prevent fistulas.

Intra-abdominal infection (IAI) is, after pneumonia, the most common cause of severe sepsis [1]. An IAI can be classified as uncomplicated IAI or as complicated IAI (cIAI) [2]. In an uncomplicated IAI, a single intra-abdominal organ is involved and the infection does not extend to the peritoneum. A cIAI proceeds beyond the affected intra-abdominal organ into the peritoneum, causing (localized or diffuse) peritonitis [3]. The term peritonitis describes infection of the abdominal cavity with the local response of the visceral peritoneum as well as the patient's reaction to bowel content containing free fluid, microorganisms and their toxins [4].

Peritonitis can be classified into primary, secondary or tertiary peritonitis [5]. Primary peritonitis is a diffuse spontaneous bacterial infection of the peritoneal cavity without loss of integrity of the gastrointestinal tract. This occurs mainly in cirrhotic patients with ascites, immunocompromised hosts or in patients with a peritoneal dialysis catheter. Secondary peritonitis, which is the most common type, describes acute peritoneal infections secondary to intra-abdominal lesions, such as perforation of the hollow viscus, anastomotic leakage (AL), bowel necrosis,

J. J. M. Claessen · F. F. van den Berg · M. A. Boermeester (✉)
Department of Surgery, Amsterdam UMC, University of Amsterdam,
Amsterdam, The Netherlands
e-mail: j.j.claessen@amsterdamumc.nl; f.f.vandenberg@amsterdamumc.nl;
m.a.boermeester@amsterdamumc.nl

© Springer Nature Switzerland AG 2021
M. Sartelli et al. (eds.), *Infections in Surgery*, Hot Topics in Acute Care Surgery
and Trauma, https://doi.org/10.1007/978-3-030-62116-2_13

143

non-bacterial peritonitis, or penetrating infectious processes. The incidence of secondary peritonitis is not entirely clear, but a global number of 19 million cases annually is estimated [6]. Tertiary peritonitis is a poorly defined entity, characterized by persistent or recurrent infections with organisms of low intrinsic virulence or with predisposition for the immunocompromised patient, usually after (successful and adequate) operative source control in the treatment of secondary peritonitis [3, 7]. In clinical practice, tertiary peritonitis is not a very useful term, and in essence simply the consequence of microbial selection and/or remnant infection after antibiotic treatment and surgery for secondary peritonitis.

Secondary peritonitis caused by a primary infection such as appendicitis or spontaneous perforation e.g. gastric ulcer perforation is termed 'community acquired', whereas secondary peritonitis as a complication of elective abdominal surgery such as iatrogenic perforation is termed 'hospital acquired' [8]. The term 'healthcare acquired' peritonitis is a relatively new term for infections acquired during the course of receiving healthcare. Not only hospital acquired infections are included, but also infections acquired in nursing institutions, having recent hospitalization within 90 days, aggressive medical therapies (intravenous therapy, wound dressing) or invasive therapies (haemodialysis, chemotherapy, radiotherapy) in outpatient departments within 30 days of the index infection [9]. The distinction is crucial with respect to underlying pathogens and related antibiotic treatment choice [8]. Patients with hospital acquired secondary peritonitis have higher mortality rates due to underlying comorbidities, atypical presentation and risk factors for multidrug-resistant microorganisms [10–15].

Postoperative peritonitis is by definition secondary peritonitis and hospital acquired. It occurs in 1–20% of patients undergoing laparotomy, depending on the type of surgery [16]. The most common cause of postoperative peritonitis is AL [17]. Other reasons are unintended injury of the gastrointestinal tract or intestinal ischemia [12].

13.1   Anastomotic Leakage

AL after gastrointestinal surgery is dreaded by all surgeons. Extensive research has been performed for AL after colon and rectal resections with reported incidences of 0.5–21% [18]. Frequencies of AL vary depending upon the tissue that is being anastomosed [19]. Low risk anastomoses comprise small bowel and right hemicolectomy anastomoses, whereas high risk anastomoses are seen after total gastrectomy, pancreatic and colorectal procedures. Table 13.1 shows ranges of incidences for different types of anastomosis that upon failure can cause (secondary) peritonitis [19–30]. Many definitions are being used for AL when reporting such results [18]. Bruce et al. have found 57 definitions in 97 studies in their systematic review and have formulated the following classification of AL [31].

- *Radiological leaks*: Leaks that are discovered only on routine imaging with none or minimal clinical signs and no specific intervention is required;

Table 13.1 Incidence of anastomotic leakage according to type or location

Location/type	Incidence (%)
Stomach	1–9
Small intestine	1–4
Ileocolic	2–6
Colon	3–5
Colorectal	3–13
Ileorectal	5–19
Pancreas	9–16
Bile ducts	10–16

- *Minor clinical leaks*: Leaks that are discovered due to clinical signs such as fever, leucocytosis, intestinal/faecal contents, amylase via drains or wounds. Some of these leaks do not require a specific intervention other than antibiotics and observation, whereas others will require radiological drainage or other forms of re-intervention, including eventual reoperation.
- *Major clinical leaks*: Major leaks having the same clinical signs as minor leaks, but with septic complications, and thus with severe disruption of the anastomosis which require intervention (usually reoperation) and are potentially life threatening with need of prompt treatment.

13.2   Risk Factors for Anastomotic Leakages

For the healing of an anastomosis, three basic requirements are needed for adequate healing; the anastomosis must be (i) tight, (ii) tension free and with (iii) a regular perfusion. Therefore, meticulous suturing or stapling, sufficient mobilization and careful preparation with special attention to the vascular supply are mandatory in avoiding AL [4]. The risk for a postoperative peritonitis from an AL depends on the surgical procedure performed, as well as other factors of which some are modifiable and others are beyond the control of the surgical team [4, 19]. Such risk factors include, but are not limited to, anastomotic tension, hypoxia, intraoperative or postoperative red blood cell transfusion, iron deficiency, ischemia, malnutrition, preoperative radiation therapy, prolonged duration of the operation, renal failure, shock, steroid therapy, cigarette smoking, zinc deficiency, alcohol abuse, anaemia, diabetes, obesity, vasopressor application, previous abdominal surgery and male gender [14, 19, 32–35].

13.3   Associated Microorganisms

Postoperative peritonitis is mainly linked to a polymicrobial infection of gram-negative, gram-positive, or anaerobes and candida (Table 13.2) [36]. Associated microorganisms depend on the location of the AL. *E. coli* and *Enterococcus* spp. are often the most prevalent of pathogens and are most often found irrespective of location of the leak in the gastrointestinal tract [37, 38]. When leakage occurs in the

Table 13.2 Microorganisms according to operative field

	Gastroduodenal	Biliary tract	Pancreas	Small intestine	Colon
Gram-positive					
Streptococcus spp.	++	–	—	—	—
Enterococcus spp.	—	++	—	—	++
Staphylococcus spp.	—	–	—	—	—
Gram-negative					
E. coli	++	++	++	++	++
Enterobacter spp.	—	–	—	—	—
Pseudomonas spp.	—	–	—	++	—
Klebsiella spp.	—	++	++	—	+
Proteus spp.	—	—	++	—	–
Anaerobes					
Bacteroides spp.	—	—	++	++	++
Clostridium spp.	—	—	–	—	++
Candida	+	–	–	–	–
Anaerobic cocci	—	—	–	—	+

Adapted from ref. [4]

++ most common, + common, – mostly not present, — rarely present

upper gastrointestinal tract (i.e. stomach or duodenum), the bacterial contamination mostly consists of *Streptococcus* spp., *E. coli* and *Candida* spp. followed by non-*E. coli* enterobacteriaceae which also found often in the small intestine. In the colon and rectum, *E. coli* and anaerobes are most frequent [37–39].

13.4 Diagnosis

Early intervention improves outcome in surgical patients with abdominal sepsis [40]. Early detection is therefore important. This remains, however, a challenge for healthcare providers, particularly after major surgery when signs and symptoms of sepsis can be unspecific and often missed on the ward [12, 41, 42]. During the early postoperative period sepsis can be difficult to distinguish from a normal postoperative inflammatory response to the surgical procedure [35]. Furthermore, clinical signs upon physical examination occur less often in postoperative (hospital acquired) peritonitis compared to community acquired secondary peritonitis of visceral perforation origin [43]. Such atypical clinical presentation may therefore be responsible for delay in diagnosis and intervention [35].

Clinical signs such as abdominal pain, distension, rigidity, fever, rebound tenderness, tachycardia, tachypnea and sudden clinical impairment are suspicious for postoperative peritonitis [3, 4, 12]. Inflammation may result in paralytic ileus resulting in nausea, obstipation and vomiting [14]. Abnormal vital signs may also be seen during an uncomplicated postoperative course. In a study of 452 patients with an uncomplicated postoperative course after bowel resection with anastomosis, 58% have experienced tachycardia, 57% tachypnea, 35% hypotension and 9% a fever on day 6 after surgery [44]. Although such findings occur more frequently in patients with AL, predictive value of these vital signs seems to be modest and insufficiently accurate. Pain relief by opiate analgesia does not alter diagnostic accuracy of bed-side physical examination or operative decision making [45–47].

Laboratory inflammatory parameters can assist in the postoperative diagnostic process, but have low positive predictive value (PPV) in itself for postoperative peritonitis [35]. With respect to AL such biomarkers have been shown to be non-specific. Several systematic reviews show that C-reactive protein (CRP) is significantly elevated in the days before AL diagnosis and has a negative predictive value (NPV) of up to 99% after colorectal surgery [48, 49]. Infectious complications after major abdominal surgery are very unlikely with a CRP level under 159 mg/L on postoperative day 3 [50]. The PPV of postoperative CRP is however modest. Therefore, the clinical value of CRP is as a negative (rule out) test. A low postoperative CRP level (day 3–5) can predict which patients are unlikely to have an AL and subsequent postoperative peritonitis [48].

Although white blood cell count (WBC) have been extensively studied in diagnosing specific intra-abdominal pathologies, much less is known about the capability of WBC to diagnose secondary peritonitis or to serve as a predictor of the need for immediate surgery [17]. About 1 in 5 uncomplicated patients have a leukocytosis (or leukopenia) on postoperative day 6 after bowel resection with anastomosis [44]. Others studies have found WBC to be a weak diagnostic marker of AL after colorectal surgery [49, 51, 52].

Procalcitonin (PCT) is also a useful negative predictor of AL following elective colorectal surgery, but not useful in demonstrating AL [53] Interleukin (IL)-6 is promising to rule out postoperative complications, having a NPV of 84% for on the first postoperative day [54]. However, a wide range of cut-off values have been used, therefore its role remains uncertain [3]. Also patients who do not develop an AL may exhibit a systemic inflammatory response with elevated inflammatory bio-marker levels, which in that case may be due to other factors such as the severity of surgical trauma, blood loss and duration of operation and depend on the infectious agent, the extent of inflammation, the disease entity, and the host immune status [55]. Nevertheless, CRP and PCT tend to normalize after few days. Therefore, prolonged increased levels of CRP or PCT should trigger further imaging to evaluate the presence of AL [56]. Conversely, low levels can select patients for safe and early discharge [50].

After recent abdominal surgery, changes of content and quantity of fluid production from an abdominal drain may be indicative for postoperative peritonitis, but normal drain contents do not exclude its presence. The level of bile, amylase or lipase in abdominal drain fluid could be helpful, specifically when distinctly elevated [4].

Once postoperative peritonitis is suspected based on vital signs, physical examination and laboratory tests, the most informative diagnostic modality is an abdominal computed tomography (CT) scan with intravenous contrast [57]. CT imaging with oral and intravenous contrast is superior to ultrasound with a sensitivity of 97.2% versus 44.3% in detecting the presence and source of postoperative peritonitis [43]. In a series of patients with early postoperative intra-abdominal sepsis after elective abdominal surgery a PPV of 71% is found for CT, resulting in quite a number of false positives, but a sensitivity of 88% and NPV of 85%, which is acceptable [58]. As mentioned previously, when AL is detected early, postoperative peritonitis can be prevented. In addition to intravenous contrast, oral contrast medium (OCM) is mostly used for more proximal anastomoses, whereas (added) rectal contrast in more distal (low colonic and rectal) anastomoses [59]. Most studies using CT scanning for detecting AL after colorectal surgery show a sensitivity and PPV around 70% and a specificity and NPV of around 90% [60, 61]. Contrast extravasation on CT is found to be the only independent predictor of diagnosing AL in colorectal surgery, and more accurate than free air [62, 63]. A CT with oral contrast only has a lower sensitivity of 60% and a lower NPV of 70% for a more proximal [59]. Enteral contrast in addition to intravenous contrast in CT improves sensitivity from 65% to 74% for anastomoses below Treitz ligament, when the contrast medium reaches the anastomosis [64]. Contrast extravasation after administration of rectal contrast enema (RCE) for rectal resections (distal anastomoses) increases sensitivity up to 90% [60, 63]. Although most studies are heterogenic and consist of small numbers, it seems that using contrast medium (orally or rectally) reduces the number of false negatives [64]. It is important, however, that the contrast medium reaches the anastomosis. Distal anastomoses are generally better reached by RCE than OCM.

However, postoperative CT has a considerable proportion of false negatives (1-sensitivity) which can lead to increased mortality related to delayed reoperation [65]. This means that in a critically ill patient, in particular with progressive organ failure, reoperation may be needed even if CT findings are negative [12].

13.5 Management

13.5.1 Initial Treatment

The cornerstones of management of secondary peritonitis due to AL are adequate source control, aggressive fluid resuscitation, organ support and broad-spectrum antibiotics [17]. Delay of diagnosis and intervention are associated with adverse outcomes [43]. Initial management is mostly dictated by an intra- or extra-peritoneal location of the leaking anastomosis and the severity of peritonitis (for flowchart see Fig. 13.1).

Goal-directed, aggressive fluid resuscitation should be given as soon as possible. There is still debate whether patients need to be partially or fully resuscitated before they are taken to the operating theatre [66, 67]. Broad-spectrum antibiotics with coverage of gram-positive, gram-negative and anaerobic bacteria are given within one hour. Decisions on the choice and duration of antibiotic treatment should be made according to local antimicrobial guidelines and in close contact with a microbiologist [68]. Infections with multidrug-resistant bacteria are on the rise and provide an additional challenge in the treatment of secondary peritonitis. Recently, new (combinations of) antibiotics have become available, but these should preferably be used as last-resort choice [69]. Addition of an antifungal is recommended for high

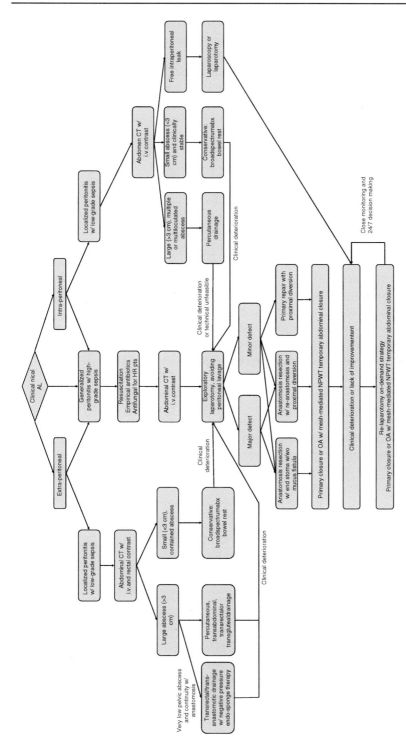

Fig. 13.1 Flowchart management of anastomotic leakage. AL anastomotic leakage, CT computer tomography, HR high risk, abx antibiotics, OA open abdomen, NPWT negative pressure wound therapy

risk patients [68], in particular in upper gastrointestinal source of peritonitis or prolonged hospitalization before current sepsis episode.

CT imaging is required for all patients that present with localized or generalized peritonitis, and for patients with signs of sepsis or septic shock preferably within the first hour after presentation. Patients with a free intraperitoneal leak need emergency surgery with end stoma or diverting stoma. A small abbess (smaller than 3 cm) in clinically stable patients can be managed conservatively with antibiotics and bowel rest. Large, or multi-located and multiple intraperitoneal abscesses require percutaneous drainage if technically feasible. For large extra-peritoneal abscesses, percutaneous transabdominal, transrectal or transgluteal drainage is done. Abscesses in the lower pelvis that are in continuity with a colorectal anastomosis can be drained trans-anal or trans-anastomotic under general anaesthesia and treated with regular endo sponge changes and delayed trans-anal surgical closure of the anastomotic leak. When patients with conservative treatment or drainage show signs of clinical deteriorate or failure to improve, an exploratory emergency reoperation is performed to achieve adequate source control, with or without a repeat CT.

The available options for surgical source control during emergency laparotomy largely depends upon the size of the defects and clinical status of the patients [70]. The safest option for major defects is resection of the anastomosis with an end stoma (e.g. Hartmann's procedure), however this increases morbidity associated with future stoma reversal. Alternatively, a re-anastomosis with a proximal diversion enterostomy can be done, but is by enlarge reserved for hemodynamically stable patients. For minor defects in hemodynamically stable patients, a primary repair with proximal diversion can be considered, however this increases the chance of inadequate source control. For a colonic anastomosis downstream washout is an option when choosing for primary repair and proximal diversion. A primary repair without proximal diversion is strongly discouraged. The use of routine and extensive peritoneal lavage remains controversial, but should be discouraged as it can promote inflammatory responses and multi-organ failure [68]. Generally, careful suction of infected peritoneal fluids during emergency laparotomy suffices. For Hinchey III complicated diverticulitis, however, laparoscopic peritoneal lavage is an effective treatment option, accepting that some patients need a delayed sigmoid resection, but overall lower stoma rates are reported [71, 72].

13.5.2 Post Emergency Surgery Treatment

For abdominal sepsis that progresses or fails to improve after emergency laparotomy, there is a need for relaparotomy, based on the "on-demand" relaparotomy strategy. Aggressive surgical approached such as radical peritoneal debridement and open abdomen treatment are associated with higher morbidity and mortality and should be abandoned [73–75]. Planned relaparotomy, where laparotomy is performed every 2 to 3 days until no intraperitoneal infection is observed, has lost popularity during the last decade. One RCT has compared planned relaparotomy with on-demand relaparotomy in patients with severe abdominal sepsis, and shows no significant difference in mortality and morbidity. However, using an on-demand strategy, a clear decrease in the number of laparotomies is seen as two-thirds of patients recovered without relaparotomy in the on-demand group, as well as shorter ICU stay and lower health care costs [76]. A strategy still popular is damage control surgery, adopted from trauma care where staged laparotomies with open abdomen are performed with the goal of treating immediate life-threatening causes, and delay of reconstructive surgery [77]. However, there is a lack of convincing evidence that damage control surgery is beneficial in non-trauma setting such as secondary peritonitis, and is therefore not preferable over on-demand treatment [8, 77]. On-demand treatment is a safe strategy and surgeons should strive for primary closure of the abdomen whenever possible. Primary open abdomen increases mortality [78]. When primary closure is not possible due to edema, the use of a temporary abdominal closure technique is recommended. A recent meta-analysis indicates that continuous mesh-mediated fascial traction with negative pressure therapy has the best results in terms of delayed closures and fistula rates [79]. Some fear abdominal compartment syndrome with progressive closure strategies, however with adequate ICU support and fluid management this is infrequently seen.

The decision to perform a relaparotomy remains difficult, since traditional scoring systems are inadequate for the prediction of ongoing peritonitis [80]. A recently developed and validated decision tool for ongoing abdominal sepsis may advise the surgeon on when to perform CT imaging in a patient who deteriorates or fails to progress [81, 82]. Furthermore, care should be provided by a multidisciplinary team with 24/7 decision making. Critically ill patients are admitted to an ICU facility with adequate set-up for complex patients (high-level ICU).

13.6   Outcome

Secondary peritonitis followed with sepsis is associated with a mortality of approximately 30%. This can be complicated by septic shock with accompanied organ failure, which increases mortality rates of up to 68% [12, 83]. Furthermore, secondary peritonitis has high morbidity rates and is associated with long-term hospital and intensive care admission [84]. Several prediction models have been validated for mortality and morbidity in peritonitis. These include general prediction models such as the Acute Physiology and Chronic Health Evaluation (APACHE-II) that predicts ICU mortality, Simplified Acute Physiology Score (SAPS), the Multiple organ dysfunction score (MODS), and the Sepsis-related Organ Failure Assessment (SOFA) [85, 86]. The Mannheim peritonitis index and Physiological and Operative Severity Score for the enumeration of Mortality and Morbidity (POSSUM) were specifically developed for operative risk assessment [87, 88]. However, it is unclear what is the preferable clinical scoring systems for the prediction of mortality and morbidity. The APACHE-II score is the most accurate outcome predictor in patients undergoing emergency laparotomy, both pre- and postoperative [89]. A recent prognostic model comprising the SOFA score and four other variables (age, lowest body temperature, highest heart rate and haematocrit) performs better than the SOFA and

APACHE-II in postoperative critically ill patients with faecal peritonitis [90]. Morbidity due to complications of secondary peritonitis after anastomotic leakage are common. These include incisional hernia, enterocutaneous fistula, recurrence of infection and/or abscesses, and stoma-associated morbidity. Also, quality of life is significantly worse compared to the general population.

References

1. Angus DC, van der Poll T. Severe sepsis and septic shock. N Engl J Med. 2013;369(21):2063.
2. Menichetti F, Sganga G. Definition and classification of intra-abdominal infections. J Chemother. 2009;21(Suppl 1):3–4.
3. Sartelli M, Chichom-Mefire A, Labricciosa FM, Hardcastle T, Abu-Zidan FM, Adesunkanmi AK, et al. The management of intra-abdominal infections from a global perspective: 2017 WSES guidelines for management of intra-abdominal infections. World J Emer Surg. 2017;12:29.
4. Herzog T, Uhl W. Postoperative peritonitis: etiology, diagnosis, and treatment. In: Sartelli M, Bassetti M, Martin-Loeches I, editors. Abdominal sepsis; 2018. p. 179–200.
5. Holzheimer RG. Management of secondary peritonitis. In: Holzheimer RG, Mannick JA, editors. Surgical treatment: evidence-based and problem-oriented. Munich: Zuckschwerdt W. Zuckschwerdt Verlag GmbH; 2001.
6. Adhikari NK, Fowler RA, Bhagwanjee S, Rubenfeld GD. Critical care and the global burden of critical illness in adults. Lancet. 2010;376(9749):1339–46.
7. Holzheimer RG, Muhrer KH, L'Allemand N, Schmidt T, Henneking K. Intraabdominal infections: classification, mortality, scoring and pathophysiology. Infection. 1991;19(6):447–52.
8. Boldingh QJ, de Vries FE, Boermeester MA. Abdominal sepsis. Curr Opin Crit Care. 2017;23(2):159–66.
9. Cardoso T, Almeida M, Friedman ND, Aragao I, Costa-Pereira A, Sarmento AE, et al. Classification of healthcare-associated infection: a systematic review 10 years after the first proposal. BMC Med. 2014;12:40.
10. Anaya DA, Nathens AB. Risk factors for severe sepsis in secondary peritonitis. Surg Infect. 2003;4(4):355–62.
11. Augustin P, Kermarrec N, Muller-Serieys C, Lasocki S, Chosidow D, Marmuse JP, et al. Risk factors for multidrug resistant bacteria and optimization of empirical antibiotic therapy in postoperative peritonitis. Crit Care. 2010;14(1):R20.
12. Hecker A, Uhle F, Schwandner T, Padberg W, Weigand MA. Diagnostics, therapy and outcome prediction in abdominal sepsis: current standards and future perspectives. Langenbeck's Arch Surg. 2014;399(1):11–22.
13. Lee DS, Ryu JA, Chung CR, Yang J, Jeon K, Suh GY, et al. Risk factors for acquisition of multidrug-resistant bacteria in patients with anastomotic leakage after colorectal cancer surgery. Int J Color Dis. 2015;30(4):497–504.
14. Pieracci FM, Barie PS. Management of severe sepsis of abdominal origin. Scand J Surg. 2007;96(3):184–96.
15. Seguin P, Fedun Y, Laviolle B, Nesseler N, Donnio PY, Malledant Y. Risk factors for multidrug-resistant bacteria in patients with post-operative peritonitis requiring intensive care. J Antimicrob Chemother. 2010;65(2):342–6.
16. Ordonez CA, Puyana JC. Management of peritonitis in the critically ill patient. Surg Clin North Am. 2006;86(6):1323–49.
17. Ross JT, Matthay MA, Harris HW. Secondary peritonitis: principles of diagnosis and intervention. BMJ. 2018;361:k1407.

18. Trencheva K, Morrissey KP, Wells M, Mancuso CA, Lee SW, Sonoda T, et al. Identifying important predictors for anastomotic leak after colon and rectal resection: prospective study on 616 patients. Ann Surg. 2013;257(1):108–13.
19. Phillips BR. Reducing gastrointestinal anastomotic leak rates: review of challenges and solutions. Open Access Surg. 2016;9:5–14.
20. Buchs NC, Gervaz P, Secic M, Bucher P, Mugnier-Konrad B, Morel P. Incidence, consequences, and risk factors for anastomotic dehiscence after colorectal surgery: a prospective monocentric study. Int J Color Dis. 2008;23(3):265–70.
21. Cong ZJ, Hu LH, Bian ZQ, Ye GY, Yu MH, Gao YH, et al. Systematic review of anastomotic leakage rate according to an international grading system following anterior resection for rectal cancer. PLoS One. 2013;8(9):e75519.
22. Damen N, Spilsbury K, Levitt M, Makin G, Salama P, Tan P, et al. Anastomotic leaks in colorectal surgery. ANZ J Surg. 2014;84(10):763–8.
23. Elton C, Makin G, Hitos K, Cohen CR. Mortality, morbidity and functional outcome after ileorectal anastomosis. Br J Surg. 2003;90(1):59–65.
24. Francone TD, Champagne B. Considerations and complications in patients undergoing ileal pouch anal anastomosis. Surg Clin North Am. 2013;93(1):107–43.
25. Gagner M, Kemmeter P. Comparison of laparoscopic sleeve gastrectomy leak rates in five staple-line reinforcement options: a systematic review. Surg Endosc. 2019;34:396–407.
26. Hyman N, Manchester TL, Osler T, Burns B, Cataldo PA. Anastomotic leaks after intestinal anastomosis: it's later than you think. Ann Surg. 2007;245(2):254–8.
27. Lee S, Carmody B, Wolfe L, Demaria E, Kellum JM, Sugerman H, et al. Effect of location and speed of diagnosis on anastomotic leak outcomes in 3828 gastric bypass cases. J Gastrointest Surg. 2007;11(6):708–13.
28. Lehmann RK, Brounts LR, Johnson EK, Rizzo JA, Steele SR. Does sacrifice of the inferior mesenteric artery or superior rectal artery affect anastomotic leak following sigmoidectomy for diverticulitis? A retrospective review. Am J Surg. 2011;201(5):623–7.
29. Leichtle SW, Mouawad NJ, Welch KB, Lampman RM, Cleary RK. Risk factors for anastomotic leakage after colectomy. Dis Colon Rectum. 2012;55(5):569–75.
30. Turrentine FE, Denlinger CE, Simpson VB, Garwood RA, Guerlain S, Agrawal A, et al. Morbidity, mortality, cost, and survival estimates of gastrointestinal anastomotic leaks. J Am Coll Surg. 2015;220(2):195–206.
31. Bruce J, Krukowski ZH, Al-Khairy G, Russell EM, Park KG. Systematic review of the definition and measurement of anastomotic leak after gastrointestinal surgery. Br J Surg. 2001;88(9):1157–68.
32. Fischer PE, Nunn AM, Wormer BA, Christmas AB, Gibeault LA, Green JM, et al. Vasopressor use after initial damage control laparotomy increases risk for anastomotic disruption in the management of destructive colon injuries. Am J Surg. 2013;206(6):900–3.
33. Lipska MA, Bissett IP, Parry BR, Merrie AE. Anastomotic leakage after lower gastrointestinal anastomosis: men are at a higher risk. ANZ J Surg. 2006;76(7):579–85.
34. Ruggiero R, Sparavigna L, Docimo G, Gubitosi A, Agresti M, Procaccini E, et al. Postoperative peritonitis due to anastomotic dehiscence after colonic resection. Multicentric experience, retrospective analysis of risk factors and review of the literature. Ann Ital Chir. 2011;82(5):369–75.
35. Sartelli M, Griffiths EA, Nestori M. The challenge of post-operative peritonitis after gastrointestinal surgery. Updat Surg. 2015;67(4):373–81.
36. Muresan MG, Balmos IA, Badea I, Santini A. Abdominal Sepsis: An Update. J Crit Care Med (Targu Mures). 2018;4(4):120–5.
37. Herzog T, Chromik AM, Uhl W. Treatment of complicated intra-abdominal infections in the era of multi-drug resistant bacteria. Eur J Med Res. 2010;15(12):525–32.
38. Steinbach CL, Topper C, Adam T, Kees MG. Spectrum adequacy of antibiotic regimens for secondary peritonitis: a retrospective analysis in intermediate and intensive care unit patients. Ann Clin Microbiol Antimicrob. 2015;14:48.

39. Wong PF, Gilliam AD, Kumar S, Shenfine J, O'Dair GN, Leaper DJ. Antibiotic regimens for secondary peritonitis of gastrointestinal origin in adults. Coch Data Sys Rev. 2005;2:Cd004539.
40. Moore LJ, Moore FA, Jones SL, Xu J, Bass BL. Sepsis in general surgery: a deadly complication. Am J Surg. 2009;198(6):868–74.
41. Poeze M, Ramsay G, Gerlach H, Rubulotta F, Levy M. An international sepsis survey: a study of doctors' knowledge and perception about sepsis. Crit Care. 2004;8(6):R409–13.
42. Robson W, Beavis S, Spittle N. An audit of ward nurses' knowledge of sepsis. Nurs Crit Care. 2007;12(2):86–92.
43. Bader FG, Schroder M, Kujath P, Muhl E, Bruch HP, Eckmann C. Diffuse postoperative peritonitis—value of diagnostic parameters and impact of early indication for relaparotomy. Eur J Med Res. 2009;14(11):491–6.
44. Erb L, Hyman NH, Osler T. Abnormal vital signs are common after bowel resection and do not predict anastomotic leak. J Am Coll Surg. 2014;218(6):1195–9.
45. Attard AR, Corlett MJ, Kidner NJ, Leslie AP, Fraser IA. Safety of early pain relief for acute abdominal pain. BMJ. 1992;305(6853):554–6.
46. Falch C, Vicente D, Haberle H, Kirschniak A, Muller S, Nissan A, et al. Treatment of acute abdominal pain in the emergency room: a systematic review of the literature. Eur J Pain. 2014;18(7):902–13.
47. Vermeulen B, Morabia A, Unger PF, Goehring C, Grangier C, Skljarov I, et al. Acute appendicitis: influence of early pain relief on the accuracy of clinical and US findings in the decision to operate—a randomized trial. Radiology. 1999;210(3):639–43.
48. Singh PP, Zeng IS, Srinivasa S, Lemanu DP, Connolly AB, Hill AG. Systematic review and meta-analysis of use of serum C-reactive protein levels to predict anastomotic leak after colorectal surgery. Br J Surg. 2014;101(4):339–46.
49. Su'a BU, Mikaere HL, Rahiri JL, Bissett IB, Hill AG. Systematic review of the role of biomarkers in diagnosing anastomotic leakage following colorectal surgery. Br J Surg. 2017;104(5):503–12.
50. Gans SL, Atema JJ, van Dieren S, Groot Koerkamp B, Boermeester MA. Diagnostic value of C-reactive protein to rule out infectious complications after major abdominal surgery: a systematic review and meta-analysis. Int J Color Dis. 2015;30(7):861–73.
51. Pedersen T, Roikjaer O, Jess P. Increased levels of C-reactive protein and leukocyte count are poor predictors of anastomotic leakage following laparoscopic colorectal resection. Dan Med J. 2012;59(12):A4552.
52. Ge W, Chen G. The value of biomarkers in early diagnosis of anastomotic leak following colorectal tumor resection: a review of the literature between 2012 and 2017. Oncotarget. 2015; https://doi.org/10.18632/oncotarget.23604.
53. Su'a B, Tutone S, MacFater W, Barazanchi A, Xia W, Zeng I, et al. Diagnostic accuracy of procalcitonin for the early diagnosis of anastomotic leakage after colorectal surgery: a meta-analysis. ANZ J Surg. 2019;90:675–80.
54. Rettig TC, Verwijmeren L, Dijkstra IM, Boerma D, van de Garde EM, Noordzij PG. Postoperative interleukin-6 level and early detection of complications after elective major abdominal surgery. Ann Surg. 2016;263(6):1207–12.
55. Welsch T, Frommhold K, Hinz U, Weigand MA, Kleeff J, Friess H, et al. Persisting elevation of C-reactive protein after pancreatic resections can indicate developing inflammatory complications. Surgery. 2008;143(1):20–8.
56. Garcia-Granero A, Frasson M, Flor-Lorente B, Blanco F, Puga R, Carratala A, et al. Procalcitonin and C-reactive protein as early predictors of anastomotic leak in colorectal surgery: a prospective observational study. Dis Colon Rectum. 2013;56(4):475–83.
57. Just KS, Defosse JM, Grensemann J, Wappler F, Sakka SG. Computed tomography for the identification of a potential infectious source in critically ill surgical patients. J Crit Care. 2015;30(2):386–9.
58. Go HL, Baarslag HJ, Vermeulen H, Lameris JS, Legemate DA. A comparative study to validate the use of ultrasonography and computed tomography in patients with post-operative intra-abdominal sepsis. Eur J Radiol. 2005;54(3):383–7.

59. Kornmann VN, van Ramshorst B, Smits AB, Bollen TL, Boerma D. Beware of false-negative CT scan for anastomotic leakage after colonic surgery. Int J Color Dis. 2014;29(4):445–51.
60. Kornmann VN, Treskes N, Hoonhout LH, Bollen TL, van Ramshorst B, Boerma D. Systematic review on the value of CT scanning in the diagnosis of anastomotic leakage after colorectal surgery. Int J Color Dis. 2013;28(4):437–45.
61. Marres CCM, van de Ven AWH, Leijssen LGJ, Verbeek PCM, Bemelman WA, Buskens CJ. Colorectal anastomotic leak: delay in reintervention after false-negative computed tomography scan is a reason for concern. Tech Coloproctol. 2017;21(9):709–14.
62. Huiberts AA, Dijksman LM, Boer SA, Krul EJ, Peringa J, Donkervoort SC. Contrast medium at the site of the anastomosis is crucial in detecting anastomotic leakage with CT imaging after colorectal surgery. Int J Color Dis. 2015;30(6):843–8.
63. Kauv P, Benadjaoud S, Curis E, Boulay-Coletta I, Loriau J, Zins M. Anastomotic leakage after colorectal surgery: diagnostic accuracy of CT. Eur Radiol. 2015;25(12):3543–51.
64. Samji KB, Kielar AZ, Connolly M, Fasih N, Doherty G, Chung A, et al. Anastomotic leaks after small- and large-bowel surgery: diagnostic performance of CT and the importance of intraluminal contrast administration. AJR Am J Roentgenol. 2018;210(6):1259–65.
65. Tamini N, Cassini D, Giani A, Angrisani M, Famularo S, Oldani M, et al. Computed tomography in suspected anastomotic leakage after colorectal surgery: evaluating mortality rates after false-negative imaging. Eur J Trauma Emerg Surg. 2019; https://doi.org/10.1007/s00068-019-01083-8.
66. Rhodes A, Evans LE, Alhazzani W, Levy MM, Antonelli M, Ferrer R, et al. Surviving sepsis campaign: international guidelines for management of sepsis and septic shock: 2016. Crit Care Med. 2017;45(3):486–552.
67. Solomkin JS, Mazuski JE, Bradley JS, Rodvold KA, Goldstein EJ, Baron EJ, et al. Diagnosis and management of complicated intra-abdominal infection in adults and children: guidelines by the Surgical Infection Society and the Infectious Diseases Society of America. Surg Infect. 2010;11(1):79–109.
68. van Ruler O, Boermeester MA. Surgical treatment of secondary peritonitis: a continuing problem. Der Chirurg; Zeitsch Geb Oper Med. 2017;88(Suppl 1):1–6.
69. Durand CR, Alsharhan M, Willett KC. New and emerging antibiotics for complicated intra-abdominal infections. Am J Ther. 2017;24(6):e763–e9.
70. Phitayakorn R, Delaney CP, Reynolds HL, Champagne BJ, Heriot AG, Neary P, et al. Standardized algorithms for management of anastomotic leaks and related abdominal and pelvic abscesses after colorectal surgery. World J Surg. 2008;32(6):1147–56.
71. Vennix S, Musters GD, Mulder IM, Swank HA, Consten EC, Belgers EH, et al. Laparoscopic peritoneal lavage or sigmoidectomy for perforated diverticulitis with purulent peritonitis: a multicentre, parallel-group, randomised, open-label trial. Lancet. 2015;386(10000):1269–77.
72. Pan Z, Pan ZH, Pan RZ, Xie YX, Desai G. Is laparoscopic lavage safe in purulent diverticulitis versus colonic resection? A systematic review and meta-analysis. Int J Surg. 2019;71:182–9.
73. Polk HC Jr, Fry DE. Radical peritoneal debridement for established peritonitis. The results of a prospective randomized clinical trial. Ann Surg. 1980;192(3):350–5.
74. Robledo FA, Luque-de-Leon E, Suarez R, Sanchez P, de-la-Fuente M, Vargas A, et al. Open versus closed management of the abdomen in the surgical treatment of severe secondary peritonitis: a randomized clinical trial. Surg Infect. 2007;8(1):63–72.
75. Kao AM, Cetrulo LN, Baimas-George MR, Prasad T, Heniford BT, Davis BR, et al. Outcomes of open abdomen versus primary closure following emergent laparotomy for suspected secondary peritonitis: a propensity-matched analysis. J Trau Acut Care Surg. 2019;87(3):623–9.
76. van Ruler O, Mahler CW, Boer KR, Reuland EA, Gooszen HG, Opmeer BC, et al. Comparison of on-demand vs planned relaparotomy strategy in patients with severe peritonitis: a randomized trial. J Am Med Assoc. 2007;298(8):865–72.
77. Weber DG, Bendinelli C, Balogh ZJ. Damage control surgery for abdominal emergencies. Br J Surg. 2014;101(1):e109–18.

78. Chen Y, Ye J, Song W, Chen J, Yuan Y, Ren J. Comparison of outcomes between early fascial closure and delayed abdominal closure in patients with open abdomen: a systematic review and meta-analysis. Gastroenterol Res Pract. 2014;2014:784056.

79. Atema JJ, Gans SL, Boermeester MA. Systematic review and meta-analysis of the open abdomen and temporary abdominal closure techniques in non-trauma patients. World J Surg. 2015;39(4):912–25.

80. van Ruler O, Kiewiet JJ, Boer KR, Lamme B, Gouma DJ, Boermeester MA, et al. Failure of available scoring systems to predict ongoing infection in patients with abdominal sepsis after their initial emergency laparotomy. BMC Surg. 2011;11:38.

81. Atema JJ, Ram K, Schultz MJ, Boermeester MA. External validation of a decision tool to guide post-operative management of patients with secondary peritonitis. Surg Infect. 2017;18(2):189–95.

82. Kiewiet JJ, van Ruler O, Boermeester MA, Reitsma JB. A decision rule to aid selection of patients with abdominal sepsis requiring a relaparotomy. BMC Surg. 2013;13:28.

83. Sartelli M, Abu-Zidan FM, Catena F, Griffiths EA, Di Saverio S, Coimbra R, et al. Global validation of the WSES Sepsis Severity Score for patients with complicated intra-abdominal infections: a prospective multicentre study (WISS Study). World J Emer Surg. 2015;10:61.

84. Kiewiet J, van Ruler O, Reitsma J, Boermeester M. Treatment of secondary peritonitis: slow progress. Ned Tijdschr Geneeskd. 2009;153:A386.

85. Legall JR, Lemeshow S, Saulnier F. A new simplified acute physiology score (Saps-Ii) based on a European North-American Multicenter Study. J Am Med Assoc. 1993;270(24):2957–63.

86. Knaus WA, Draper EA, Wagner DP, Zimmerman JE. APACHE II: a severity of disease classification system. Crit Care Med. 1985;13(10):818–29.

87. Linder MM, Wacha H, Feldmann U, Wesch G, Streifensand RA, Gundlach E. The Mannheim Peritonitis Index—an instrument for the intraoperative prognosis of peritonitis. Der Chirurg; Zeitsch Geb Oper Med. 1987;58(2):84–92.

88. Copeland GP, Jones D, Walters M. POSSUM: a scoring system for surgical audit. Br J Surg. 1991;78(3):355–60.

89. Oliver CM, Walker E, Giannaris S, Grocott MP, Moonesinghe SR. Risk assessment tools validated for patients undergoing emergency laparotomy: a systematic review. Br J Anaesth. 2015;115(6):849–60.

90. Tridente A, Bion J, Mills GH, Gordon AC, Clarke GM, Walden A, et al. Derivation and validation of a prognostic model for postoperative risk stratification of critically ill patients with faecal peritonitis. Ann Intensive Care. 2017;7(1):96.

Management of Necrotizing Fasciitis 14

Saleh Abdel-Kader, Massimo Sartelli,
and Fikri M. Abu-Zidan

14.1 Introduction

Necrotizing fasciitis is an infection of the soft tissue which starts in the superficial fascia and progresses rapidly into the deep facia resulting in occlusion of the small blood vessels that supply the overlying skin. Eventually skin necrosis will occur [1].

It may have serious effects when progresses to necrosis that initiates a systemic inflammatory response syndrome (SIRS) and septic shock [2]. The main diagnostic dilemma is distinguishing superficial from deep soft-tissue infection, the latter is more serious. Delaying the diagnosis is associated with an increased mortality rate [3]. Therefore, any spreading infection in one of the layers of the soft tissue (skin, subcutaneous tissue, superficial fascia, deep fascia and muscles) which is associated with necrosis of these layers should be considered a necrotizing fasciitis and hence requires an urgent surgical debridement [4, 5].

14.2 Epidemiology

Approximately 500 cases of necrotizing fasciitis are diagnosed every year in the United Kingdom (UK). Trauma was directly attributed to 26.1% of cases while 4.3% are related to surgical wounds [1]. The risk factors for necrotizing fasciitis

S. Abdel-Kader
Department of Surgery, NMC Specialty Hospital, Al Ain, United Arab Emirates and
Department of Surgery, Ain Shams University Hospital, Cairo, Egypt

M. Sartelli
Department of Surgery, Macerata Hospital, Macerata, Italy

F. M. Abu-Zidan (✉)
Department of Surgery, College of Medicine and Health Sciences, UAE University,
Al-Ain, UAE
e-mail: fabuzidan@uaeu.ac.ae

© Springer Nature Switzerland AG 2021
M. Sartelli et al. (eds.), *Infections in Surgery*, Hot Topics in Acute Care Surgery
and Trauma, https://doi.org/10.1007/978-3-030-62116-2_14

include diabetes mellitus, severe peripheral vascular disease, alcoholism, trauma, malignancy (particularly leukaemia and lymphoma), reduced immunity, organ transplantation, injection drug use and the use of non-steroidal anti-inflammatory drugs [6]. The mortality rate of necrotizing fasciitis is about 25%, however when sepsis occurs the mortality raises up to 80% of cases [6].

14.3   Classification

Necrotizing fasciitis is classified by the Society of Infectious Disease, into two groups depending on the infectious pathogen. Type I necrotizing fasciitis is caused by polymicrobial organisms (aerobic and anaerobic organisms) which commonly originates from the bowel flora. Type II necrotizing fasciitis is most commonly caused by group A *Streptococcus* (*Streptococcus pyogenes*), *Staphylococcus aureus*, *Vibrio vulnificus*, *Vibrio damsel*, *Aeromonas hydrophila* and anaerobic *Streptococci* [7]. Toxic shock syndrome, which is caused by release of exotoxins A, B and C, may occur following infection with *Staphylococcus aureus* [8].

14.4   Pathogenesis of Necrotizing Fasciitis

M-proteins of group A *Streptococci* produce collagenase and hyaluronidase enzymes which cause liquefactive necrosis of the fascia and fat [9]. This leads to the separation of the skin from the underlying tissues, thrombosis of the small blood vessels, tissue necrosis, decreased oxygen saturation and growth of anaerobics [10]. Diabetic microangiopathy may reduce the tissue oxygenation [1]. Synergism between aerobes and anaerobic infection releases heparinase, streptokinase and streptodornase enzymes which further destroy the tissues. The spread of infection along the fascial planes is attributed to the diminished phagocytic activity of the leucocytes in the necrotic tissue [11].

Diminished venous return from the overlying skin are caused initially by fat and fascial thrombophlebitis. With more necrosis and liquefaction, thrombosis occurs in the nutrient arteries that are passing through the involved fascia and skin. Finally, ischemia and compression of the cutaneous innervation eventually occurs [12].

14.5   Clinical Presentation

Early diagnosis of necrotizing fasciitis is challenging because of the rarity of the disease and because of the lack of early pathognomonic signs. Pain out of proportion to physical findings is the earliest symptom of necrotizing fasciitis which disappears with disease progression [6]. Fever exists in only 40% of patients. Absence of fever will not exclude the diagnosis of necrotizing fasciitis. It is not infrequent to misdiagnose the disease as cellulitis or abscess formation [13].

Skin manifestations may be minimal relative to systemic findings. Three levels of skin manifestations are recognized; stage I (early stage) presented by warmness, tenderness, erythema, swelling and indurated wooden skin; stage II (intermediate stage) presented by blisters and bullae and stage III (late stage) presented by haemorrhagic bullae, crepitus, skin anaesthesia and necrosis (Fig. 14.1) [7]. At the late stages, patients may have septicaemia [14].

On clinical examination, necrotizing fasciitis is different from simple soft-tissue infection. It has skin tenderness beyond the involved area, ill-defined skin margins, absence of lymphangitis and the patient's condition deteriorate despite the use of antibiotics [13].

Equivocal cases need repeated physical examination with pain scoring and marking the area of skin involvement. Late clinical signs include fever, hypotension, tachycardia, altered mental status and signs of organ dysfunction.

Necrotizing fasciitis may occur in a wide range of anatomical locations including the external genitalia and perineum (Fournier's gangrene) or the submandibular region. Fournier's gangrene is an extensive, rapidly progressive necrosis affecting

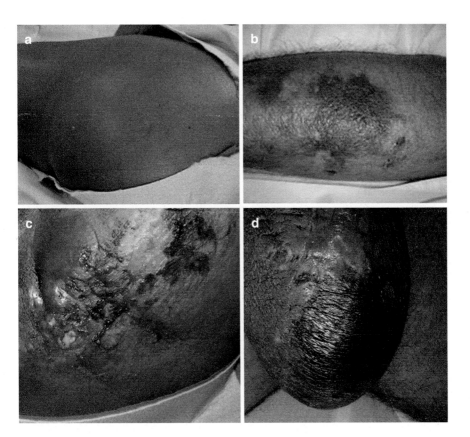

Fig. 14.1 The clinical picture of necrotizing fasciitis can be very deceiving. There may be unnoticeable skin changes (**a**), changes mimicking cellulitis (**b**), skin bullae that rupture (**c**), or skin necrosis (**d**) (Courtesy of Professor Fikri Abu-Zidan, College of Medicine and Health Sciences, UAE University, Al-Ain, UAE)

the fascia and perifascial planes of the external genitalia and perineum. It frequently extends to the abdominal wall, into the perirectal and gluteal spaces, and, occasionally, into the retroperitoneum. The early diagnosis of Fournier's gangrene depends on the clinical symptoms of genital discomfort and pruritus, which is followed by scrotal pain, genital oedema and erythema. If the condition is not treated adequately, it will progress to partial scrotal necrosis, induration, crepitation, feculent odour and fever.

Necrotizing fasciitis of the head and neck is rare because of their rich blood supply. It includes cranial, facial and/or cervical infection. The most common source of infection is odontogenic (47%), particularly the second and third lower molar teeth, because their roots are positioned below the mylohyoid line. Other sources of infection include pharyngitis, supraglotitis, tonsillitis, salivary gland infection, otitis media and mastoiditis. Malignancy and radiotherapy reduces the immunity and predisposes to necrotizing fasciitis. In 5% of the cases, no primary source can be identified.

14.6 Diagnosis

The diagnosis of necrotizing fasciitis is primarily clinical. There is no particular laboratory test for diagnosing necrotizing fasciitis. However, certain blood investigations may help differentiating necrotizing fasciitis form other soft-tissue infections, such as a white blood cell count of more than 14,000 cells per mm^3, a raised C-reactive protein exceeding 13 mg/dl, a serum sodium level less than 135 mEq per L, a blood urea nitrogen level greater than 15 mg per dL, and a creatinine kinase level over 700 units per L [1, 6, 15]. The most accurate diagnostic scoring system present is the Laboratory Risk Indicator for Necrotizing Fasciitis (LRINEC scoring system). It is a useful adjunct for the clinical diagnosis of necrotizing fasciitis. A score of ≥ 6 was 93% sensitive and 92% specific for diagnosing necrotizing fasciitis in Singapore but had 74% sensitivity and 81% specificity in a validation study done in the UK [13, 16].

In severely toxic patients, immediate surgical debridement has priority over radiological imaging. Plain radiographs, ultrasound, computed tomography (CT), and magnetic resonance imaging (MRI) can be used for diagnosing necrotizing fasciitis. In early stages of necrotizing fasciitis radiographic findings are nonspecific and similar to those of cellulitis. It includes soft-tissue opacity and thickness. In advanced stages, plain X-rays may show soft-tissue emphysema tracking along fascial planes [17]. Ultrasound can be done at bedside in critically-ill patients. Subcutaneous air will appear as shiny hyperechoic white dots in the facial planes while oedema will be hypoechoic spreading the tissue layers. Muscle tissue can be oedematous (Fig. 14.2) [18].

CT findings can be correlated with the pathological findings of soft-tissue inflammation or liquefactive necrosis. This will appear as dermal thickening, increased soft-tissue attenuation, inflammatory fat stranding, and possible superficial or deep crescentic gas or fluid collections that expand along fascial planes. CT is the most

Fig. 14.2 The ultrasound findings of necrotizing fasciitis include shiny hyperechoic white dots in the facial planes representing air (yellow arrows) inter-fascial hypoechoic collections (arrow head) representing dishwater pus, and muscle tissue oedema (M). (Courtesy of Professor Fikri Abu-Zidan, College of Medicine and Health Sciences, UAE University, Al-Ain, UAE)

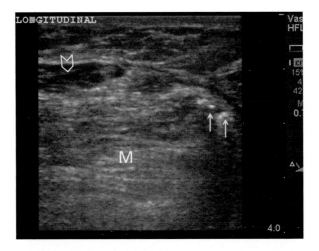

Fig. 14.3 CT scan findings of necrotizing fasciitis include dermal thickening, increased soft-tissue attenuation (arrow heads), and soft-tissue gas (white arrows). (Courtesy of Dr Saleh Abdel-Kader, Department of Surgery, NMC Specialty Hospital, Al-Ain, UAE)

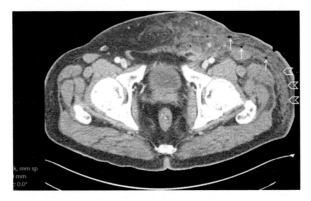

sensitive modality for soft-tissue gas detection (Fig. 14.3). However, in early stages of the disease the gas may not be present or detected. CT may demonstrate the underlying source of infection or reveal serious complications such as vascular rupture complicating tissue necrosis [19].

MRI is the modality of choice for detailed evaluation of soft-tissue infections. It is often not performed in emergency situations because it is time consuming and will delay management [17]. The MRI key finding of necrotizing fasciitis is the high T2 signal intensity along the deep fascia. It is characterized by an extensive involvement of the deep inter-muscular fascia, thickening of fascia measuring 3 mm or more at STIR or fat-suppressed T2-weighted imaging, involvement of three or more compartments, and low signal intensity with fat-suppressed T2-weighted imaging in the deep fascia with corresponding non-enhancement on post contrast images. It shows circumferential dermal and soft-tissue thickening that have variable signal intensity on T1-weighted sequences and increased signal intensity on fluid-sensitive sequences. Subcutaneous edema in necrotizing fasciitis is typically less-prominent feature compared with cellulitis [20].

Patients with negative or nonspecific imaging findings and a high clinical suspicion of necrotizing fasciitis should be promptly surgically explored. Follow-up imaging can be performed in relatively stable patients. Late-stage gas collections are seen as punctate or curvilinear T1- and T2-hypointense foci on MRI. Intravenous gadolinium contrast material increases sensitivity for tissue necrosis and can be used for more detailed evaluation of soft-tissue involvement. The abnormal fascia generally enhances and may be surrounded by non-enhancing islands of tissue. However, patients with necrotizing fasciitis may also present with renal failure, and thus administration of intravenous gadolinium may not be possible [21].

During surgical debridement, if the index finger easily dissects the subcutaneous tissue off the deep fascia along the facial plane, then the 'finger test' is positive. Other operative findings that confirm the diagnosis include; grey necrotic tissue; fascial oedema; thrombosed vessels; thin watery foul-smelling fluid (dishwater pus), and finally non-contracting muscles [1, 13].

Deep tissue culture and biopsy are essential in guiding further antibiotic therapy even if it takes longer time to get their results. Histopathological findings of necrotizing fasciitis include oedema of inter and intrafascicular fibrous septa surrounding the skeletal muscle bundles, infiltration of inflammatory cells (plasma cells, lymphocytes, neutrophils, and rarely eosinophils), and early fibroblastic proliferation. Gram staining of the tissue fluid and exudate often suggests the infective pathogen [6, 22].

14.7 Treatment

Immediate and aggressive surgical debridement of all necrotic tissue is the cornerstone to achieve successful treatment of necrotizing fasciitis (Fig. 14.4). It is the sole most important treatment modality for determining the patient's clinical outcome. Surgery that controls the source of infection hinders the spread of necrotizing fasciitis and prevents the release of inflammatory mediators responsible for systemic sepsis [13, 23].

An empirical broad-spectrum antimicrobial therapy with coverage of gram-negative and gram-positive anaerobes and aerobes should be started immediately before surgical debridement and should be changed according to the culture findings and clinical progress [24]. Debridement alone does not bring about a rapid change in the condition of patients with systemic sepsis. There are multiple factors that indicate that patients should be managed in the intensive care unit, including the need for fluid resuscitation, strict monitoring, appropriate wound dressing and frequent extensive debridement [11].

Successful management of severe necrotizing fasciitis necessitates a multidisciplinary team approach for repeated evaluation, supportive critical care, nutritional support, and reconstruction/rehabilitation when needed [14].

In individual cases with cervical necrotizing fasciitis, immediate airway control is crucial. Consideration for early tracheostomy is necessary to avoid the need for a difficult intubation following repeated debridement [10]. In selected patients with

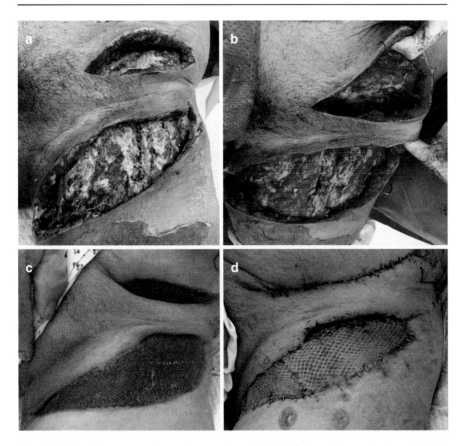

Fig. 14.4 Immediate, aggressive and repeated surgical debridement of necrotic tissue (**a–b**) is essential to control the source of infection, stop the spread of the disease and achieve successful clinical outcome. Clean wound defects (**c**) can be closed by primary closure or skin grafts (**d**). (Courtesy of Dr Saleh Abdel-Kader, Department of Surgery, NMC Specialty Hospital, Al-Ain, UAE)

urethral or penile involvement, urinary diversion in the form of suprapubic cystostomy may be indicated. Usually urinary catheterization provides adequate urine diversion. Patients with involvement of the anorectal region having a high risk of faecal contamination may need a colostomy [24]. Orchidectomy and penile amputations are extremely rarely required in patients with Fournier's gangrene [11].

The debrided wounds are usually kept to heel by secondary intention, or delayed primary wound closure. Vacuum-assisted closure has shown successful results. However, patients with large clean wound defects are referred for reconstructive surgery with skin grafts or local skin flaps [23, 25].

Hyperbaric oxygen therapy (HBOT) is a recognized adjunct treatment for necrotizing fasciitis, which is officially accepted by the Undersea and Hyperbaric Medical Society. HBOT entails providing 100% oxygen at 2.5 absolute atmosphere (2.5 ATA) of pressure for 90–120 min [26]. HBOT improves leukocyte function, inhibits anaerobic growth, inhibits toxin production, enhances the penetration of some antibiotics into the bacterial cells and has a synergistic effect with certain antimicrobial agents [27]. HBOT promotes wound healing, angiogenesis, stimulation of fibroblasts and the production of granulation tissues. The role of HBO as an adjunct treatment has been debated, and no prospective randomized clinical trials have been published. HBO could be beneficial, if available, but it should not delay surgical management, particularly if the patient needs to be transferred to another unit [28].

Intravenous immunoglobulin therapy (IVIG) is another adjunct therapy which is suggested to improve the outcome in a selected group of patients of necrotizing fasciitis. Its mechanism of action involves inhibition of super-antigen activity of secreted exotoxins, reversal of the hyperproliferation of T-cells, and downregulation of the production of tumour necrosis factor. Furthermore, it reduces mortality in patients with severe group A streptococcal infection [29]. Recent studies have shown no difference between IVIG and placebo in terms of hospital stay and mortality [30].

14.8   Learning Points

- Necrotizing fasciitis is an uncommon, rapidly progressive, and often fatal soft-tissue infection. Clinicians should have a high index of suspicion of necrotizing fasciitis for its diagnosis.
- Patients usually present with pain and swelling from skin infection that is out of proportion to the physical findings. Diabetes, liver cirrhosis and other pathologies associated with immune-suppression increase the incidence of this disease.
- The LRINEC score is a useful adjunct in the clinical diagnosis of necrotising fasciitis particularly with the addition of clinical parameters such as pain, pyrexia and comorbidities. Laboratory investigations are not specific and may aid in determining the severity of the disease.
- Imaging showing gas tracking along fascial planes in septic patients is virtually pathognomonic. CT and MRI are the most important radiological investigations. The CT hallmark of necrotizing fasciitis is soft-tissue air associated with fluid collections within the deep fascia. MRI is more useful in detecting the degree and extent of tissue involvement.
- Early decision to explore and extensively debride the necrotic tissue is important for successful clinical outcome.
- Proper antibiotics therapy, fluid resuscitation and adequate wound care are crucial.
- Patients with generalized sepsis should be carefully monitored in the intensive care unit, and managed by a multidisciplinary team.
- HBOT and IVIG are adjuncts to treatment. Some centres advocate them; however, their benefit is still unproven.

References

1. Goh T, Goh LG, Ang CH, Wong CH. Early diagnosis of necrotizing fasciitis. Br J Surg. 2014;10:119–25.
2. May AK, Stafford RE, Bulger EM, Heffernan D, Guillamondegui O, Bochicchio G, Eachempati SR, Surgical Infection Society. Treatment of complicated skin and soft tissue infections. Surg Infect. 2009;10:467–99.
3. Elliott DC, Kufera JA, Myers RA. Necrotizing soft tissue infections. Risk factors for mortality and strategies for management. Ann Surg. 1996;224:672–83.
4. Stevens DL, Bisno AL, Chambers HF, Dellinger EP, Goldstein EJ, Gorbach SL, et al. Practice guidelines for the diagnosis and management of skin and soft tissue infections: 2014 update by the Infectious Diseases Society of America. Clin Infect Dis. 2014;59:147–59.
5. Sartelli M, Guirao X, Hardcastlem T, et al. Recommendations for the management of skin and soft-tissue infections. World J Emerg Surg. 2018;13:58.
6. Richard P, Usatine MD, Sandy N. Dermatologic emergencies. American Family Physician. 2010;82:773–80.
7. Wong CH, Chang HC, Pasupathy S, Khin LW, Tan JL, Low CO. Necrotizing fasciitis: clinical presentation, microbiology, and determinants of mortality. J Bone Joint Surg Am. 2003;85-A:1454–60.
8. Pasternack MS, Swartz MN. Skin and soft tissue infections: cellulitis, necrotizing fasciitis, and subcutaneous tissue infections. In: Mandell GL, Bennett JE, Dolin R, editors. Principles and practices of infectious diseases. 7th ed. Philadelphia, PA: Elsevier; 2010. p. 1307–9.
9. Darenberg J, Luca-Harari B, Jasir A, et al. Molecular and clinical characteristics of invasive group A streptococcal infection in Sweden. Clin Infect Dis. 2007;45:450–8.
10. Oguz H, Yilmaz MS. Diagnosis and management of necrotizing fasciitis of the head and neck. Curr Infect Dis Rep. 2012;14:161–5.
11. Sroczyński M, Sebastian M, Rudnicki J, Sebastian A, Agrawal AK. Complex approach to the treatment of Fournier's gangrene. Adv Clin Exp Med. 2013;22:131–5.
12. Howell GM, Rosengart MR. Necrotizing soft tissue infections. Surg Infect. 2011;12:185–90.
13. Sultan HY, Boyle AA, Sheppard N. Necrotising fasciitis. BMJ. 2012;345:4274–9.
14. Gunaratne DA, Tseros EA, Hasan Z, et al. Cervical necrotizing fasciitis: systematic review and analysis of 1235 reported cases from the literature. Head Neck. 2018;40:2094–102.
15. Usatine R, Smith MA, Mayeaux EJ Jr, Chumley H, Tysinger J. The Color Atlas of family medicine, vol. 128. New York, NY: McGraw-Hill; 2009. p. 1–2.
16. Bechar J, Sepehripour S, Hardwicke J, Filobbos G. Laboratory risk indicator for necrotising fasciitis (LRINEC) score for the assessment of early necrotising fasciitis: a systematic review of the literature. Ann R Coll Surg Engl. 2017;99:341–6.
17. Schurr C, Burghartz M, Miethke T, Kesting M, Hoang N, Staudenmaier R. Management of facial necrotizing fasciitis. Eur Arch Otorhinolaryngol. 2009;266:325–31.
18. Yen ZS, Wang HP, Ma HM, Chen SC, Chen WJ. Ultrasonographic screening of clinically-suspected necrotizing fasciitis. Acad Emerg Med. 2002;9:1448–51.
19. Struk DW, Munk PL, Lee MJ, Ho SG, Worsley DF. Imaging of soft tissue infections. Radiol Clin N Am. 2001;39:277–303.
20. Hayeri MR, Ziai MP, Shehata ML, Teytelboym OM. Soft-tissue infections and their imaging mimics: from cellulitis to necrotizing fasciitis. Rad Graph. 2016;36:1888–910.
21. Kim KT, Kim YJ, Won Lee J, Kim YJ, Park SW, Lim MK, Suh CH. Can necrotizing infectious fasciitis be differentiated from non-necrotizing infectious fasciitis with MR imaging? Radiology. 2011;259:816–24.
22. Chaudhry AA, Baker KS, Gould ES, Gupta R. Necrotizing fasciitis and its mimics: what radiologists need to know. Musculoskel Imag: AJR. 2015;204:128–39.
23. Ord R, Coletti D. Cervico-facial necrotizing fasciitis. Oral Dis. 2009;15:133–41.
24. Yanar H, Taviloglu K, Ertekin C, Guloglu R, Zorba U, Cabioglu N, Baspinar I. Fournier's gangrene: risk factors and strategies for management. World J Surg. 2006;30:1750–4.

25. Huang WS, Hsieh SC, Hsieh CS, Schoung JY, Huang T. Use of vacuum-assisted wound closure to manage limb wounds in patients suffering from acute necrotizing fasciitis. Asian J Surg. 2006;29:135–9.
26. Levett DZ, Bennett MH, Millar I. Adjunctive hyperbaric oxygen for necrotizing fasciitis. Cochrane Database Syst Rev. 2015;1:CD007937.
27. Faunø Thrane J, Ovesen T. Scarce evidence of efficacy of hyperbaric oxygen therapy in necrotizing soft tissue infection: a systematic review. Infect Dis (Lond). 2019;51:485–92.
28. Memara MY, Yekania M, Alizadehd N, Baghi HB. Hyperbaric oxygen therapy: antimicrobial mechanisms and clinical application for infections. Biomed Pharmacother. 2019;109:440–7.
29. Norrby-Teglund A, Ihendyane N, Darenberg J. Intravenous immunoglobulin adjunctive therapy in sepsis, with special emphasis on severe invasive group A streptococcal infections. Scand J Infect Dis. 2003;35:683–9.
30. Madsen MB, Hjortrup PB, Hansen MB, et al. Immunoglobulin G for necrotising soft tissue infections (INSTINCT): a randomised, blinded, placebo-controlled trial. Intensive Care Med. 2017;43:1585–93.

Infections in Elderly Patients

15

Mario Improta, Fausto Catena, Luca Ansaloni,
Massimo Chiarugi, Massimo Sartelli,
and Federico Coccolini

15.1 Background

Emergency abdominal surgery is associated with poorer outcome compared to elective surgery, particularly in aged patients.

In the elderly, the emergent laparotomy for peritonitis is a high-risk procedure graved with elevated mortality and morbidity [1, 2].

The improvement in the overall care and the aging of the global population, along with the increase in life expectancy, led to an increasing number of elderly patients accepted to the emergency department suffering from acute peritonitis, therefore the number of patients who require surgery is rising although the disease pattern and the epidemiology underneath the intra-abdominal sepsis is very different in the geriatric population [3].

15.2 Elderly Patients and Acute Peritonitis Outcomes

Notwithstanding advance in the care of the critically ill, patients older than 65 years experience worse outcome after emergent abdominal surgery with mortality rates up to 44% in some series. Recently has been advised that the real operative mortality of the elderly patient is underestimated since the majority of studies describe the

M. Improta · L. Ansaloni
General, Emergency and Trauma Surgery Department, Bufalini Hospital, Cesena, Italy
e-mail: mario.improta@studio.unibo.it; lansaloni@asst-pg23.it

F. Catena
Emergency Surgery Department, Maggiore Hospital, Parma, Italy

M. Chiarugi · F. Coccolini (✉)
General, Emergency and Trauma Surgery Department, Pisa University Hospital, Pisa, Italy

M. Sartelli
Department of Surgery, Macerata Hospital, Macerata, Italy

© Springer Nature Switzerland AG 2021
M. Sartelli et al. (eds.), *Infections in Surgery*, Hot Topics in Acute Care Surgery
and Trauma, https://doi.org/10.1007/978-3-030-62116-2_15

in-hospital or 30-day mortality outcome, while the elderly have a prolonged recovery period with increased risk of death in long-term follow-up. Rangel et al. in a retrospective survey of 390 patients older than 70 years who underwent emergency surgery, described a mortality of 16.2% at 30 days and 32.5% at 1 year, reflecting that in this cohort the outcome drastically worsened over a 1-year timeframe [4].

Patient age was found to be an independent variable predictive of mortality (OR = 1.1; 95%CI = 1.0–1.1; $p < 0.0001$) in a recent global prospective observational study (CIAOW Study) designed by the World Society of Emergency Surgery (WSES) [4–6].

15.3 Stratification of Elderly Patients with Acute Peritonitis

The sepsis response due to peritonitis in association with the preexisting comorbidities places the elderly patient ad higher risk, furthermore, older patients with deranged physiological ability to react to the insult, may present with fewer signs of peritonitis and this combines the risk of delays to definitive treatment that further enhances risk of mortality [7].

Aging is an inevitable natural process; the diminished homeostasis and enhanced organism frailty causes a reduction in the ability to withstand environmental insults and is associated with an increased inclination to disability and mortality.

Numerous studies examined aging physiopathology and report that older age is accompanied by a low-grade inflammatory process, which may be upregulated throughout sepsis and surgical insults [8].

Frailty is proposed to be as a deterioration in the physiological reserves that make the person exposed to dramatic consequences in response to minor insults. The assessment of the frailty of a patient can be challenging, and often relies on the physicians' clinical judgment or on measurements such as the ability to walk that hardly can be estimated in an emergency setting.

To overcome this issue, sarcopenia has been proposed as a valid surrogate for estimating the frailty of patients [9]. One way to assess sarcopenia, and thus frailty has been proposed recently. The total psoas area measured at a single slice at the level of L3 in CT images obtained in the emergency department and then normalized for height of the patient was evaluated and sarcopenia was defined as a "Total Psoas Index (TPI)" less than 1.50 cm^2/m^2 for women and less than 2.16 cm^2/m^2 for men. (total psoas index = ((left + right psoas area cm^2)/height m^2))). Sarcopenic patient identified with this rapid, easy-to-use tool, showed higher mortality in a 1-year follow-up after emergency surgery (49% sarcopenic vs 27% non-sacropenic; $p < 0.01$) [10].

A lot of validated risk score such as the Physiological Operative Severity Score for enUmeration of Morbidity and Mortality (POSSUM) have been proposed to predict mortality in the postoperative period, but those are not specific for the geriatric population and their aim is to predict the 30-days mortality, which is recently been questioned since it appears that in the elderly the mortality after emergent surgery continue extending in a 12-months period [4].

Table 15.1 WSES Sepsis Severity Score for patients with complicated intra-abdominal infections (Range: 0–18)

Clinical condition at admission	
• Severe sepsis (acute organ dysfunction) at the admission	**3 score**
• Septic shock (acute circulatory failure characterized by persistent arterial hypotension. It always requires vasopressor agents) at admission	**5 score**
Setting of acquisition	
• Healthcare-associated infection	**2 score**
Origin of the IAIs	
• Colonic non-diverticular perforation peritonitis	**2 score**
• Small bowel perforation peritonitis	**3 score**
• Diverticular diffuse peritonitis	**2 score**
• Postoperative diffuse peritonitis	**2 score**
Delay in source control	
• Delayed initial intervention [preoperative duration of peritonitis (localized or diffuse) > 24 h)]	**3 score**
Risk factors	
• Age > 70	**2 score**
• Immunosuppression (chronic glucocorticoids, immunosuppressant agents, chemotherapy, lymphatic diseases, virus)	**3 score**

Other scores, like the WSES Sepsis Severity Score for patients with complicated intra-abdominal infections, have been advocated to help in the assessment of the severity of the patients with a good ability to recognize those who survived the surgical procedure from those who died. The overall mortality was 0.63% for those who had a score of 0–3, 6.3% for those who had a score of 4–6, 41.7% for those who had a score of ≥ 7. In patients who had a score of ≥ 9, the mortality rate was 55.5%, those who had a score of ≥ 11 the mortality rate was 68.2% and those who had a score ≥ 13 the mortality rate was 80.9% [11]. The main limit to this score is the need of multiple information to complete the assessment as well as the definitive diagnosis sub standing the peritonitis which sometimes can be obtained only after surgical exploration, hence lowering its utility in preoperative decisions (Table 15.1).

Some indicators such as low serum albumin and low BMI were recognized as predictors in long-term mortality up to 1 year after surgery, with albumin greater than 3.5 g/dl being associated with 59.8% of survival vs. 40.2% (in the population with albumin less than 3.5 g/dl) in the univariate analysis ($p < 0.001$) [4].

15.4 Conclusions

Elderly patients with acute peritonitis are a great challenge and an adequate organization of emergency care system is mandatory in order to improve outcomes. At the time of the admission of an elderly patient with severe peritonitis, the surgeon needs to determine whether a surgical procedure is justified comparing benefits and surgical hazards that are increased in the older population because of intrinsic frailty and comorbidities. The surgeon should use all the bedside, laboratory and radiologic tools to improve his ability to provide the best counsel even in emergency settings in order to help the patient and family to reach informed conclusions as well as establishing realistic expectations about long-term outcomes.

References

1. Arenal JJ, Bengoechea-Beeby M. Mortality associated with emergency abdominal surgery in the elderly. Can J Surg. 2003;46(2):111–6.
2. Zerbib Ph, Kuick JF, Lebuffe G, Khoury-Helou A, Pleiner I, Chamnbon JP. Emergency major abdominal surgery in patients over 85 years of age. World J Surg. 2005;29(7):820–5.
3. Thorsen K, Soreide JA, Kvaloy JT, Glomsaker T, Soreide K. Epidemiology of perforated peptic ulcer: age and gender-adjusted analysis of incidence and mortality. World J Gastroenterol. 2013;19(3):347–54.
4. Rangel EL, Cooper Z, et al. Mortality after emergency surgery continues to rise after discharge in the elderly: predictors of 1-year mortality. J Trauma Acute Care Surg. 2015;79:349–58.
5. Sartelli M, Catena F, Ansaloni L, Leppaniemi A, Taviloglu K, van Goor H, et al. Complicated intra-abdominal infections in Europe: a comprehensive review of the CIAO study. World J Emerg Surg. 2012;7(1):36. https://doi.org/10.1186/1749-7922-7-36.5.
6. Sartelli M, Catena F, Ansaloni L, Coccolini F, Corbella D, Moore EE, et al. Complicated intra-abdominal infections worldwide: the definitive data of the CIAOW study. World J Emerg Surg. 2014;9:37.
7. Søreide K, Desserud KF. Emergency surgery in the elderly: the balance between function, frailty, fatality, and futility. Scand J Trauma Resusc Emerg Med. 2015;23:10.
8. Candore G, Caruso C, Jirillo E, Magrone T, Vasto S. Low-grade inflammation as a common pathogenetic denominator in age-related diseases: novel drug targets for anti-aging strategies and successful aging achievement. Curr Pharm Des. 2010;16(6):584–96.
9. Fried LP, Ferrucci L. DarerJ et al. untangling of the concepts of disability, frailty, and comorbidity: implication for improved tageting care. J Gerontol. 2004;59(3):255–63.
10. Erika LR, Arturo JRD, Jennifer W, et al. Sarcopenia increases risk of long-term mortality in elderly patients undergoing emergency abdominal surgery. J Trauma Acute Care Surg. 2017;83:1179–86.
11. Sartelli M, Abu-Zidan FM, Catena F, Griffiths EA, Di Saverio S, Coimbra R, et al. Global validation of the WSES sepsis severity score for patients with complicated intra-abdominal infections: a prospective multicentre study (WISS study). World J Emerg Surg. 2015 Dec 16;10:61.

How to Use Antibiotics in Critically Ill Patients with Sepsis and Septic Shock

16

Morgan Collom and Therese M. Duane

16.1 Introduction

Starting in 1991, a consensus conference developed an initial perspective that sepsis resulted from the body's systemic inflammatory response syndrome to an underlying infection. Sepsis plus organ dysfunction was defined as severe sepsis, which could lead to septic shock. Septic shock was noted to be persistent hypotension despite fluid resuscitation [1]. Later, in 2001, a task force noticed limitations with the 1991 definitions, but lacked the necessary evidence to alter the current guidelines [2]. In 2014, the European Society of Intensive Care Medicine and the Society of Critical Care Medicine created a task force of 19 different specialties to reexamine the current definitions [3]. The task force came forth with terms and altered definitions, known as the Sepsis-3 guidelines.

Sepsis is a life threatening organ dysfunction that is initiated by a deregulated response in the host to infection. Organ dysfunction is recognized as a change in the total Sequential (sepsis-related) Organ Failure Assessment (SOFA) score ≥ 2 points as a result of the infection among patients who are critically ill, assuming a SOFA of 0 points for patients not known to have preexisting organ dysfunction [4]. The formal SOFA score can be replaced by the qSOFA (Quick SOFA) score, which can be done quickly at the bedside in patients with presumed infections outside of the intensive care unit, who are predicted to become critically ill. The qSOFA score, which is significant if two or more factors are present, includes: alteration in mental

M. Collom
Envision Healthcare, Nashville, TN, USA

Medical city Plano, Plano, TX, USA

T. M. Duane (✉)
Envision Healthcare, Nashville, TN, USA

Texas Health Resources Fort Worth, Fort Worth, TX, USA

© Springer Nature Switzerland AG 2021
M. Sartelli et al. (eds.), *Infections in Surgery*, Hot Topics in Acute Care Surgery and Trauma, https://doi.org/10.1007/978-3-030-62116-2_16

status (Glasgow Coma Scale score of 13 or less), systolic blood pressure $\leq$ 100 mmHg, or respiratory rate $\geq$ 22 breaths/min [5].

Septic shock is a subgroup of sepsis in which mortality is significantly increased due to circulatory, cellular, and metabolic abnormalities [4]. Clinical identification of septic shock involves a vasopressor requirement to maintain a mean arterial pressure of 65 mmHg or greater, and serum lactate level greater than 2 mmol/L despite adequate fluid resuscitation [6].

Surviving Sepsis Campaign initially published guidelines in 2004, revised in 2008 and 2012, and the current 2016 version was released at the same time as the sepsis-3 definitions were published. A vital recommendation put forth by the Surviving Sepsis Campaign includes that hospitals have a performance improvement system for sepsis [7]. Performance improvement systems are linked to improved patient outcomes and should include representation from all disciplines [8]. A cornerstone of this has been early recognition of sepsis via a formal screening effort and implementation of bundles, which are a core set of recommendations [9, 10]. Compliance with the Surviving Sepsis Campaign has proved to be beneficial through multiple studies, one being a study of 1794 patients from 62 different countries with sepsis or septic shock. There was a 36–40% risk reduction of death when the 3- or 6-h bundles were utilized [11].

Along with performance improvement systems, routine microbiologic cultures (including blood) are recommended by the campaign to be obtained prior to starting antimicrobial therapy in patients with suspected sepsis or septic shock [7].

If time allows for cultures to be obtained, the results can make identification of a pathogen more successful, which then allows for appropriate de-escalation of antimicrobial therapy, resulting in lower resistance and fewer side effects [12]. The type of microbiologic culture can vary per patient, but should include two or more sets of blood cultures (aerobic and anaerobic), drawn together on the same occasion. In patients with an intravascular catheter (placed over 48 h) with a suspicion of catheter-associated infection, one culture should be taken from the catheter and the other from a peripheral site via venipuncture. The guidelines suggest that no more than 1-h elapse in obtaining cultures before antimicrobial therapy is initiated [7].

16.2   Timing of Antimicrobials

Time to administration of antimicrobials is of vital importance in the presence of sepsis and septic shock. In these situations, each hour delay in antimicrobial treatment is associated with a significant mortality increase [13, 14]. Although timing is of utmost importance when delivering antimicrobials, the initiation of the appropriate therapy is also an important facet in the management of sepsis and septic shock [7]. Failure to choose the correct empiric antibiotic therapy can be associated with an increase in morbidity and mortality in patients with sepsis or septic shock [15]. The initial empiric regimen selected should be broad enough to cover all likely pathogens. This decision is multifactorial and should consider certain factors, including: site of infection, medical history, chronic organ failure, current medications, indwelling devices, the state of the immune system, recent infections/colonization, recent antimicrobial treatments, patient location at time of infection, prevalence of local pathogens, and the potential for intolerance and toxicity [7].

16.3 De-escalation of Antimicrobials

Empiric broad-spectrum antimicrobial therapy is warranted for patients with sepsis and septic shock until the causative agent and the antimicrobial sensitivities are delineated. Once sensitivities have resulted, removing unnecessary antimicrobials will narrow the coverage to include more specific antimicrobials [16]. The only caveat with de-escalation of antibiotics is when the cultures are negative, in which circumstance; empiric narrowing should be tailored to a good clinical response [7].

Due to the possibility of antimicrobial resistance, the duration of treatment with antimicrobial therapy should be vigilantly monitored. Along with resistance, antimicrobial-associated secondary infections such as *Clostridium difficile* colitis and super infections with multidrug-resistant pathogens are possibilities [17]. Treatment duration of 7–10 days is recommended to be adequate for serious infections in patients with sepsis and septic shock. Data even supports that serious infections can be treated with a shorter duration of therapy in the setting of successful source control [18]. A prolonged course with antimicrobial therapy is necessary when there is an undrainable area of infection, slow clinical response by a patient, *S aureus* bacteremia, some viral and/or fungal infections, and immunological diseases [19, 20]. Ultimately the decision to stop therapy or continue should be made on the basis of sound clinical judgment. There are many different clinical scenarios that can imitate infectious etiologies, but are related to inflammation, drug use, corticosteroid utilization, etc. Due to the unpredicted nature and possible adverse effects that antimicrobials can cause, it is imperative to perform daily assessments for de-escalation of therapy, especially in patients with sepsis and septic shock. Studies report that daily assessments of antimicrobials are associated with improved mortality rates [21].

Biomarkers can also play a role in de-escalation of antimicrobial therapy. The Surviving Sepsis Campaign suggests with low quality of evidence that procalcitonin levels can be used and interpreted to support shortening the length of therapy in patients with sepsis. The biomarker could also be used to discontinue antibiotics in patients who appeared to have sepsis, but had no clinical evidence to support the diagnosis. Procalcitonin should be considered in treatment decisions, but should not be relied upon exclusively to guide management [7].

16.4 Antibiograms

Resistance to antibiotics is a significant problem, making the decision of which empiric antimicrobial therapy to use, exceedingly difficult. Hospital-acquired and community-acquired infections have variable differences in susceptibility, which influence the selection of empiric antibiotics [22]. Hospital-wide antibiograms aide in the initial selection of antibiotics based on the differences in organisms and susceptibility patterns per hospital [23].

16.5   Pharmacokinetic and Pharmacodynamics Principles

A thorough understanding of drug pharmacokinetics can improve the overall outcome of patients with severe infection. Patients with sepsis and septic shock have metabolic differences compared to the general infected patient and these differences can affect the overall management strategy. The main differences include a predisposition to infection with organisms that are resistant, increased likelihood of hepatic and/or renal dysfunction, immune dysfunction, and an increased volume of distribution due to aggressive fluid resuscitation [7].

Plasma targets vary per antimicrobial; therefore failure to reach peak plasma targets has correlated with clinical failure in aminoglycosides [24]. Comparably, clinical failure for severe MRSA infections have been linked to insufficient early vancomycin trough levels [25]. Higher peak blood levels, especially in relation to pathogen minimum inhibitory concentration (MIC), have been linked with the clinical success rate in regards to fluoroquinolones [26] and aminoglycosides [24]. Beta-lactams differ in that clinical and microbiologic success rates have been associated with a longer duration of plasma concentration above the pathogen MIC, especially in the critically ill [27]. Optimizing peak drug plasma concentrations is directly related to the dosing strategy in aminoglycosides and fluoroquinolones. For aminoglycosides, once daily dosing (5–7 mg/kg/day gentamicin) produces analogous efficacy and less risk of renal toxicity when compared to multiple daily dosing [28]. In regards to fluoroquinolones, a dosing approach that optimizes the dose within a nontoxic range (ciprofloxacin 600 mg every 12 h or levofloxacin 750 mg every 24 h) should provide the best clinical and microbiologic response [29, 30]. Vancomycin is an antibiotic whose effectiveness is concentration dependent and therefore, a targeted trough of 15–20 mg/L is needed to achieve adequate pharmacodynamics, increase tissue penetration and augment clinical outcomes [31]. In patient populations with sepsis and septic shock, the recommended intravenous loading dose is 25–30 mg/kg to reach the target trough. Loading doses of certain antibiotics with low volumes of distribution are necessary in critical patients to achieve therapeutic drug levels, because of the effect that fluid resuscitation has on the body's extracellular volume [32, 33]. In the beta-lactam group, pharmacodynamics coincides with the time the plasma concentration of the drug is above the pathogen MIC relative to the dosing interval (T > MIC). In the critically ill patient, especially those with sepsis, the best response is with a T > MIC of 100% [34]. The easiest way to do this is to increase the frequency of the dosing. Loading doses are also utilized for beta-lactams and are administered as continuous or extended infusions to rapidly obtain therapeutic blood levels [35]. Some studies even suggest that after the initial loading dose, extended and continuous infusions of beta-lactams may be more effective in critically ill patients with sepsis [36, 37].

The data supports the pharmacokinetic driven dosing of antimicrobials, but the problem is much greater. Patient's in this target group that are critically ill and septic have multiple physiologic alterations that can alter the pharmacokinetics of the antimicrobials. These physiologic derangements include: unstable hemodynamics, increased extracellular volume, increased cardiac output, variations of kidney and hepatic perfusion leading to changes in drug clearance, reduced serum albumin, which can affect drug binding [38]. Therapeutic drug monitoring for multiple antimicrobials is therefore difficult to perform, specifically in critically ill patients with sepsis.

16.6   Double Coverage

Antimicrobial resistance is becoming a more prevalent issue in many parts of the world today. In order to obtain adequate coverage initially, broad-spectrum multidrug empiric therapy should be utilized. Combination therapy implies the use of two different classes of antimicrobials targeted toward a single sensitive pathogen, specifically to aide in accelerating pathogen clearance [7].

Studies have shown that combination therapy results in reduced mortality in patients with septic shock [39, 40]. Even though multiple meta-analyses have shown this to be accurate, there are no randomized controlled trials to support this approach conclusively [7]. Severely ill patients, such as those with bacteremia and sepsis without shock, should be treated with combination therapy subjectively, as there is low quality of evidence to support its benefit [41, 42]. High-risk neutropenic patients with sepsis should not be administered combination therapy routinely [43]. Early de-escalation of antimicrobial therapy has not been well studied in the setting of combination therapy, but an approach that emphasizes early de-escalation is favored according to Surviving Sepsis Campaign. There are no criteria for early de-escalation, but rather it is based on clinical progress, resolution of infection based on biomarkers, and/or a fixed duration of combination therapy [7].

16.7   Antifungal Coverage

When deciding about initial empiric coverage, it is important to assess whether *Candida* is a likely pathogen. Risk factors that could predispose a patient to an invasive *Candida* infection include: immunocompromised state, prolonged invasive vascular devices, total parenteral nutrition, necrotizing pancreatitis, prolonged hospital/ICU stay, recent fungal infection, recent major abdominal surgery, prolonged antibiotic exposure, or multisite colonization [44, 45].

Once the risk for *Candida* has been assessed, the selection of the antifungal agent should be selected according to the severity of the infection, recent exposure to an antifungal, and the local pattern of the *Candida* species. Use of echinocandin empirically is the drug of choice in patients who are severely ill, specifically those in septic shock, who have been recently treated with other antifungals, or there is a suspicion for *Candida glabrata* or *Candida krusei* [7]. If there is echinocandin toxicity or intolerance, than liposomal amphotericin B is an alternative [46]. Triazoles are more appropriate in less ill patients, with no previous exposure/colonization. B-D-glucan or rapid polymerase chain reaction assays can be used for rapid diagnostic testing to direct therapy, but the negative predictive value of these tests are not substantial enough to definitively utilize them [7].

16.8 Conclusion

This chapter sets forth the major contributions from both the Surviving Sepsis Campaign and the Sepsis-3 guidelines. It is imperative that clinicians understand the role and utility of antimicrobials in patients with sepsis and septic shock. The key to antimicrobial use is early initiation and broad coverage, along with continuous reassessment and eventual de-escalation of the therapy, eventually tailoring the treatment to the specific pathogen. Antimicrobial overuse or misuse can often lead to unfavorable outcomes. Furthermore, antibiograms and biomarkers should be utilized and studied to aid in the appropriate de-escalation of antibiotics.

References

1. Bone RC, Balk RA, Cerra FB, et al. American College of Chest Physicians/Society of Critical Care Medicine Consensus Conference: definitions for sepsis and organ failure and guidelines for the use of innovative therapies in sepsis. Crit Care Med. 1992;20(6):864–74.
2. Levy MM, Fink MP, Marshall JC, et al. International sepsis definitions conference. 2001 SCCM/ESICM/ACCP/ATS/SIS international sepsis definitions conference. Intensive Care Med. 2003;29(4):530–8.
3. Vincent J-L, Opal SM, Marshall JC, Tracey KJ. Sepsis definitions: time for change. Lancet. 2013;381(9868):774–5.
4. Singer M, Deutschman CS, Seymour CW, et al. The third international consensus definitions for sepsis and septic shock (sepsis-3). JAMA. 2016;315:801–10.
5. Seymour CW, Liu VX, Iwashyna TJ, et al. Assessment of clinical criteria for Sepsis: for the third international consensus definitions for sepsis and septic shock (sepsis-3). JAMA. 2016;315:762–74.
6. Shankar-Hari M, Phillips GS, Levy ML, et al. Sepsis definitions task force: developing a new definition and assessing new clinical criteria for septic shock: for the third international consensus definitions for sepsis and septic shock (sepsis-3). JAMA. 2016;315:775–87.
7. Rhodes A, Evans L, Alhazzani W, et al. Surviving sepsis campaign: international guidelines for management of sepsis and septic shock: 2016. Critical Care Med. 2017;45(3):486–552.
8. Dellinger RP. Foreword. The future of sepsis performance improvement. Crit Care Med. 2015;43:1787–9.
9. Jones SL, Ashton CM, Kiehne L, et al. Reductions in sepsis mortality and costs after design and implementation of a nurse-based early recognition and response program. Jt Comm J Qual Patient Saf. 2015;41:483–91.
10. Levy MM, Pronovost PJ, Dellinger RP, et al. Sepsis change bundles: converting guidelines into meaningful change in behavior and clinical outcome. Crit Care Med. 2004;32:S595–7.
11. Rhodes A, Phillips G, Beale R, et al. The surviving sepsis campaign bundles and outcome: results from the international multicentre prevalence study on Sepsis (the IMPreSS study). Intensive Care Med. 2015;41:1620–8.

12. Pollack LA, van Santen KL, Weiner LM, et al. Antibiotic stewardship programs in U.S. acute care hospitals: findings from the 2014 National Healthcare Safety Network annual hospital survey. Clin Infect Dis. 2016;63:443–9.
13. Kumar A, Roberts D, Wood KE, et al. Duration of hypotension before initiation of effective antimicrobial therapy is the critical determinant of survival in human septic shock. Crit Care Med. 2006;34:1589–96.
14. Ferrer R, Martin-Loeches I, Phillips G, et al. Empiric antibiotic treatment reduces mortality in severe sepsis and septic shock from the first hour: results from a guideline-based performance improvement program. Crit Care Med. 2014;42:1749–55.
15. Barie PS, Hydo LJ, Shou J, et al. Influence of antibiotic therapy on mortality of critical surgical illness caused or complicated by infection. Surg Infect. 2005;6:41–54.
16. Guo Y, Gao W, Yang H, et al. De-escalation of empiric antibiotics in patients with severe sepsis or septic shock: a meta-analysis. Heart Lung. 2016;45:454–9.
17. Garnacho-Montero J, Gutiérrez-Pizarraya A, Escoresca-Ortega A, et al. De-escalation of empirical therapy is associated with lower mortality in patients with severe sepsis and septic shock. Intensive Care Med. 2013;40(1):32–40.
18. Sawyer RG, Claridge JA, Nathens AB, et al. Trial of short-course antimicrobial therapy for intraabdominal infection. N Engl J Med. 2015;372:1996–2005.
19. Liu C, Bayer A, Cosgrove SE, et al.; Infectious Diseases Society of America. Clinical practice guidelines by the Infectious Diseases Society of America for the treatment of methicillin-resistant Staphylococcus aureus infections in adults and children. Clin Infect Dis. 2011;52:e18–55.
20. Pappas PG, Kauffman CA, Andes DR, et al. Clinical practice guideline for the management of candidiasis: 2016 update by the Infectious Diseases Society of America. Clin Infect Dis. 2016;62:e1–50.
21. Weiss CH, Moazed F, McEvoy CA, et al. Prompting physicians to address a daily checklist and process of care and clinical outcomes: a single-site study. Am J Respir Crit Care Med. 2011;184:680–6.
22. Kaufman D, Haas CE, Edinger R, et al. Antibiotic susceptibility in the surgical intensive care unit compared with the hospital-wide antibiogram. Arch Surg. 1998;133:1041–5.
23. Moellering RC. Principles of antiinfective therapy. In: Mandell GL, Bennett JE, Dolin R, editors. Principles and practice of infectious disease. 4th ed. New York, NY: Churchill Livingstone; 1995. p. 199–212.
24. Moore RD, Smith CR, Lietman PS. Association of aminoglycoside plasma levels with therapeutic outcome in gram-negative pneumonia. Am J Med. 1984;77:657–62.
25. Men P, Li HB, Zhai SD, et al. Association between the AUC0-24/MIC ratio of vancomycin and its clinical effectiveness: a systematic review and meta-analysis. PLoS One. 2016;11:e0146224.
26. Forrest A, Nix DE, Ballow CH, et al. Pharmacodynamics of intra-venous ciprofloxacin in seriously ill patients. Antimicrob Agents Chemother. 1993;37:1073–81.
27. Schentag JJ, Smith IL, Swanson DJ, et al. Role for dual individualization with cefmenoxime. Am J Med. 1984;77:43–50.
28. Barza M, Ioannidis JP, Cappelleri JC, et al. Single or multiple daily doses of aminoglycosides: a meta-analysis. BMJ. 1996;312:338–45.
29. van Zanten AR, Polderman KH, van Geijlswijk IM, et al. Ciprofloxacin pharmacokinetics in critically ill patients: a prospective cohort study. J Crit Care. 2008;23:422–30.
30. Dunbar LM, Wunderink RG, Habib MP, et al. High-dose, short- course levofloxacin for community-acquired pneumonia: a new treatment paradigm. Clin Infect Dis. 2003;37:752–60.
31. Rybak MJ, Lomaestro BM, Rotschafer JC, et al. Vancomycin therapeutic guidelines: a summary of consensus recommendations from the infectious diseases Society of America, the American Society of Health-System Pharmacists, and the Society of Infectious Diseases Pharmacists. Clin Infect Dis. 2009;49:325–7.
32. Pea F, Viale P. Bench-to-bedside review: appropriate antibiotic therapy in severe sepsis and septic shock–does the dose matter? Crit Care. 2009;13:214.

33. Wang JT, Fang CT, Chen YC, et al. Necessity of a loading dose when using vancomycin in critically ill patients. J Antimicrob Chemother. 2001;47:246.
34. McKinnon PS, Paladino JA, Schentag JJ. Evaluation of area under the inhibitory curve (AUIC) and time above the minimum inhibitory concentration (T>MIC) as predictors of outcome for cefepime and ceftazidime in serious bacterial infections. Int J Antimicrob Agents. 2008;31:345–51.
35. Rhodes NJ, MacVane SH, Kuti JL, et al. Impact of loading doses on the time to adequate predicted beta-lactam concentrations in prolonged and continuous infusion dosing schemes. Clin Infect Dis. 2014;59:905–7.
36. Falagas ME, Tansarli GS, Ikawa K, et al. Clinical outcomes with extended or continuous versus short-term intravenous infusion of carbapenems and piperacillin/tazobactam: a systematic review and meta-analysis. Clin Infect Dis. 2013;56:272–82.
37. Yusuf E, Spapen H, Piérard D. Prolonged vs intermittent infusion of piperacillin/tazobactam in critically ill patients: a narrative and systematic review. J Crit Care. 2014;29:1089–95.
38. Roberts JA, Abdul-Aziz MH, Lipman J, et al.; International Society of Anti-Infective Pharmacology and the Pharmacokinetics and Pharmacodynamics Study Group of the European Society of Clinical Microbiology and Infectious Diseases. Individualised antibiotic dosing for patients who are critically ill: challenges and potential solutions. Lancet Infect Dis. 2014;14:498–509.
39. Kumar A, Safdar N, Kethireddy S, et al. A survival benefit of combination antibiotic therapy for serious infections associated with sepsis and septic shock is contingent only on the risk of death: a meta-analytic/meta-regression study. Crit Care Med. 2010;38:1651–64.
40. Kumar A, Zarychanski R, Light B, et al.; Cooperative Antimicrobial Therapy of Septic Shock (CATSS) Database Research Group. Early combination antibiotic therapy yields improved survival compared with monotherapy in septic shock: a propensity-matched analysis. Crit Care Med. 2010;38:1773–85.
41. Safdar N, Handelsman J, Maki DG. Does combination antimicrobial therapy reduce mortality in Gram-negative bacteraemia? A meta-analysis. Lancet Infect Dis. 2004;4:519–27.
42. Paul M, Silbiger I, Grozinsky S, Soares-Weiser K, Leibovici L. Beta lactam antibiotic monotherapy versus beta lactam-aminoglycoside antibiotic combination therapy for sepsis. Cochrane Database Syst Rev. 2006;1:CD003344.
43. Freifeld AG, Bow EJ, Sepkowitz KA, et al. Infectious Diseases Society of America: clinical practice guideline for the use of anti-microbial agents in neutropenic patients with cancer: 2010 update by the infectious diseases society of America. Clin Infect Dis. 2011;52:e56–93.
44. Pittet D, Monod M, Suter PM, et al. Candida colonization and subsequent infections in critically ill surgical patients. Ann Surg. 1994;220:751–8.
45. Blumberg HM, Jarvis WR, Soucie JM, et al.; National Epidemiology of Mycoses Survey (NEMIS) Study Group. Risk factors for candidal bloodstream infections in surgical intensive care unit patients: the NEMIS prospective multicenter study. The National Epidemiology of Mycosis Survey. Clin Infect Dis. 2001;33:177–86.
46. Bow EJ, Evans G, Fuller J, et al. Canadian clinical practice guidelines for invasive candidiasis in adults. Can J Infect Dis Med Microbiol. 2010;21:e122–50.

Acute Gastrointestinal Injury

17

Francesco Cortese, Margherita Loponte, Stefano Rossi,
Biagio Picardi, Simone Rossi Del Monte,
and Pietro Fransvea

Bacteria use antibiotics judiciously. Humans do not

Matt McCarthy

17.1 Introduction

The stratification of mortality and morbidity risk plays a crucial role in the management of critical and *precritical* patient [1–3]. Before the creation of the Score Systems many of the physician's decision-making process were based on the clinical instinct, what the Anglo-Saxons call "gut-feeling." The ASA (American Society of Anesthesiologists) was one of the first classification developed by anesthesiologists, starting from exclusively clinical evaluations and designated in order to provide a preoperative patient assessment [4, 5]. Later, many other index and scores were developed, with most rating pulmonary, cardiovascular, and renal function and many also rating neurologic, hepatic, and hematologic functions. The scoring systems describe the extent of organ dysfunction and the number of organ failures to predict mortality, among these scores, dramatically raised during the years, and the best known and used is the Sofa and qSOFA [6, 7].

Despite its pathophysiological role, the gastrointestinal tract (GIT) has not been sufficiently valued and investigated for the potential failure as both a consequence and a potential driver of the critical illness state has not figured in standard scoring systems even if it may portend worse prognosis among ICU patients [8–10]. Recently, in conjunction with an grooving of scientific interest on the concept of bacterial intestinal translocation, Enterobacteriaceae origin, post-infection or over-infection

F. Cortese (✉) · M. Loponte · S. Rossi · B. Picardi · S. Rossi Del Monte
Emergency Surgery and Trauma Care Unit, St Filippo Neri Hospital, Rome, Italy

P. Fransvea
Emergency Surgery and Trauma, Fondazione Policlinico Universitario A. Gemelli IRCCS, Rome, Italy

© Springer Nature Switzerland AG 2021
M. Sartelli et al. (eds.), *Infections in Surgery*, Hot Topics in Acute Care Surgery
and Trauma, https://doi.org/10.1007/978-3-030-62116-2_17

sepsis, multiple organ deficiency syndrome in critically ill patients, the role of intestinal microbiota, the GIT has risen to its proper importance, an organ that first initiates the immune response, with the largest component of lymphatic tissue, involved in a series of processes such as digestive process, endogenous metabolic and exogenous process, endocrine and homeostatic immune system [11, 12]. Related to these concepts Manu Malbrain released a new mantra "It's all in the gut" [13]. In light of all this, the acknowledgment and the understanding of mechanisms of gastrointestinal pathophysiology has led to the codification of the concept of gastrointestinal failure and the definition of Acute Gastrointestinal Injury (AGI) [14–16].

17.2 Hints of Anatomy and Physiology

17.2.1 Peritoneum and Mesentery

The human GI tract is composed of multiple different organs and can be divided into the upper and lower GI tract. The upper GI tract refers to the mouth, esophagus, stomach duodenum, jejunum, and ileum, while the colon, rectum, and anus make up the lower GI tract. The anatomic formation of the esophagus, stomach, intestine, liver, and pancreas are achieved in the fourth fetal week through a series of evaginations, elongations, and dilatations. Anatomic development progresses through cell proliferation, growth, and morphogenesis. The supportive elements that will provide the vascular supply, the neural and hormonal regulation, and the host defenses of the GI tract evolve concurrently with its anatomic development. The arterial bed develops as three ventral outbuddings from the aorta to form the celiac axis and the superior and inferior mesenteric arteries. To accomplish the digestive processes in a coordinated manner, the GI tract has a functional anatomy that in general terms is composed of a series of layers including the inner mucosal layer of the GI tract composed of absorptive and secretory epithelial cells. The remaining layers of the GI tract include the submucosal layer containing nerves, lymphatics, and connective tissue; the smooth muscle layer composed of longitudinal and circular smooth muscle; and the outer serosal layer.

Peritoneum: The peritoneal cavity is a complex anatomical structure with multiple attachments and connections. The peritoneum is a large and complex serous membrane. It consists of two continuous transparent layers: the parietal and visceral peritoneum. It is situated directly beneath the abdominal musculature (*rectus abdominis* and *transversus abdominis*) and comprises a thin layer of loose connective tissue covered by a single layer of mesothelial cells. The *parietal* peritoneum lines the internal surface of the abdominopelvic cavity with multiple attachments to the abdominal wall, while the *visceral* layer lines the abdominal viscera. The narrow space within these two layers is referred to as the peritoneal cavity. The peritoneum contains the peritoneal fluid, approximately 100 ml. This fluid is continually produced, circulated and resorbed. The PF facilitates frictionless movement of abdominal organs (e.g. during peristalsis), permits the exchange of nutrients, removes pathogens and cells ascending from the female genital tract, and allows reparative events. More over growth factors, nutrients, cytokines, and chemokines, as well as leukocytes, are continuously exchanged between the PF and the blood. The peritoneal membrane contributes to the protection of the abdominal cavity, providing an environment that facilitates response to mechanical stresses and in which organs are kept separate and slide on one another. The peritoneum provides a route for entry of nerves, blood, and lymphatic vessels. Pathogens and bacterial toxins are also readily absorbed and cause inflammation. Its response to damage includes the recruitment, proliferation, and activation of a variety of hematopoietic and stromal cells. A thorough understanding of peritoneal cavity can aid interpretation of a wide variety of common human diseases.

Mesentery: it is a continuous folded band of membranous tissue (peritoneum) that is attached to the wall of the abdomen and encloses the viscera. In humans, the mesentery wraps around the pancreas and the small intestine and extends down around the colon and the upper portion of the rectum. One of its major functions is to hold the abdominal organs in their proper position. Because the mesentery is a continuous tissue and possesses clear anatomical and functional properties, some researchers consider it to be a distinct organ. Whether the mesentery should be viewed as part of the intestinal, vascular, endocrine, cardiovascular, or immunological systems is so far unclear, as it has important roles in them all. Mesenteric mesothelial plasticity and transformation contribute to several disorders, including adhesion and hernia formation. Connective tissue contiguity could explain the development of musculoskeletal, ocular, and cutaneous abnormalities in intestinal diseases, such as ulcerative colitis and Crohn's disease, and might also account for so far unexplained patterns of pathogen and disease spread. Armed with this knowledge, the diagnosis and assessment of a wide range of common intra-abdominal diseases becomes straightforward [17–22]. All these concepts are also reinforced by the fact that since 2016, the mesentery has acquired the dignity of organ, with therefore specific and unique features and functions [17].

17.2.2 Gastrointestinal Tract Function

The gastrointestinal (GI) tract is a complex organ system that next to the digestive functions, carries out endocrine, immune, and barrier functions [23–26]. In broad terms, the gut is composed of three entities: the epithelium, the mucosal immune system, and the commensal flora. These are each innervated by the enteric nervous system and each of these components interact in a complex ecosystem that is under constant surveillance and is tightly regulated. Luminal contents move along the GI tract via smooth muscle peristalsis, while smooth muscle segmentation ensures adequate contact time and exposure to the absorptive epithelial mucosal surface. The peptides released from the stomach and/or intestine modulate motility, secretion, absorption, mucosal growth, and immune function of the gastrointestinal tract. These hormones also have effects outside the gastrointestinal tract particularly in relation to the regulation of energy intake and glycemia. It also serves to prevent intestinal microbial invasion through the epithelial barrier and mucosal immune system. These absorptive and protective factors of the intestinal mucosa are reconciled in a selectively permeable epithelium that adapts to luminal nutrients, cytokines, and infectious organisms. Intestinal motility is of critical importance in the maintenance of the digestive and protective functions of the GI tract. The epithelium performs the digestive functions of the gastrointestinal tract that is critical both for absorbs food necessary for host well-being and to preserve intestinal integrity. The mucosal surface of the gut represents the largest body surface in contact with the outside world (approximately 300 m^2, roughly the area of a tennis court). Small and large intestinal motility is under multiple levels of control including the ENS and CNS, as well as GI hormones and paracrine agents. Approximately 20,000 protein coding genes are expressed in human cells and 75% of these genes are expressed in at least one of the different parts of the digestive organ system. Over 600 of these genes are more specifically expressed in one or more parts of the GI tract and the corresponding proteins have functions related to digestion of food and uptake of nutrients. Examples of specific proteins with such functions are pepsinogen PGC and the lipase LIPF, expressed in chief cells, and gastric ATPase ATP4A and gastric intrinsic factor GIF, expressed in parietal cells of the stomach mucosa. To ensure effective digestion and proper GI tract health requires a complex series of coordinated neural events accomplished by the central nervous system (CNS), the nerve network within the gut itself known as the enteric nervous system (ENS), and a whole host of GI endocrine peptides that target specific cells and tissues that make up the GI tract [27–31].

17.2.3 Role of Microbiota: Victim and Actor

The human body consists of around 10 trillion cells, whereas 100 trillion bacteria colonize our surfaces and intestinal tract which directly interact with the host and participate in health homeostasis. This cohabitation in the GI tract is both beneficial and essential to the human host by providing digestion of foods, nutrient processing, and immune functions. Microbiota refers to the entire population of microorganisms that colonizes a particular location. Several high quality data from the US Human Microbiome Project (HMP), European Meta-genomics of the Human Intestinal Tract (MetaHIT), and several other studies have now demonstrated the beneficial functions of the normal gut flora on health down to the genetic level.

At birth, the gut is first colonized and then stabilized through adaptation with four dominant phyla: Firmicutes, Bacteriodetes, Proteobacteria, and Actinobacteria. Depending on environmental conditions, genetics, the host's immune system, diet, and early exposure to infection or antibiotics, the presence and dominance of these species becomes highly varied among healthy individuals. The gut microbiota maintains a symbiotic relationship with the gut mucosa and imparts substantial metabolic, immunological and gut protective functions in the healthy individual. Hippocrates self has been quoted as saying "death sits in the bowels" and "bad digestion is the root of all evil" in 400 B.C., showing that the importance of the intestines in human health has been long recognized. Gut microbiota have a complex influence on metabolism, nutrition, and immune function in the host, and therefore disruption or alteration of the microbiota plays a pivotal role in GI. Significant interest have evolved on the gut microbiota in the recent years within the scientific community; and the gut microbiota have been associated with a large array of human diseases. Gut microbiota now appears to influence the host at nearly every level and in every organ system, highlighting our interdependence and coevolution [32–41].

17.3 Definition

The definition of gastrointestinal failure or dysfunction has evolved over the years. The term "intestinal failure" was originally defined by Fleming and Remington as "a reduction in the functioning gut mass below the minimal amount necessary for adequate digestion and absorption of food." [42] Although this definition was subsequently modified to include failure of the intestinal tract to maintain adequate hydration and electrolyte balance in the absence of artificial fluid and electrolyte support. The *European Society for Clinical Nutrition and Metabolism (ESPEN) Special Interest Group* define this condition as "a reduction in gut function below the minimum necessary for the absorption of macronutrients and/or water and electrolytes, such that intravenous supplementation is required to maintain health and/ or growth." Intestinal failure may be acquired or congenital, and of gastrointestinal or systemic, benign or malignant origin. It may have an abrupt onset, or be the slow, progressive evolution of a chronic illness, and it may be a self-limiting short-term or a long-lasting condition (chronic intestinal failure, CIF). The term **"Acute Gastrointestinal Injury" (AGI)** has been proposed to address GI dysfunction as part of the multiple organ dysfunction syndrome in critically ill patients, whether or not they have primary abdominal pathology [43–47].

17.4 Classification

From a function point of view based on onset, and metabolic and expected outcome criteria, IF has been classified as:

- Type I—Acute, short-term and usually self-limiting condition; this is a common feature, occurring in the perioperative setting after abdominal surgery and/or in association with critical illnesses; it recedes when those illnesses subside; IVS is required over a period of days or a few weeks
- Type II—Prolonged acute condition, often in metabolically unstable patients, requiring complex multidisciplinary care and IVS over periods of weeks or months
- Type III—Chronic condition, in metabolically stable patients, requiring IVS over months or years; it represents the chronic intestinal failure (CIF), that may be reversible or irreversible.

In 2012, the Working Group on Abdominal Problems of the European Society of Intensive Care Medicine (ESICM) defined acute gastrointestinal injury (AGI) as the malfunctioning of the GI tract in critically ill patients due to their acute illness.

Type I and type II Intestinal failure form the **Acute Gastrointestinal Injury** group. In turn AGI is classified as:

- **Primary:** AGI is associated with primary disease or direct injury to organs of the GI system.
- Rationale—Condition may usually be observed early (during the first day) after the insult to the GI system. Examples: Peritonitis, pancreatic or hepatic pathology, abdominal surgery, abdominal trauma, etc.
- **Secondary:** AGI develops as the consequence of a host response in critical illness without primary pathology in the GI system.

Rationale—Condition develops without direct insult to the GI tract. Examples: GI malfunction in a patient with pneumonia (Fig. 17.1), pulmonary critical conditions (Fig. 17.2), cardiac pathology, non-abdominal surgery or trauma, post-resuscitation [43, 48–50].

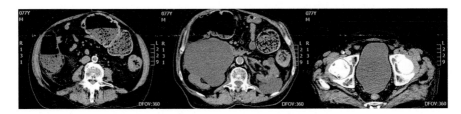

Fig. 17.1 AGI II/76-year-old man with COPD in acute exacerbation. Note the right kidney cyst and the acute urine retention. Treated with urinary catheterization and percutaneous cyst drainage. Discharged 6 days later

Fig. 17.2 Abdominal compartment syndrome in an obese 34-year-old man with pulmonary embolism— Decompression 3 days later after admittance. Total colectomy for tertiary abdominal compartment syndrome 3 days later. Alive at 2 years

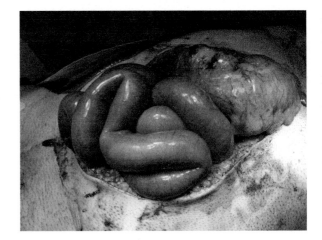

17.5   Epidemiology

Type I AIF is a common, short-lived, and in most cases self-limiting condition, diagnosed in approximately 15% patients in the perioperative setting after abdominal surgery, or in association with critical illness such as head injury, pneumonia, or acute pancreatitis, or after cardiac surgery.

Type II AIF is an uncommon clinical condition accompanied by septic, metabolic, and complex nutritional complications. It generally develops as a consequence of trauma; it may follow an acute event (such as intestinal volvulus, strangulated hernia, mesenteric thrombosis, or abdominal trauma) necessitating massive bowel resections, or occur as a complication of intestinal surgery (anastomotic leak, unrecognized intestinal injury, fistula formation, abdominal wall dehiscence, laparostomy/open abdomen), often in a setting of considerable preexisting comorbidity. Data on the type II-prolonged AIF were provided by British study in 2006, which estimated an annual incidence of nine patients per million population. The meta-analysis of Zhang D et al. estimated the prevalence of AGI in these critically ill patients at 40% (95% CI: 27–54%). Because clinical evaluation of the intestinal function is difficult, radiological signs are not specific, subtle or absent and there is lack of universally accepted criteria for gut failure in ICU patients, gut dysfunction often goes unrecognized.

The epidemiology of Type III is based on the data from home parenteral nutrition (HPN) which often include patients with either benign or malignant diseases. In Europe, the prevalence of HPN for Type III IF has been estimated to range from 5 to 80 per million population, with the incidence ranging from 7.7 to 15 IF/HPN patients/million inhabitants/year. Around 10% of patients were in the pediatric age group [50, 51].

17.6   Grading

Reintam et al. [52] proposed a 5-grade GI failure scoring system for ICU patients, based on the presence of feeding intolerance and/or intra-abdominal hypertension (IAH), which correlated with ICU mortality. In 2012, the Working Group on Abdominal Problems (WGAP) of the European Society of Intensive Care Medicine (ESICM) proposed a definition of AGI in intensive care patients as malfunctioning of the GI tract in critically ill patients due to their acute illness. Four grades of severity were identified: AGI grade I, a self-limiting condition with future risk of GI dysfunction or failure; AGI grade II (GI dysfunction), interventions are required to restore GI function; AGI grade III (GI failure), interventions cannot restore GI function; AGI grade IV, GI failure that is immediately life-threatening disturbances in the gut's barrier functions, increased virulence of the gut microbiome, and post-antibiotic abrogation of the gut microbiome's ability to promote immune autoregulation may play a role in the development and progression of MOF. Both selective gastrointestinal decontamination and replenishment of the nonpathogenic microbiome with probiotics have shown positive effects Treatment of persistent sepsis-associated MOF with fecal microbiota transplant (after eradication of the inciting infection) is an intriguing concept that needs further evaluation.

Though an element of the SOFA score and other MOF scores, the implications of sepsis-associated cholestasis are poorly understood. Management is conservative. Frank hepatic failure is rare as a result of sepsis-associated MOF and should raise concern for an alternative diagnosis [52–55].

17.7 Etiology

Berg and Garlington in 1979 first defined the phenomenon of bacterial passage through the gut wall as "bacterial translocation." [56] However, the gut was first hypothesized to be the "motor" of MODS in 1985. In the decades since, numerous studies have tried to define the role of the gut in the origin and propagation of sepsis and MODS. Recently, it has been recognized that, apart from the intestinal ischemia-reperfusion injury, gut luminal contents, including the mucus gel layer, pancreatic proteases and gut flora, as well as the luminal response to splanchnic ischemia play also an important role in modulating gut injury. Acute gastrointestinal injuries usually presents following an acute traumatic event such as a traffic accident, following surgical procedures associated with anastomotic leaks, vascular or viscous injury during other surgery creation of laparostomy (open abdominal wound), and acute unpredictable events such as enterocutaneous fistulae, intestinal volvulus, and mesenteric infarction. For example, luminal pancreatic proteases appear to be crucial for the development of gut-derived sepsis following hemorrhagic shock, while bile-derived tumor necrosis factor-αseems to act on the luminal side of the mucosa in the endotoxin-induced gut injury model, causing intestinal damage. The exact nature of the relationship between gut and sepsis, SIRS, and MODS remains to be elucidated. It seems clear that bacterial translocation plays a role but is certainly not the sole cause. Alteration of all the components of the GI tract the mucosal surface, the gut associated lymphoid, the gut flora and hormone secretion are involved.

The mucosal surface of the gut represents the largest body surface in contact with the outside world. The intestinal epithelium is a single layer of columnar epithelial cells constantly renewed from stem cells originating in the crypts of Lieberkühn. Integrity of the layer is assured by apical junction complexes [12], creating a dynamic barrier keeping the internal milieu sterile. Sepsis and inflammation disrupt the anatomical structures, increase apoptosis in the gut epithelium and decrease cell proliferation [13–16], resulting in loss of this barrier function and bacterial translocation. The gut-associated lymphoid tissue (GALT) is the largest lymphatic organ in the body, the surface area of the digestive tract is estimated to be about 32 square meters. With such a large exposure (more than three times larger than the exposed surface of the skin), these immune components function to prevent pathogens from entering the blood and lymph circulatory systems It is composed of four distinct compartments: Peyer patches, mesenteric lymph nodes, the lamina propria, and intraepithelial lymphocytes (IELs). Enterocytes are also capable of producing cytokines after an inflammatory stimulus in the absence of bacteremia or translocation. Critical illness has a profound effect upon the number of cells in the mucosal immune system, the main phenomenon being loss of lymphocytes; this can be encountered after ischemia/reperfusion or after sepsis, which increases apoptosis in lamina propria lymphocytes. Recent studies re-appraise the role of intestinal microflora in critical illness and gut-origin sepsis. The gut flora acts as an effective barrier against opportunistic and pathogenic microorganisms with its "colonization resistance." The gut flora can be divided into benign/beneficial and potentially harmful species. Several factors are believed to modify gut microflora during critical illness: changes in circulating stress hormones, gut ischemia, immunosuppression, the use of antibiotics and other drugs, and the lack of nutrients. Changes in local milieu may induce the expression of virulence genes. Notably, a hierarchical system of virulence gene expression in bacteria has recently been described, known as quorum sensing (QS). Ischemia, hypoxia, and intestinal epithelium injury induce the release of molecules that activate QS circuitry in the opportunistic pathogens, which interact with mucosal epithelium and trigger the expression of a particular pro inflammatory mediator in a susceptible host.

In ICU patients, modifications in hormonal secretions can be observed. "Endocrine failure" of the gastrointestinal tract may be considered alongside other endocrine insufficiencies in critically ill patients, such as sympatho-adrenal insufficiency, and it needs to be included in a more generalized definition of gut failure [56–59].

Deitch proposed the three hit model. According to this, an initial insult causes visceral hypoperfusion (First Hit) and the gut responds by producing and releasing proinflammatory factors. Hemodynamic resuscitation leads to reperfusion, resulting in ischemia-reperfusion injury to the intestine (Second Hit), loss of gut barrier function and an augmented gut inflammatory response, without the need for translocation of bacteria or toxins. Once bacteria and endotoxin cross the mucosal barrier, they further enhance the immune response with the release of chemokines, cytokines, and other inflammatory mediators, which affect the immune system both locally and systemically (Third Hit), leading to SIRS and MODS [60, 61]. Clark and Coopersmith in 2007 suggested the "intestinal crosstalk" theory which assumes a three-way partnership among the intestinal epithelium, the immune tissue and the endogenous microflora of the gut [62]. In this partnership, each element modifies the others via crosstalk, within a state where all components of the gut interact, concluding that the intestine is a complex organ which can even crosstalk with extra-intestinal tissues. In critically ill patients, loss of the balance between these highly interrelated systems results in the development of systemic manifestations of disease, whose repercussions extend far beyond the intestine.

Undoubtedly, the intestine plays an important role in the development of sepsis syndrome and MOF. Modification of the gut barrier seems to occur clinically and to be responsible for the increased prevalence of infectious complications in critically ill patients [63–67].

17.8 Clinical Presentation and Diagnosis

Several studies show that critically ill patients with an expected duration of mechanical ventilation of more than 6 h have GI symptoms during the first week of admission. Some specific symptoms, including absent BS, GI bleeding, and bowel distension, as well as the total number of GI symptoms, were associated with 28 day mortality. In most cases, gastrointestinal dysfunction is suspected because of feeding intolerance, ileus, diarrhea, digestive bleeding, or intestinal ischemia.

In 2012, the Working Group on Abdominal Problems (WGAP) of the European Society of Intensive Care Medicine (ESICM) proposed a definition of AGI in intensive care patients as malfunctioning of the GI tract in critically ill patients due to their acute illness.

Four grades of severity were identified: AGI grade I, a self-limiting condition with future risk of GI dysfunction or failure; AGI grade II (GI dysfunction), interventions are required to restore GI function; AGI grade III (GI failure), interventions cannot restore GI function; AGI grade IV, GI failure that is immediately life threatening.

- *AGI grade I* (risk of developing GI dysfunction or failure)—The function of the GI tract is partially impaired, expressed as GI symptoms related to a known cause and perceived as transient. Rationale: Condition is clinically seen as occurrence of GI symptoms after an insult, which expectedly has temporary and self-limiting nature. Examples: postoperative nausea and/or vomiting during the first days after abdominal surgery, postoperative absence of bowel sounds, diminished bowel motility in the early phase of post-acute event or shock.
- *AGI grade II* (gastrointestinal dysfunction)—The GI tract is not able to perform digestion and absorption adequately to satisfy the nutrient and fluid requirements. The clinical condition of the patient could worsen related to GI problems. Rationale: The condition is characterized by acute occurrence of GI symptoms requiring therapeutic interventions for achievement of nutrient and fluid requirements. This condition occurs without previous GI interventions or is more severe than might be expected in relation also, but not only (Figs. 17.3 and 17.4), to the course of preceding abdominal procedures. Examples: gastroparesis with high gastric residuals or reflux, stop-bowel, diarrhea, intra-abdominal hypertension (IAH), visible bile in gastric content or blood in the stool, feeding intolerance could be present if at least 20 kcal/kg BW/day via enteral route cannot be reached within 72 h of feeding attempt.
- *AGI grade III* (gastrointestinal failure)—Loss of GI function, where restoration of GI function is not achieved despite interventions and the general condition is not improving. Rationale: Clinically seen as sustained intolerance to enteral feeding without improvement after treatment (e.g. erythromycin, post-pyloric tube placement), leading to persistence or worsening of MODS. Examples: despite treatment, feeding intolerance is persisting-high gastric residuals, persisting GI paralysis, occurrence or worsening of bowel dilatation, progression of IAH to grade II (IAP 15–20 mmHg), low abdominal perfusion pressure (APP)

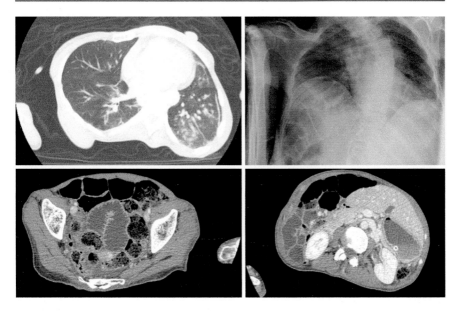

Fig. 17.3 AGI II in acute pneumonia in a 63-year-old woman with *post-natal cerebral damage with Chilaiditi sign*

Fig. 17.4 AGI II in myocardial infarction in cocaine abuse

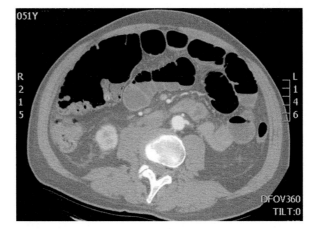

(below 60 mmHg). Feeding intolerance is present and possibly associated with persistence or worsening of MODS.

- *AGI grade IV* (gastrointestinal failure with severe impact on distant organ function)—AGI has progressed to become directly and immediately life-threatening, with worsening of MODS and shock. Rationale: Situation when AGI has led to an acute critical deterioration of the general condition of the patient with distant organ dysfunction. Examples: bowel ischemia with necrosis, GI bleeding leading to hemorrhagic shock, Abdominal Compartment Syndrome (ACS) requiring decompression.

This definition mainly depends on the symptoms and signs of AGI, which are usually not sufficient to diagnose the underlying disease. Moreover, evaluating the small bowel is difficult for two reasons: it is a deep organ, far from the mouth, anus, and abdominal wall, and critically ill patients are frequently not able to inform clinicians about a digestive complaint. This explains why its dysfunction may sometimes be occult or misdiagnosed, and the fact that it is not clearly integrated into the overall approach used to treat ICU patients [49, 52].

Reintam et al. created a gastrointestinal failure (GIF) score in critically ill patients, based upon the occurrence of feeding intolerance and IAH, ranging from level 0 (normal gastrointestinal function) to level 4 (ACS) [49]. They showed that GIF score was correlated with ICU mortality and improved the prognostic value of the sequential organ failure assessment (SOFA) score. Some biomarkers, for example, blood intestinal fatty acid binding protein (i-FABP), D-lactate (D-la), and lipopolysaccharide (LPS), have been proposed as possible markers for intestinal barrier function and the detection of AGI. However, their clinical validity in the diagnosis and classification of AGI is still unclear. Another interesting biomarker is the plasma citrulline. The link between low plasma citrulline concentration and loss of gut barrier function was suggested by Herbers et al. who showed that after high-dose chemotherapy low plasma citrulline concentration is linked to bacteremia [68]. In addition, low plasma citrulline concentration has been clearly correlated with clinical and biological evidence of mucosal barrier injury after chemotherapy in pediatric patients. Because small bowel ischemia is often related to an acute reduction of enterocyte mass, it could be a third context of interest for using plasma citrulline concentration [69–72].

AGI grading is a strong predictor for mortality. FI within the first week of ICU stay has an independent and incremental prognostic value for mortality, suggesting that the combination of the AGI grade on the first day of ICU admission and persistent FI within the first week of ICU stay could improve risk stratification in critically ill patients.

It is therefore easy to consider the GI involved in the development of different pathological processes. More over the GI system is considered critical to the development of multiple organ failure (MOF), with bacterial translocation in intensive care unit (ICU) patients supporting the concept of the gut having a role in MOF [73, 74].

17.9 Abdominal Compartment Syndrome: An Overview

The Abdominal Compartment Syndrome (ACS) represents the most famous, despite until today not well known in the medical world [75, 76], AGI-related clinical picture. The basic pathophysiology is very simple to the detrimental final effects: an increase in the abdominal internal pressure. The abdomen is a close compartment by the diaphragm, the abdominal muscular layers and the pelvic muscle. The standard pressure is around 6–8 mmHg. Any pathological condition able to increase this pressure can determine an ACS. Obesity and pregnancy also lead to an increase in abdominal pressure without pathological results.

ACS was recognized and described in the end of the '800 and was reported in the literature in an erratic mode until across the new millennium. In the last twenty years, ACS was revaluated as a very dangerous problem in every critical or subcritical patient independently from the origin of the recovery, medical, surgical, cardiological, and infective. Any clinical problem at any age is a potential trigger for an ACS. Any clinician in any area could be aware of the possible rising problem called ACS with a mortality rate when unrecognized rounding 50%. The ACS is the final result of an increasing pressure value not promptly recognized and treated. There is an important "intermediate window" between a normal AP and the ACS called Intra-Abdominal-Hypertension (IAH) with mean values between 12 and 19 mmHg. In this window a correct approach reduces the clinical damages for the patient before the configuring ACS (Abdominal Pressure 20 mmHg).

The likely of ACS is related to the deep modifications and the relationship with the meso and macro-circulation in the pressure values of the microcirculation of the single district, intestinal tract or parenchyma of the abdomen also in the kidneys.

A correct and continue perfusion of the gastrointestinal tract is mandatory in the maintenance of the anatomical, biological and functional status and for its homeostasis. In this evaluation is created the term of abdominal perfusion pressure (AAP) determined by the mean arterial pressure (MAP) less intra-abdominal pressure with a normal and correct value of over 60 mmHg. It's obvious to consider that an increase of the AP associated with a reduced MAP as in critical patients can start a vicious circle with critical damages in the abdominal viscera. In this situation the attempts to increase the MAP can become very dangerous because this maneuver reduce the microcirculation in a derangement between the two regimens of circulation as described [77–79]. The same problem of microcirculation happen as in the abdominal organs in the cortex of the kidney were the glomerular filtrate (GF) is the result of this simple formula GF = MAP − [2 × IAP] [80].

We can grade the IAH/ACS as follow:

- Grade I 12–15 mmHg Physiological compensated
- Grade II 16–20 mmHg Abdominal Hypertension
- Grade III 20–25 mmHg Visceral dysfunction, anuria
- Grade IV 25 mmHg MODS

ACS can be also divided into primary, secondary, and tertiary:

- Primary—When is sustained by a pathology or a pathological process arising in the peritoneal space (bowel ischemia, infection, visceral aneurysms, acute pancreatitis, hematomas, hematological disorders or neoplasms, solid neoplasms).
- Secondary—When is sustained by a pathological process not arising in the peritoneal space (myocardial infarction, pulmonary embolism, sepsis, pneumonia, leukemia, solid neoplasm in other district, infections, massive transfusion) (Fig. 17.5). Rarely ACS can be considered chronic in particular patient (Fig. 17.6).
- Tertiary—(Persistent or ongoing) ACS persistent despite some treatments).

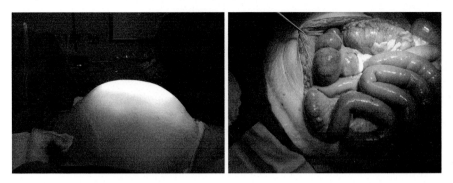

Fig. 17.5 Acute abdominal compartment syndrome in CPR for acute myocardial infarction 36 h before. Dead after 24 h after decompression

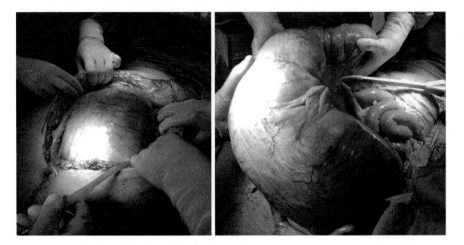

Fig. 17.6 Chronic ACS in a 42-year-old-man with severe obesity, BMI of 55.5,with a history of diabetes and hypertension and BDZ treatment

Some clinical characterizations have to be described. The ACS arising during the recovery has a worse prognosis than if present at admittance. The developing of ACS is a critical element in the clinical course of the patient. It means that the patient is getting weak. Little variations in the grading of the abdominal pressure can determine strong variations in the clinical status of the patient. Clinical diagnosis is very simple. The devices for the measurement of the bladder pressure, insertable to the urinary catheter, are cheap and very useful for any patient also if not in ICU (Fig. 17.7).

It exists also an electronic device much less compliant in the clinical practice. In patients without or impracticable bladder, radiology has stated seven TC-related issues for diagnosing of abdominal compartment syndrome (Table 17.1).

The ACS is so called for the district involved, the abdomen itself. Clinical impact is so strong for the whole body that a multicompartment syndrome has been

Fig. 17.7 UnoMeter™—
Abdo-Pressure™ by
ConvaTec©

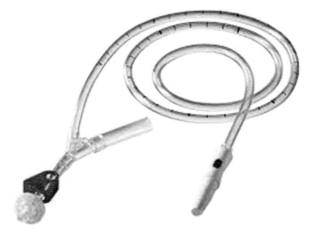

Table 17.1 CT scan features in intra-abdominal hypertension		
	1	Narrowing of upper intrahepatic inferior vena cava
	2	Small/large bowel wall thickening (>3 mm)
	3	Round belly signs (ratio > 0.80)
	4	Direct renal displacement or compression
	5	Compression and/or displacement of solid organ
	6	Bilateral femoral/inguinal hernation
	7	Elevation of the diaphragm

described [81–83]. Thoracic and cerebral districts can be involved, both or single, in this very dangerous "pressures storm".

The treatment of ACS is the decompressive laparotomy (DL). Very rarely, a medical reduction and/or resolution of the syndrome is possible by adequate fluid management, diuretics, or hemodialysis. Anecdotic episodes of surgical lateral incisions of the abdominal wall muscles have no scientific or literature support. With an abdominal pressure rounding 20 mmHg increasing and persisting DL is mandatory also without organ dysfunction or MODS. The surgical procedure is very simple and applicable also in hypercritic patients in ICU [84, 85] (Fig. 17.8).

After this maneuver the challenge is: close or not close the abdomen? We're completely agree with De Laet affirming "open up and keep the lymphatic open: they're the hydraulics of the body" [86] The peritoneal stomata play a pivotal role in the physiopathology of the peritonitis, their normal diameter of 4–12 cm in any acute abdominal condition arise to 23 cm. In a critical patient 24/48 h with a completely open abdomen can result in a dramatic improvement of the clinical status. The successive option are (1) Open abdomen with negative pressure (ABThera®) device in order to evacuate any infected or suspected fluid. (2) Single skin closure to avoid a dangerous increase in the abdominal pressure. In this phase all the peritoneal spaces, districts and organ and the patient as a "biological-system" are very sensible to any minimal dramatic oscillation of the internal abdominal pressures. (3) Definitive abdominal wall reconstruction with or without specific and dedicated protheses. The real enemy is the hurry in close the abdomen. These clinical critical

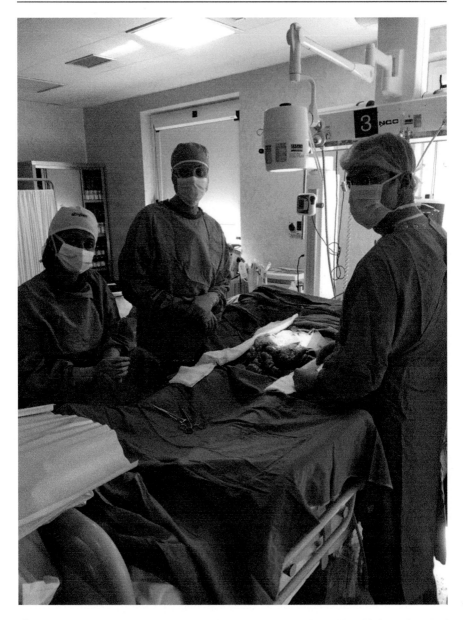

Fig. 17.8 Decompressive laparotomy in an ICU's hypercritic patient with ACS due to intestinal ischemia. (Courtesy of Mrs Maria Brisichella)

condition as AGI/ACS requires right times. We need to care, not simply cure, the patient, not its abdomen. The blind standard application of rigid protocols or guidelines is very dangerous, and any patient has its own story.

Acute Gastrointestinal Injury represents an old clinical situation recently recognized and described as syndrome in the literature. No specific therapy exists because it is nonspecific pathology. The cornerstones in the treatment are two: the diagnosis and the comprehension of its physiopathology.

It's absolutely necessary recognize AGI, any clinician could think to this clinical picture in any patient because as above reported "all is in the gut."

The second item is to treat the patient critical pathology (lung, heart, soft tissue, circulatory district, invasive infections, sepsis). Only the when AGI arises from a specific abdominal process the treatment is specific with the source control strategy. The ACS has a surgical way with the decompressive laparotomy. AGI is the expression of a man-failure as the cardiac arrhythmias, the Acute Kidney Injury (AKI), the Acute Lung Injury (ALI), and the ARDS. The different is in the structure of the gastrointestinal tube totally colonized by bacteria with a joint-venture essential for the life. Any pathological condition able to derange this equilibrium protected by a very thin layer called mucosa create a pathological condition with bacterial translocation, deep modifications in the bacterial burdens, shift in pathological condition of the saprophytic flora as trigger of the inflammatory and infective processes.

The precision medicine, the genomic, the proteomics, nanotechnology, the relationship between sepsis and infection phenotypes, and the microbiome knowledge are bringing to a therapy "tailored" for any critical clinical situation in any patient in any condition.

References

1. Mooneesinghe SR, Mythen MG, Das P, Rowan KM, Grocott MP. Risk stratification tools for predicting morbidity and mortality in adult patients undergoing major surgery: qualitative systematic review. Anesthesiology. 2013;119(4):959–81.
2. Knaus WA, Wagner DP, Draper EA, Zimmerman JE, Bergner M, Bastos PG, Sirio CA, Murphy DJ, Lotring T, Damiano A, et al. The APACHE III prognostic system. Risk prediction of hospital mortality for critically ill hospitalized adults. Chest. 1991;100(6):1619–36.
3. Copeland CC, Young A, Grogan T, Gabel E, Dhillon A, Gudzenko V. Preoperative risk stratification of critically ill patients. J Clin Anesth. 2017;39:122–7.
4. Mayhew D, Mendonca V, Murthy BVS. A review of ASA physical status - historical perspectives and modern developments. Anaesthesia. 2019;74(3):373–9.
5. Sankar A, Johnson SR, Beattie WS, Tait G, Wijeysundera DN. Reliability of the merican Society of Anesthesiologists physical status scale in clinical practice. Br J Anaesth. 2014;113(3):424–32.
6. García-Gigorro R. Sáez-de la Fuente I, Marín Mateos H, Andrés-Esteban EM, Sanchez-Izquierdo JA, Montejo-González JC. Utility of SOFA and Δ-SOFA scores for predicting outcome in critically ill patients from the emergency department. Eur J Emerg Med. 2018;25(6):387–93.
7. Wang H, Chen T, Wang H, Song Y, Li X, Wang J. A systematic review of the Physiological and Operative Severity Score for the enUmeration of Mortality and morbidity and its Portsmouth modification as predictors of post-operative morbidity and mortality in patients undergoing pancreatic surgery. Am J Surg. 2013;205(4):466–72.
8. Li H, Chen Y, Huo F, Wang Y, Zhang D. Association between acute gastrointestinal injury and biomarkers of intestinal barrier function in critically ill patients. BMC Gastroenterol. 2017;17(1):45.

9. Elke G, Felbinger TW, Heyland DK. Gastric residual volume in critically ill patients: a dead marker or still alive? Nutr Clin Pract. 2015;30(1):59–71.
10. Reintam Blaser A, Starkopf J, Malbrain ML. Abdominal signs and symptoms in intensive care patients. Anaesthesiol Intensive Ther. 2015;47(4):379–87.
11. Reintam Blaser A, Malbrain ML, Starkopf J, Fruhwald S, Jakob SM, De Waele J, Braun JP, Poeze M, Spies C. Gastrointestinal function in intensive care patients: terminology, definitions and management. Recommendations of the ESICM Working Group on Abdominal Problems. Intensive Care Med. 2012;38(3):384–94.
12. Taylor RW. Gut motility issues in critical illness. Crit Care Clin. 2016;32(2):191–201.
13. Malbrain ML, De Laet I. It's all in the gut: introducing the concept of acute bowel injury and acute intestinal distress syndrome.... Crit Care Med. 2009;37(1):365–6.
14. Chen H, Zhang H, Li W, Wu S, Wang W. Acute gastrointestinal injury in the intensive care unit: a retrospective study. Ther Clin Risk Manag. 2015;11:1523–9.
15. Zhang D, Li Y, Ding L, Fu Y, Dong X, Li H. Prevalence and outcome of acute gastrointestinal injury in critically ill patients: a systematic review and meta-analysis. Medicine (Baltimore). 2018;97(43):e12970.
16. Li H, Zhang D, Wang Y, Zhao S. Association between acute gastrointestinal injury grading system and disease severity and prognosis in critically ill patients: a multicenter, prospective, observational study in China. J Crit Care. 2016;36:24–8.
17. Coffey JC, O'Leary DP. The mesentery: structure, function, and role in disease. Lancet Gastroenterol Hepatol. 2016;1(3):238–47.
18. Capobianco A, Cottone L, Monno A, Manfredi AA, Rovere-Querini P. The peritoneum: healing, immunity, and diseases. J Pathol. 2017;243(2):137–47.
19. Coffey JC, Dillon M, Sehgal R, et al. Mesenteric-based surgery exploits gastrointestinal, peritoneal, mesenteric and fascial continuity from duodenojejunal fl exure to the anorectal junction—a review. Dig Surg. 2015;32:291–300.
20. Culligan K, Coffey JC, Kiran RP, Kalady M, Lavery IC, Remzi FH. The mesocolon: a prospective observational study. Color Dis. 2012;14:421–8.
21. Heel KA, Hall JC. Peritoneal defences and peritoneum-associated lymphoid tissue. Br J Surg. 1996;83:1031–6.
22. Healy JC, Reznek RH. The peritoneum, mesenteries and omenta: normal anatomy and pathological processes. Eur Radiol. 1998;8:886–900.
23. Di Paolo N, Sacchi G. Atlas of peritoneal histology. Perit Dial Int. 2000;20(Suppl 3):S5–S96.
24. Mais DD. Quick compendium of clinical pathology. 2nd ed. Chicago: American Society for Clinical Pathology Press; 2009.
25. Blackburn SC, Stanton MP. Anatomy and physiology of the peritoneum. Semin Pediatr Surg. 2014;23:326–30.
26. Standring S. Gray's anatomy: the anatomical basis of clinical practice. London: Elsevier Health Sciences; 2015.
27. Garside P, Millington O, Smith KM. The anatomy of mucosal immune responses. Ann N Y Acad Sci. 2004;1029:9–15.
28. Bilsborough J, Viney JL. Getting to the guts of immune regulation. Immunology. 2002;106(2):139–43.
29. Deane A, Chapman MJ, Fraser RJL, Horowitz M. Bench-to-bedside review: the gut as an endocrine organ in the critically ill. Crit Care. 2010;14:228.
30. Kang W, Kudsk KA. Is there evidence that the gut contributes to mucosal immunity in humans? J Parenter Enter Nutr. 2007;31:246–58.
31. Schmidt WE. The intestine, an endocrine organ. Digestion. 1997;58(Suppl 1):56–8.
32. Alverdy JC. Microbiome medicine: this changes everything. J Am Coll Surg. 2018;226(5):719–29.
33. Eckerle M, Ambroggio L, Puskarich MA, et al. Metabolomics as a driver in advancing precision medicine in sepsis. Pharmacotherapy. 2017;37:1023–32.
34. Allen-Vercoe E. Petrof EO the microbiome: what it means for medicine. Br J Gen Pract. 2014;64(620):118–9.

35. Amedei A, Boem F. I've gut a feeling: microbiota impacting the conceptual and experimental perspectives of personalized medicine. Int J Mol Sci. 2018;19(12):3756.
36. Chang CS, Kao CY. Current understanding of the gut microbiota shaping mechanisms. J Biomed Sci. 2019;26(1):59.
37. Lederer AK, Pisarski P, Kousoulas L, Fichtner-Feigl S, Hess C, Huber R. Postoperative changes of the microbiome: are surgical complications related to the gut flora? A systematic review. BMC Surg. 2017;17(1):125.
38. van Praagh JB, de Goffau MC, Bakker IS, van Goor H, Harmsen HJM, Olinga P, Havenga K. Mucus microbiome of anastomotic tissue during surgery has predictive value for colorectal anastomotic leakage. Ann Surg. 2019;269(5):911–6.
39. Guyton K, Alverdy JC. The gut microbiota and gastrointestinal surgery. Nat Rev Gastroenterol Hepatol. 2017;14(1):43–54.
40. Gershuni VM, Friedman ES. The microbiome-host interaction as a potential driver of anastomotic leak. Curr Gastroenterol Rep. 2019;21(1):4.
41. Skowron KB, Shogan BD, Rubin DT, Hyman NH. The new frontier: the intestinal microbiome and surgery. J Gastrointest Surg. 2018;22(7):1277–85.
42. Fleming CR, Remington M. Intestinal failure. In: Hill GL, editor. Nutrition and the surgical patient. Edinburgh: Churchill Livingstone; 1981. p. 219–35.
43. Pironi L, Arends J, Baxter J, Bozzetti F, Peláez RB, Cuerda C, Forbes A, Gabe S, Gillanders L, Holst M, Jeppesen PB, Joly F, Kelly D, Klek S, Irtun Ø, Olde Damink SW, Panisic M, Rasmussen HH, Staun M, Szczepanek K, Van Gossum A, Wanten G, Schneider SM, Shaffer J; Home Artificial Nutrition & Chronic Intestinal Failure; Acute Intestinal Failure Special Interest Groups of ESPEN. ESPEN endorsed recommendations. Definition and classification of intestinal failure in adults. Clin Nutr. 2015;34(2):171–80.
44. O'Keefe SJD, Buchman AL, Fishbein TM, Jeejeebhoy KN, Jeppesen PB, Shaffer J. Short bowel syndrome and intestinal failure: consensus definitions and overview. Clin Gastroenterol Hepatol. 2006;4:6–10.
45. Nightingale JMD, Small M, Jeejeebhoy K. Intestinal failure definition and classification comments: good in parts but could be better. Clin Nutr. 2016;35(2):536.
46. Pironi L. Definitions of intestinal failure and the short bowel syndrome. Best Pract Res Clin Gastroenterol. 2016;30(2):173–85.
47. Ukleja A. Altered GI motility in critically ill patients: current understanding of pathophysiology, clinical impact, and diagnostic approach. Nutr Clin Pract. 2010;25(1):16–25.
48. Pironi L, Corcos O, Forbes A, Holst M, Joly F, Jonkers C, Klek S, Lal S, Blaser AR, Rollins KE, Sasdelli AS, Shaffer J, Van Gossum A, Wanten G, Zanfi C, Lobo DN. ESPEN Acute and Chronic Intestinal Failure Special Interest Groups. Intestinal failure in adults: recommendations from the ESPEN expert groups. Clin Nutr. 2018;37(6 Pt A):1798–809.
49. Reintam Blaser A, Malbrain ML, Starkopf J, Fruhwald S, Jakob SM, De Waele J, Braun JP, Poeze M, Spies C. Gastrointestinal function in intensive care patients: terminology, definitions and management. Recommendations of the ESICM Working Group on Abdominal Problems. Intensive Care Med. 2012;38(3):384–94.
50. Lal S, Teubner A, Shaffer JL. Review article: intestinal failure. Aliment Pharmacol Therapeut. 2006;24:19–31.
51. Zhang D, Li Y, Ding L, Fu Y, Dong X, Li H. Prevalence and outcome of acute gastrointestinal injury in critically ill patients: a systematic review and meta-analysis. Medicine (Baltimore). 2018;97(43):e12970.
52. Reintam A, Parm P, Kitus R, Starkopf J, Kern H. Gastrointestinal failure score in critically ill patients: a prospective observational study. Crit Care. 2008;12(4):R90.
53. Zhang D, Fu R, Li Y, Li H, Li Y, Li H. Comparison of the clinical characteristics and prognosis of primary versus secondary acute gastrointestinal injury in critically ill patients. J Intensive Care. 2017;5:26.
54. Li H, Zhang D, Wang Y, Zhao S. Association between acute gastrointestinal injury grading system and disease severity and prognosis in critically ill patients: a multicenter, prospective, observational study in China. J Crit Care. 2016;36:24–8.

55. Hu B, Sun R, Wu A, Ni Y, Liu J, Guo F, Ying L, Ge G, Ding A, Shi Y, Liu C, Xu L, Jiang R, Lu J, Lin R, Zhu Y, Wu W, Xie B. Severity of acute gastrointestinal injury grade is a predictor of all-cause mortality in critically ill patients: a multicenter, prospective, observational study. Crit Care. 2017;21(1):188.

56. Berg RD, Garlington AW. Translocation of certain indigenous bacteria from the gastrointestinal tract to the mesenteric lymph nodes and other organs in the gnotobiotic mouse model. Infect Immun. 1979;23:403–11.

57. Meng M, Klingensmith NJ, Coopersmith CM. New insights into the gut as the driver of critical illness and organ failure. Curr Opin Crit Care. 2017;23(2):143–8.

58. Sertaridou E, Papaioannou V, Kolios G, Pneumatikos I. Gut failure in critical care: old school versus new school. Ann Gastroenterol. 2015;28(3):309–22.

59. Assimakopoulos SF, Triantos C, Thomopoulos K, Fligou F, Maroulis I, Marangos M, Gogos CA. Gut-origin sepsis in the critically ill patient: pathophysiology and treatment. Infection. 2018;46(6):751–60.

60. Deitch EA. Bacterial translocation or lymphatic drainage of toxic products from the gut: what is important in human beings? Surgery. 2002;131:241–4.

61. Deitch EA. Gut-origin sepsis: evolution of a concept. Surgeon. 2012;10:350–6.

62. Clark JA, Coopersmith CM. Intestinal crosstalk: a new paradigm for understanding the gut as the "motor" of critical illness. Shock. 2007;28(4):384–93.

63. Chang JX, Chen S, Ma LP, et al. Functional and morphological changes of the gut barrier during the restitution process after hemorrhagic shock. World J Gastroenterol. 2005;11:5485–91.

64. Fay KT, Ford ML, Coopersmith CM. The intestinal microenvironment in sepsis. Biochim Biophys Acta Mol Basis Dis. 2017;1863(10 Pt B):2574–83.

65. Lyons JD, Coopersmith CM. Pathophysiology of the gut and the microbiome in the host response. Pediatr Crit Care Med. 2017;18(3_suppl Suppl 1):S46–9.

66. Klingensmith NJ, Coopersmith CM. The gut as the motor of multiple organ dysfunction in critical illness. Crit Care Clin. 2016;32(2):203–12.

67. Otani S, Coopersmith CM. Gut integrity in critical illness. J Intensive Care. 2019;7:17.

68. Herbers AH, Feuth T, Donnelly JP, Blijlevens NM. Citrulline-based assessment score: first choice for measuring and monitoring intestinal failure after high-dose chemotherapy. Ann Oncol. 2010;21(8):1706–11.

69. Piton G, Manzon C, Monnet E, Cypriani B, Barbot O, Navellou JC, Carbonnel F, Capellier G. Plasma citrulline kinetics and prognostic value in critically ill patients. Intensive Care Med. 2010;36(4):702–6.

70. Piton G, Manzon C, Cypriani B, Carbonnel F, Capellier G. Acute intestinal failure in critically ill patients: is plasma citrulline the right marker? Intensive Care Med. 2011;37(6):911–7.

71. Reintam Blaser A, Jakob SM, Starkopf J. Gastrointestinal failure in the ICU. Curr Opin Crit Care. 2016;22(2):128–41.

72. Klek S, Forbes A, Gabe S, Holst M, Wanten G, Irtun Ø, Damink SO, Panisic-Sekeljic M, Pelaez RB, Pironi L, Blaser AR, Rasmussen HH, Schneider SM, Thibault R, RGJ V, Shaffer J. Management of acute intestinal failure: a position paper from the European Society for Clinical Nutrition and Metabolism (ESPEN) Special Interest Group. Clin Nutr. 2016;35(6):1209–18.

73. Madl C, Druml W. Gastrointestinal disorders of the critically ill. Systemic consequences of ileus. Best Pract Res Clin Gastroenterol. 2003;17(3):445–56.

74. Baue AE. The role of the gut in the development of multiple organ dysfunction in cardiothoracic patients. Ann Thorac Surg. 1993;55(4):822–9.

75. Balogh ZJ, Leppäniemi A. The neglected (abdominal) compartment: what is new at the beginning of the 21st century? World J Surg. 2009;33(6):1109.

76. Kaussen T, Otto J, Steinau G, Höer J, Srinivasan PK, Schachtrupp A. Recognition and management of abdominal compartment syndrome among German anesthetists and surgeons: a national survey. Ann Intensive Care. 2012;5(2, Suppl 1):S7.

77. Arnold RC, Dellinger RP, Parrillo JE, Chansky ME, Lotano VE, McCoy JV, Jones AE, Shapiro NI, Hollenberg SM, Trzeciak S. Discordance between microcirculatory alterations and arterial pressure in patients with hemodynamic instability. J Crit Care. 2012;27(5):531.e1–7.

78. Trzeciak S, Dellinger RP, Parrillo JE, Guglielmi M, Bajaj J, Abate NL, Arnold RC, Colilla S, Zanotti S, Hollenberg SM. Microcirculatory alterations in resuscitation and shock investigators. Early microcirculatory perfusion derangements in patients with severe sepsis and septic shock: relationship to hemodynamics, oxygen transport, and survival. Ann Emerg Med. 2007;49(1):88–98, 98.e1–98.e2.
79. Edul VS, Ince C, Navarro N, Previgliano L, Risso-Vazquez A, Rubatto PN, Dubin A. Dissociation between sublingual and gut microcirculation in the response to a fluid challenge in postoperative patients with abdominal sepsis. Ann Intensive Care. 2014;4:39.
80. Olofsson PH, Berg S, Ahn HC, Brudin LH, Vikström T, Johansson KJ. Gastrointestinal microcirculation and cardiopulmonary function during experimentally increased intra-abdominal pressure. Crit Care Med. 2009;37(1):230–9.
81. Malbrain ML, Wilmer A. The polycompartment syndrome: towards an understanding of the interactions between different compartments! Intensive Care Med. 2007;33(11):1869–72.
82. Scalea TM, Bochicchio GV, Habashi N, McCunn M, Shih D, McQuillan K, Aarabi B. Increased intra-abdominal, intrathoracic, and intracranial pressure after severe brain injury: multiple compartment syndrome. J Trauma. 2007;62(3):647–56; discussion 656.
83. Youssef AM, Hamidian Jahromi A, Vijay CG, Granger DN, Alexander JS. Intra-abdominal hypertension causes reversible blood-brain barrier disruption. J Trauma Acute Care Surg. 2012;72(1):183–8.
84. Piper GL, Maerz LL, Schuster KM, Maung AA, Luckianow GM, Davis KA, Kaplan LJ. When the ICU is the operating room. J Trauma Acute Care Surg. 2013;74(3):871–5.
85. Seternes A, Fasting S, Klepstad P, Mo S, Dahl T, Björck M, Wibe A. Bedside dressing changes for open abdomen in the intensive care unit is safe and time and staff efficient. Crit Care. 2016;20(1):164.
86. De Laet IE, Ravyts M, Vidts W, Valk J, De Waele JJ, Malbrain ML. Current insights in intra-abdominal hypertension and abdominal compartment syndrome: open the abdomen and keep it open! Langenbeck's Arch Surg. 2008;393(6):833–47.

Infections in Trauma Patients

18

Inge A. M. Van Erp, Sarah Y. Mikdad, and April E. Mendoza

18.1 Introduction

Over $80 billion dollars are spent each year for hospital costs associated with injuries, with septic complications being the main reason for excess costs in care [1]. Trauma patients have increased complications when compared to elective surgical patients with the most common being surgical site infections, urinary tract infections, and pneumonia [1]. For the trauma patients that survive their initial injury and develop hospital-acquired complications, sepsis is the most common cause of in-patient mortality [1]. It is therefore imperative to develop ways to prevent, identify, and provide effective treatments to improve outcomes and reduce costs.

Posttraumatic shock alters the immune response fundamentally with a shift toward a heavy reliance on innate immunity [2]. An exaggerated innate immune response is likely responsible for the so-called persistent inflammation, immunosuppression and catabolism syndrome (PICS), which drives the observed susceptibility to nosocomial infections and multiple organ dysfunction [3]. This undoubtedly complex response involves the interaction of pathogen-associated molecular patterns (PAMPs), damage-associated molecular proteins (DAMPs), and immune cellular receptors [4, 5].

In this chapter, we focus on the most common infections after traumatic injury such as healthcare-associated infections, but also injury-specific infections, which include surgical sites, infections complicating embolization and the rare overwhelming postsplenectomy sepsis (OPSI).

I. A. M. Van Erp
Department of Neurosurgery, Leiden University Medical Center, Leiden, The Netherlands

Division of Trauma, Emergency Surgery, and Surgical Critical Care, Department of Surgery, Massachusetts General Hospital, Boston, MA, USA

S. Y. Mikdad · A. E. Mendoza (✉)
Division of Trauma, Emergency Surgery, and Surgical Critical Care, Department of Surgery, Massachusetts General Hospital, Boston, MA, USA
e-mail: AEMENDOZA@mgh.harvard.edu

© Springer Nature Switzerland AG 2021
M. Sartelli et al. (eds.), *Infections in Surgery*, Hot Topics in Acute Care Surgery and Trauma, https://doi.org/10.1007/978-3-030-62116-2_18

18.2   Common Postoperative Complications: Healthcare-Associated Infections

Healthcare-associated infections (HAIs) are a major burden in patients admitted to the intensive care unit as they are associated with increased mortality, length of stay, costs, and bacterial resistance [6]. Trauma patients are especially at high risk for the development of infections due to disruption in tissue integrity and impaired host defense mechanisms [7]. Trauma patients have an infection rate ranging from 2–37% [8]. If diagnosed with sepsis, trauma patients have a six-fold higher risk of mortality, whereas HAIs complicating other inpatients result in nearly 1.5–2-fold higher risk [7]. Furthermore, infections complicating a trauma admission worsen functional status and increase healthcare usage up to a year after injury [9]. Catheter-associated urinary tract infections (CAUTIs), ventilator-associated pneumonias (VAPs), central line-associated bloodstream infections (CLABSIs), and surgical site infections (SSIs) remain the most common and therefore the most important HAIs in trauma patients [10].

18.2.1 Urinary Tract Infections

UTI is the most common nosocomial infection (40%) and approximately 80% of the healthcare-related UTIs are associated with urinary catheter use [11]. Trauma patients are particularly prone to CAUTIs as the degree of injury severity independently correlates with the risk of developing an UTI [11]. The risk of developing a CAUTI increases with the duration of catherization and may reach 50% with each day of use [12]. In the trauma population, UTI does result in significant morbidity and has been associated with an increase in mortality, especially in older patients [11]. Injuries that require chronic catheter usage such as injuries of the spinal cord, sacrum, sacral nerve roots, and pelvic nerves are associated with increased UTI. Additionally, undiagnosed or misdiagnosed urethral injuries can also result in chronic UTI [13]. In 2008, the Centers for Medicare & Medicaid Services (CMS) stopped reimbursing hospitals for the care of CAUTIs. Initially, the CMS policy had no measurable effect on the rate of CAUTIs, however, recent studies demonstrate a decline in incidence of CAUTIs and also CLABSIs [14, 15]. There is some evidence that nurse-driven protocols have improved CAUTI rates after implementation of an education program and a urinary catheter protocol [16, 17].

18.2.2 Hospital-Acquired Pneumonias

Important risk factors for development of hospital-acquired pneumonias (HAP) in trauma patients include aspiration, chest or upper abdominal surgery, frequent transport for imaging, polytrauma, supine position (for logroll precautions), and prolonged intubation [18–20]. Patients with severe traumatic brain injury (TBI) are prone to develop HAP for a multitude reasons ranging from a decreased level of consciousness, need for frequent patient transport, and prolonged ventilatory support [19]. Halperin et al. have suggested that the use of a mobile CT for such neurologic patients was associated with a reduction in HAPs [19].

VAP can develop ≥48 h after endotracheal intubation and has a reported incidence ranging from 8–44% in trauma patients [21]. As the oral flora of critically ill patients differs from normal healthy adults, lack of effective oral hygiene was thought to introduce respiratory pathogens resulting in VAP. However, the evidence of oral hygiene has remained controversial. While there is some evidence that oral hygiene with chlorhexidine may decrease VAP, this does not appear to reduce mortality, ventilatory-days or ICU length of stay [22]. Early tracheostomy has long been advocated to improve pulmonary toilet and possibly reduce the incidence of VAP. However, this benefit also remains unclear as the data regarding the incidence of pneumonia is conflicting [23, 24]. Two randomized trials failed to show an effect on mortality, prevalence of VAP or hospital length of stay with early tracheostomy [25, 26]. Data remains insufficient to show clear benefit to early tracheostomy (within four days) for mechanically ventilated patients in the ICU [27].

VAP prevention bundles, involving the implementation of various measures attempting to reduce the incidence of VAP amongst high-risk patients, appear promising. The effectiveness of these interventions in a coordinated way seems promising but remains under investigation [28]. High-quality evidence with compliance is needed [29].

18.2.3 Central-Line-Associated Bloodstream Infection

Studies have estimated CLABSIs account for 84,000–204,000 infection per year at a cost of up to 21 billion dollars per year [30]. CLABSI rates among trauma patients are considered 1.5–2-fold higher than in the general ICU population [28].

Peripherally inserted central venous catheters (PICC) are gaining in popularity due to their perceived safety and longevity as an access option. In both centrally inserted central catheters (CICC) and PICC, the rate of bloodstream infection increases with the higher number of lumens and catheter diameter. The incidence rate of CLABSI after PICC placement varies from 16–29% [31]. With regard to the insertion site, a multicenter trial showed that subclavian vein catheterization was associated with a lowest risk of bloodstream infection compared to femoral-vein catheterization [32]. The most recent Institute for Healthcare Improvement (IHI) guidelines recommend avoiding the femoral vein but the risk of CLABSI for femoral insertion sites remains inconclusive [33]. There appears no benefit in antibiotic prophylaxis for central venous catheter placement, and a meta-analysis showed no significant difference in infection rate comparing antibiotics versus no antibiotics [34].

Several systematic reviews have demonstrated that antimicrobial-impregnated dressings and catheters reduce CLABSI and colonization, but none have shown a reduction in sepsis or mortality [35, 36]. The implementation of central line bundles which include a set of evidence-based interventions intended to be implemented together, have been proposed as another method to reduce CLABSI [37]. However, variability in compliance exists at the national level [37].

18.2.4 Surgical Site Infections

Important procedure-related risk factors that increase the prevalence of SSI include emergency settings and wound classification [38].

Damage control procedures are highly associated with wound infections where 1 out of 5 trauma laparotomies develop an deep organ space surgical site infection [39]. Timely closure and serial abdominal wound lavage or irrigation are believed to reduce this risk. However, there is little high-quality evidence that supports any intracavitary lavage or antimicrobial irrigation for the reduction of SSI [40, 41].

Negative pressure wound therapy (NPWT) is increasingly being used prophylactically on closed incision wounds and wounds healing by secondary intention in case of contaminated wounds to prevent SSI [42, 43]. NPWT is thought to promote wound healing and prevent infection by reducing bacterial contamination [44]. Although many trials support NPWT, the role of NPWT in trauma patients, and especially in contaminated wounds, remains under investigation [45, 46]. NPWT does appear to promote wound healing and reduce infectious complications, but large studies are warranted [47].

18.3 Solid Organ Infectious Complications

18.3.1 Liver

The liver is the most commonly injured abdominal organ, with the majority of injuries occurring secondary to blunt force trauma during motor vehicle collisions [48]. Complications following operative management are common and the incidence of complications increases with the grade of liver injury. Over the past four decades, advances in diagnostic management and treatment have led to a shift in paradigm. Currently, the standard of care for hemodynamically stable patients has evolved toward an emphasis on nonoperative management (NOM) [49]. This has resulted in decreased mortality [50], with success rates greater than 90% [51, 52]. However, injury grade is an important risk factor for complications in that grade IV and V liver injuries have higher bile leaks, hemobilia, hepatic necrosis, and abscess, and delayed hemorrhage [53–56]. Hepatic abscesses occur in 4% of the nonoperatively managed liver injuries and have a 10% mortality rate [57].

Hepatic angioembolization (AE) is often used as a valuable tool to assist in successful NOM. It is often employed in conjunction with damage control packing to assist in hemorrhage control. AE is associated with hepatic necrosis, and its resultant complications such as hepatic abscess, sepsis, bacteremia, liver dysfunction and coagulopathy. The rate of hepatic necrosis after AE is reported from 0–42% [52].

Gallbladder necrosis can occur after AE of the right hepatic artery, and has a reported incidence of 0–7% after AE [58].

Postoperative perihepatic abscess and bile collections are frequently managed by parenteral antibiotics and drainage [59]. Occasionally, surgical debridement is required for source control if conservative management fails.

18.3.2 Spleen

Splenic preservation is believed to offer an immunologic advantage to the host especially in regard to encapsulated microbial infections. For hemodynamically stable splenic injury patients, the standard of care is nonoperative management and 90% of splenic trauma patients are treated successfully in this manner [60]. Splenic AE is frequently employed for splenic salvage in a hemodynamically stable patient [61]. In this section we will discuss the risk and management of OPSI after splenectomy and infectious complications associated with splenic preservation particularly after AE.

Splenectomy is an independent risk factor for postoperative infectious complications, such as intraabdominal abscesses, wound infections, pneumonia, and sepsis [62]. Nonetheless, asplenic patients have a unique risk for overwhelming postsplenectomy infection (OPSI). Although rare, with an incidence of 0.05–2%, it is associated with significant morbidity and mortality [63]. Mortality after OPSI has been reported at 50–70% and most deaths occur within 24 h [64]. Symptoms of OPSI can initially present as flu-like symptoms, but this can progress to the rapid development of septic shock, multiorgan failure, and death [65].

Multiple interventions are considered to prevent the development of OPSI. Appropriate and timely vaccination is imperative, but prophylactic antibiotic therapy, early management of animal bites, and malaria prophylaxis for patients travelling to endemic countries should also be considered. Patient- and family-counselling is pivotal in order to educate for the signs and symptoms as the risk is considered lifelong [66].

Current guidelines highly recommend that patients receive either 13-valent or 23-valent pneumococcal vaccine and vaccines for *Haemophilus influenzae* type B and *Neisseria meningitidis* [53, 67]. Timing of vaccination after an emergency splenectomy is favorable at 14 days postoperatively, as there is evidence that the antibody response is optimal at this time [54–56]. However, this is not always an option and therefore immunization upon discharge is acceptable. Yearly influenza vaccination is recommended in all asplenic adults and in children older than 6 months [68].

Immunization requirements after AE remains undetermined [69, 70]. In vitro studies suggest that patients remain immunocompetent after splenic embolization [70–73], and currently there are no cases that have reported the development of OPSI in this population.

18.4   Pelvic Trauma Infections

Complex pelvic trauma carries a significant morbidity and mortality, and typically requires a coordinated approach involving a team of surgical specialists [74]. Priorities of initial management include hemorrhage control and resuscitation. Common maneuvers for hemorrhage control involve fracture stabilization with a pelvic binder, angioembolization, preperitoneal packing, and less commonly, resuscitative endovascular balloon occlusion (REBOA). These hemorrhage control techniques can produce extensive tissue necrosis and result in unique infectious complications. The proximity and high-energy mechanisms that produce complex pelvic trauma can frequently result in associated injuries involving the bladder, urethra, vagina, nerves, anal sphincter, and rectum [74]. Management of open pelvic fractures involving these organ spaces require a thoughtful and often aggressive approach. These injuries are often associated with substantial tissue contamination with an elevated risk of pelvic sepsis. The standard management of concomitant rectal trauma includes proximal diversion of the fecal stream [75]. Performance of distal rectal washout and presacral drainage for the prevention of pelvic or presacral infections after open pelvic fractures has not been shown to improve survival and reduce infectious complications [76, 77].

Damage control angiography for pelvic bleeding often involves selective or nonselective embolization of pelvic arteries [78]. The rate of complications has ranged from 0–24% after AE [78–80]. However, there are reports of bilateral internal iliac artery embolization producing ischemic complications such as gluteal ischemia, bladder necrosis, and deep pelvic space infections [81]. However, AE does appear preferable over operative internal iliac artery ligation with fewer infections observed after AE [82].

Preperitoneal pelvic packing (PPP) is a common approach to control severe pelvic hemorrhage. However, pelvic infections remain a major morbidity varying from 10 to over 20% [83, 84]. Subsequent repacking results in a significant increase in pelvic space infections [85]. Early removal of packed materials should be considered within 1–2 days to reduce the risk of infection [86].

REBOA is a more recent, albeit underutilized form of pelvic hemorrhage control [87]. The true incidence of ischemic complications and subsequent deep space infections following REBOA remains largely unknown. In a recent study evaluating outcomes after REBOA within a national database, REBOA patients had higher incidence of acute kidney injury and amputation which is likely the result of profound tissue ischemia and necrosis [88]. However, whether these patients have a higher risk for infection remains unknown, and further studies are warranted to investigate the incidence of infections after REBOA placement.

18.5   Open Fractures

The development of infection after open fractures remains a serious complication. The rate of infection ranges from less than 1% in grade I open fractures to 50% in grade III fractures [43]. Infectious complications can be classified as acute, which include superficial and deep soft tissue infections, and chronic infections. Chronic infections can result in nonunion, flap failure, and osteomyelitis [43]. Deep infections leading to osteomyelitis and intramedullary sepsis are difficult to manage. The rate of secondary amputation from chronic osteomyelitis ranges from 4 to 10% [89]. This section will point out the proper management of open fracture wounds to reduce infection rates, including irrigation and debridement (I&D), tetanus and antibiotic prophylaxis, and early tissue coverage with plastic surgery assistance.

The initial management of open fractures requires thorough I&D to prevent infection and promote wound and bone healing. Standard practice of I&D within 6 h of injury remains controversial as time to I&D does not affect the development of local infectious complications if performed within 24 h [90]. Soft tissue reconstruction in more severe injuries should be performed early, within the first week after injury, because delays have been associated with increased infectious complications [91].

Any patient presenting with an open fracture or tetanus prone wound should be interrogated for tetanus toxoid immunization. If tetanus immunization status is unknown, the patient should be given a tetanus toxoid booster or human tetanus immune globin (HTIG). If the patient has completed vaccination and the last dose is less than 5 years prior, vaccination is not warranted [92]. Tetanus vaccination older than 5 years warrants tetanus toxoid administration. HTIG is indicated if the patient is immunocompromised or if the last dose is more than 10 years prior [92].

Choice of antibiotic prophylaxis is guided by the Gustilo and Anderson classification [93, 94] and the tenth edition of the Advanced Trauma Life Support (ATLS) [95] (Table 18.1). In patients with open fractures, antibiotics need to be administered as soon as possible, as delay of antibiotic administration beyond 3 h is related to an increased risk of infection [95].

Patients with type I and II open fractures should be given a first-generation, gram-positive cephalosporin (cefazolin). In patients with serious β lactam allergy, clindamycin is an appropriate alternative [96]. Type III open fractures benefit from gram-positive and gram-negative coverage. A broad-spectrum gram-positive and negative should be considered for fractures associated with fecal or clostridial contamination. Nevertheless, clinicians often overuse broad-spectrum antibiotics rather than guideline antibiotic recommendations regardless of the injury severity [97]. Most guidelines support early systemic antibiotics, but local antibiotic regimens remain poorly studied and optimal practice guidelines remain elusive [97].

The Eastern Association for the Surgery of Trauma (EAST) Practice Management Guidelines recommend antibiotics to be discontinued 24 h after successful wound closure for type I and type II fractures. For type III fractures, antibiotics should be continued for 72 h subsequent to the injury, but not >24 h subsequent to successful soft tissue coverage of the wound [98].

Weight-based dosing in open fracture infection treatment is of great importance as underdosing of antibiotics has been found to be relatively common in trauma patients [99].

In conclusion, patients with open fractures should be treated as soon as possible with intravenous antibiotics and irrigation and debridement. Further management decisions, like tetanus prophylaxis, should be based on the patient history.

Table 18.1 Intravenous antibiotic weight-based dosing guidelines [95]

Open fracture type	Recommended systemic antibiotic prophylaxis	Weight-based dosing
Gustilo and Anderson type I	First-generation cephalosporin (cefazolin) *β lactam allergy:* clindamycin if anaphylactic penicillin allergy	*Cefazolin:* <50 kg: 1 g Q 8 h 50–100 kg: 2 g Q 8 h >100 kg: 3 g Q 8 h *Clindamycin:* <80 kg: 600 mg Q h >80 kg: 900 mg Q h
Gustilo and Anderson type II	First-generation cephalosporin (cefazolin) *β lactam allergy:* clindamycin if anaphylactic penicillin allergy	*Cefazolin:* <50 kg: 1 g Q 8 h 50–100 kg: 2 g Q 8 h >100 kg: 3 g Q 8 h *Clindamycin:* <80 kg: 600 mg Q h >80 kg: 900 mg Q h
Gustilo and Anderson type III	First-generation cephalosporin (*β lactam allergy:* clindamycin if anaphylactic penicillin allergy) **plus** aminoglycoside (gentamicin)	*Cefazolin:* <50 kg: 1 g Q 8 h 50–100 kg: 2 g Q 8 h >100 kg: 3 g Q 8 h *Clindamycin:* <80 kg: 600 mg Q h >80 kg: 900 mg Q h *Gentamicin:* 2.5 mg/kg for child (or <50 kg) 5 mg/kg for adult
Farmyard, soil, or standing water, irrespective of wound size or severity	Third-generation cephalosporin (piperacillin/tazobactam) *β lactam allergy:* consult Infectious Disease Department	*Piperacillin/tazobactam:* <100 kg: 3.375 g Q 6 h >100 kg: 4.5 g Q 6 h

18.6   Conclusion

Infections after major injury remain a critical challenge for the trauma population. Alterations in the immune response and compromised integrity of normal tissue barriers likely make these patients especially susceptible. Prompt surgical control of contamination, restoration of physiologic derangements, and adherence to best practices with sterile techniques remain critical to infection prevention. Effective treatment of infections requires timely recognition and a high-index of suspicion.

References

1. Haider AH, Gupta S, Zogg CK, Kisat MT, Schupper A, Efron DT, et al. Beyond incidence: costs of complications in trauma and what it means for those who pay. Surgery. 2015;158(1):96–103.
2. Xiao W, Mindrinos MN, Seok J, Cuschieri J, Cuenca AG, Gao H, et al. A genomic storm in critically injured humans. J Exp Med. 2011;208(13):2581–90.

3. Gentile LF, Cuenca AG, Vanzant EL, Efron PA, McKinley B, Moore F, et al. Is there value in plasma cytokine measurements in patients with severe trauma and sepsis? Methods (San Diego, Calif). 2013;61(1):3–9.

4. Mollen KP, Anand RJ, Tsung A, Prince JM, Levy RM, Billiar TR. Emerging paradigm: toll-like receptor 4-sentinel for the detection of tissue damage. Shock (Augusta, Ga). 2006;26(5):430–7.

5. Zhang Q, Raoof M, Chen Y, Sumi Y, Sursal T, Junger W, et al. Circulating mitochondrial DAMPs cause inflammatory responses to injury. Nature. 2010;464(7285):104–7.

6. Rosenthal VD. International nosocomial infection control consortium (INICC) resources: INICC multidimensional approach and INICC surveillance online system. Am J Infect Control. 2016;44(6):e81–90.

7. Glance LG, Stone PW, Mukamel DB, Dick AW. Increases in mortality, length of stay, and cost associated with hospital-acquired infections in trauma patients. Arch Surg (Chicago, Ill: 1960). 2011;146(7):794–801.

8. Lazarus HM, Fox J, Burke JP, Lloyd JF, Snow GL, Mehta RR, et al. Trauma patient hospital-associated infections: risks and outcomes. J Trauma. 2005;59(1):188–94.

9. Czaja AS, Rivara FP, Wang J, Koepsell T, Nathens AB, Jurkovich GJ, et al. Late outcomes of trauma patients with infections during index hospitalization. J Trauma. 2009;67(4):805–14.

10. Rosenthal VD, Maki DG, Mehta Y, Leblebicioglu H, Memish ZA, Al-Mousa HH, et al. International nosocomial infection control consortium (INICC) report, data summary of 43 countries for 2007–2012. Device-associated module. Am J Infect Control. 2014;42(9):942–56.

11. Monaghan SF, Heffernan DS, Thakkar RK, Reinert SE, Machan JT, Connolly MD, et al. The development of a urinary tract infection is associated with increased mortality in trauma patients. J Trauma. 2011;71(6):1569–74.

12. Mota EC, Oliveira AC. Catheter-associated urinary tract infection: why do not we control this adverse event? Rev Esc Enferm U S P. 2019;53:e03452.

13. Tezval H, Tezval M, von Klot C, Herrmann TR, Dresing K, Jonas U, et al. Urinary tract injuries in patients with multiple trauma. World J Urol. 2007;25(2):177–84.

14. Thirukumaran CP, Glance LG, Temkin-Greener H, Rosenthal MB, Li Y. Impact of Medicare's nonpayment program on hospital-acquired conditions. Med Care. 2017;55(5):447–55.

15. Waters TM, Daniels MJ, Bazzoli GJ, Perencevich E, Dunton N, Staggs VS, et al. Effect of Medicare's nonpayment for hospital-acquired conditions: lessons for future policy. JAMA Intern Med. 2015;175(3):347–54.

16. Sampathkumar P. Reducing catheter-associated urinary tract infections in the ICU. Curr Opin Crit Care. 2017;23(5):372–7.

17. Reisinger JD, Wojcik A, Jenkins I, Edson B, Pegues DA, Greene L. The project protect infection prevention fellowship: a model for advancing infection prevention competency, quality improvement, and patient safety. Am J Infect Control. 2017;45(8):876–82.

18. Walaszek M, Kosiarska A, Gniadek A, Kolpa M, Wolak Z, Dobros W, et al. The risk factors for hospital-acquired pneumonia in the intensive care unit. Przegl Epidemiol. 2016;70(1):15–20, 107–110.

19. Halperin JJ, Moran S, Prasek D, Richards A, Ruggiero C, Maund C. Reducing hospital-acquired infections among the neurologically critically ill. Neurocrit Care. 2016;25(2):170–7.

20. Wang L, Li X, Yang Z, Tang X, Yuan Q, Deng L, et al. Semi-recumbent position versus supine position for the prevention of ventilator-associated pneumonia in adults requiring mechanical ventilation. Cochrane Database Syst Rev. 2016;1(1):Cd009946.

21. Lewis RH, Sharpe JP, Swanson JM, Fabian TC, Croce MA, Magnotti LJ. Reinventing the wheel: impact of prolonged antibiotic exposure on multidrug-resistant ventilator-associated pneumonia in trauma patients. J Trauma Acute Care Surg. 2018;85(2):256–62.

22. Hua F, Xie H, Worthington HV, Furness S, Zhang Q, Li C. Oral hygiene care for critically ill patients to prevent ventilator-associated pneumonia. Cochrane Database Syst Rev. 2016;10:Cd008367.

23. Ibrahim EH, Tracy L, Hill C, Fraser VJ, Kollef MH. The occurrence of ventilator-associated pneumonia in a community hospital: risk factors and clinical outcomes. Chest. 2001;120(2):555–61.
24. Nseir S, Di Pompeo C, Jozefowicz E, Cavestri B, Brisson H, Nyunga M, et al. Relationship between tracheotomy and ventilator-associated pneumonia: a case control study. Eur Respir J. 2007;30(2):314–20.
25. Terragni PP, Antonelli M, Fumagalli R, Faggiano C, Berardino M, Pallavicini FB, et al. Early vs late tracheotomy for prevention of pneumonia in mechanically ventilated adult ICU patients: a randomized controlled trial. JAMA. 2010;303(15):1483–9.
26. Young D, Harrison DA, Cuthbertson BH, Rowan K. Effect of early vs late tracheostomy placement on survival in patients receiving mechanical ventilation: the TracMan randomized trial. JAMA. 2013;309(20):2121–9.
27. Andriolo BN, Andriolo RB, Saconato H, Atallah AN, Valente O. Early versus late tracheostomy for critically ill patients. Cochrane Database Syst Rev. 2015;1:Cd007271.
28. Major JS, Welbourne J. Nosocomial infection in trauma intensive care. J Intensive Care Soc. 2015;16(3):193–8.
29. Pileggi C, Mascaro V, Bianco A, Nobile CGA, Pavia M. Ventilator bundle and its effects on mortality among ICU patients: a meta-analysis. Crit Care Med. 2018;46(7):1167–74.
30. Umscheid CA, Mitchell MD, Doshi JA, Agarwal R, Williams K, Brennan PJ. Estimating the proportion of healthcare-associated infections that are reasonably preventable and the related mortality and costs. Infect Control Hosp Epidemiol. 2011;32(2):101–14.
31. Duwadi S, Zhao Q, Budal BS. Peripherally inserted central catheters in critically ill patients - complications and its prevention: a review. Int J Nurs Sci. 2019;6(1):99–105.
32. Parienti JJ, Mongardon N, Megarbane B, Mira JP, Kalfon P, Gros A, et al. Intravascular complications of central venous catheterization by insertion site. N Engl J Med. 2015;373(13):1220–9.
33. Arvaniti K, Lathyris D, Blot S, Apostolidou-Kiouti F, Koulenti D, Haidich AB. Cumulative evidence of randomized controlled and observational studies on catheter-related infection risk of central venous catheter insertion site in ICU patients: a pairwise and network meta-analysis. Crit Care Med. 2017;45(4):e437–e48.
34. Johnson E, Babb J, Sridhar D. Routine antibiotic prophylaxis for totally implantable venous access device placement: meta-analysis of 2,154 patients. JVIR. 2016;27(3):339–43; quiz 44.
35. Wei L, Li Y, Li X, Bian L, Wen Z, Li M. Chlorhexidine-impregnated dressing for the prophylaxis of central venous catheter-related complications: a systematic review and meta-analysis. BMC Infect Dis. 2019;19(1):429.
36. Lai NM, Chaiyakunapruk N, Lai NA, O'Riordan E, Pau WS, Saint S. Catheter impregnation, coating or bonding for reducing central venous catheter-related infections in adults. Cochrane Database Syst Rev. 2016;3:Cd007878.
37. Furuya EY, Dick AW, Herzig CT, Pogorzelska-Maziarz M, Larson EL, Stone PW. Central line-associated bloodstream infection reduction and bundle compliance in intensive care units: a National Study. Infect Control Hosp Epidemiol. 2016;37(7):805–10.
38. Ban KA, Minei JP, Laronga C, Harbrecht BG, Jensen EH, Fry DE, et al. American College of Surgeons and surgical infection society: surgical site infection guidelines, 2016 update. J Am Coll Surg. 2017;224(1):59–74.
39. Mueller TC, Nitsche U, Kehl V, Schirren R, Schossow B, Goess R, et al. Intraoperative wound irrigation to prevent surgical site infection after laparotomy (IOWISI): study protocol for a randomized controlled trial. Trials. 2017;18(1):410.
40. Norman G, Atkinson RA, Smith TA, Rowlands C, Rithalia AD, Crosbie EJ, et al. Intracavity lavage and wound irrigation for prevention of surgical site infection. Cochrane Database Syst Rev. 2017;10(10):CD012234-CD.
41. Mashbari H, Hemdi M, Chow KL, Doherty JC, Merlotti GJ, Salzman SL, et al. A randomized controlled trial on intra-abdominal irrigation during emergency trauma laparotomy; time for yet another paradigm shift. Bull Emerg Trauma. 2018;6(2):100–7.

42. De Vries FE, Wallert ED, Solomkin JS, Allegranzi B, Egger M, Dellinger EP, et al. A systematic review and meta-analysis including GRADE qualification of the risk of surgical site infections after prophylactic negative pressure wound therapy compared with conventional dressings in clean and contaminated surgery. Medicine. 2016;95(36):e4673.

43. Zalavras CG. Prevention of infection in open fractures. Infect Dis Clin N Am. 2017;31(2):339–52.

44. Braakenburg A, Obdeijn MC, Feitz R, van Rooij IA, van Griethuysen AJ, Klinkenbijl JH. The clinical efficacy and cost effectiveness of the vacuum-assisted closure technique in the management of acute and chronic wounds: a randomized controlled trial. Plast Reconstr Surg. 2006;118(2):390–7; discussion 8–400.

45. Iheozor-Ejiofor Z, Newton K, Dumville JC, Costa ML, Norman G, Bruce J. Negative pressure wound therapy for open traumatic wounds. Cochrane Database Syst Rev. 2018;7(7):CD012522-CD.

46. Webster J, Liu Z, Norman G, Dumville JC, Chiverton L, Scuffham P, et al. Negative pressure wound therapy for surgical wounds healing by primary closure. Cochrane Database Syst Rev. 2019;3:Cd009261.

47. Frazee R, Manning A, Abernathy S, Isbell C, Isbell T, Kurek S, et al. Open vs closed negative pressure wound therapy for contaminated and dirty surgical wounds: a prospective randomized comparison. J Am Coll Surg. 2018;226(4):507–12.

48. Tinkoff G, Esposito TJ, Reed J, Kilgo P, Fildes J, Pasquale M, et al. American Association for the Surgery of Trauma organ injury scale I: spleen, liver, and kidney, validation based on the national trauma data bank. J Am Coll Surg. 2008;207:646–55.

49. Stassen NA, Bhullar I, Cheng JD, Crandall M, Friese R, Guillamondegui O, et al. Nonoperative management of blunt hepatic injury: an Eastern Association for the Surgery of Trauma practice management guideline. J Trauma Acute Care Surg. 2012;73:S288–93.

50. David Richardson J, Franklin GA, Lukan JK, Carrillo EH, Spain DA, Miller FB, et al. Evolution in the management of hepatic trauma: a 25-year perspective. Ann Surg. 2000;232:324–30.

51. Hurtuk M, Reed RL, Esposito TJ, Davis KA, Luchette FA. Trauma surgeons practice what they preach: the NTDB story on solid organ injury management. J Trauma. 2006;61:243–54; discussion 54–55.

52. Green CS, Bulger EM, Kwan SW. Outcomes and complications of angioembolization for hepatic trauma: a systematic review of the literature. J Trauma Acute Care Surg. 2016;80:529–37.

53. Alvarado AR, Udobi K, Berry S, Assmann J, McDonald T, Winfield RD. An opportunity for improvement in trauma care: 8-week booster vaccination adherence among patients after trauma splenectomy. Surgery. 2018;163(2):415–8.

54. Shatz DV, Schinsky MF, Pais LB, Romero-Steiner S, Kirton OC, Carlone GM. Immune responses of splenectomized trauma patients to the 23-valent pneumococcal polysaccharide vaccine at 1 versus 7 versus 14 days after splenectomy. J Trauma. 1998;44(5):760–5; discussion 5–6.

55. Konradsen HB, Rasmussen C, Ejstrud P, Hansen JB. Antibody levels against Streptococcus pneumoniae and Haemophilus influenzae type b in a population of splenectomized individuals with varying vaccination status. Epidemiol Infect. 1997;119(2):167–74.

56. Shatz DV, Romero-Steiner S, Elie CM, Holder PF, Carlone GM. Antibody responses in postsplenectomy trauma patients receiving the 23-valent pneumococcal polysaccharide vaccine at 14 versus 28 days postoperatively. J Trauma. 2002;53(6):1037–42.

57. Yoon W, Jeong YY, Kim JK, Seo JJ, Lim HS, Shin SS, et al. CT in blunt liver trauma. Radiographics. 2005;25(1):87–104.

58. Dabbs DN, Stein DM, Scalea TM. Major hepatic necrosis: a common complication after angioembolization for treatment of high-grade liver injuries. J Trauma. 2009;66(3):621–7; discussion 7–9.

59. Kozar RA, Moore JB, Niles SE, Holcomb JB, Moore EE, Cothren CC, et al. Complications of nonoperative management of high-grade blunt hepatic injuries. J Trauma. 2005;59(5):1066–71.

60. Coccolini F, Montori G, Catena F, Kluger Y, Biffl W, Moore EE, et al. Splenic trauma: WSES classification and guidelines for adult and pediatric patients. WJES. 2017;12:40.
61. Aiolfi A, Inaba K, Strumwasser A, Matsushima K, Grabo D, Benjamin E, et al. Splenic artery embolization versus splenectomy: analysis for early in-hospital infectious complications and outcomes. J Trauma Acute Care Surg. 2017;83(3):356–60.
62. Demetriades D, Scalea TM, Degiannis E, Barmparas G, Konstantinidis A, Massahis J, et al. Blunt splenic trauma. J Trauma Acute Care Surg. 2012;72:229–34.
63. Cullingford GL, Watkins DN, Watts ADJ, Mallon DF. Severe late postsplenectomy infection. Br J Surg. 1991;78:716–21.
64. Okabayashi T, Hanazaki K. Overwhelming postsplenectomy infection syndrome in adults - a clinically preventable disease. World J Gastroenterol. 2008;14(2):176–9.
65. Sinwar PD. Overwhelming post splenectomy infection syndrome - review study. Int J Surg (London, England). 2014;12(12):1314–6.
66. Rubin LG, Schaffner W. Clinical practice. Care of the asplenic patient. N Engl J Med. 2014;371(4):349–56.
67. Centers for Disease Control and Prevention (CDC). Use of 13-valent pneumococcal conjugate vaccine and 23-valent pneumococcal polysaccharide vaccine for adults with immunocompromising conditions: recommendations of the advisory committee on immunization practices (ACIP). MMWR Morb Mortal Wkly Rep. 2012;61(40):816–9.
68. Rubin LG, Levin MJ, Ljungman P, Davies EG, Avery R, Tomblyn M, et al. 2013 IDSA clinical practice guideline for vaccination of the immunocompromised host. Clin Infect Dis. 2014;58(3):309–18.
69. Crooker KG, Howard JM, Alvarado AR, McDonald TJ, Berry SD, Green JL, et al. Splenic embolization after trauma: an opportunity to improve best immunization practices. J Surg Res. 2018;232:293–7.
70. Skattum J, Titze TL, Dormagen JB, Aaberge IS, Bechensteen AG, Gaarder PI, et al. Preserved splenic function after angioembolisation of high grade injury. Injury. 2012;43(1):62–6.
71. Walusimbi MS, Dominguez KM, Sands JM, Markert RJ, McCarthy MC. Circulating cellular and humoral elements of immune function following splenic arterial embolisation or splenectomy in trauma patients. Injury. 2012;43(2):180–3.
72. Foley PT, Kavnoudias H, Cameron PU, Czarnecki C, Paul E, Lyon SM. Proximal versus distal splenic artery embolisation for blunt splenic trauma: what is the impact on splenic immune function? Cardiovasc Intervent Radiol. 2015;38(5):1143–51.
73. Pirasteh A, Snyder LL, Lin R, Rosenblum D, Reed S, Sattar A, et al. Temporal assessment of splenic function in patients who have undergone percutaneous image-guided splenic artery embolization in the setting of trauma. JVIR. 2012;23(1):80–2.
74. Coccolini F, Stahel PF, Montori G, Biffl W, Horer TM, Catena F, et al. Pelvic trauma: WSES classification and guidelines. WJES. 2017;12:5.
75. Lavenson GS, Cohen A. Management of rectal injuries. Am J Surg. 1971;122(2):226–30.
76. Ahmed N, Thekkeurumbil S, Mathavan V, Janzen M, Tasse J, Chung R. Simplified management of low-energy projectile extraperitoneal rectal injuries. J Trauma. 2009;67(6):1270–1.
77. Bosarge PL, Como JJ, Fox N, Falck-Ytter Y, Haut ER, Dorion HA, et al. Management of penetrating extraperitoneal rectal injuries: an Eastern Association for the Surgery of Trauma practice management guideline. J Trauma Acute Care Surg. 2016;80(3):546–51.
78. Awwad A, Dhillon PS, Ramjas G, Habib SB, Al-Obaydi W. Trans-arterial embolisation (TAE) in haemorrhagic pelvic injury: review of management and mid-term outcome of a major trauma Centre. CVIR Endovasc. 2018;1(1):32.
79. Travis T, Monsky WL, London J, Danielson M, Brock J, Wegelin J, et al. Evaluation of short-term and long-term complications after emergent internal iliac artery embolization in patients with pelvic trauma. JVIR. 2008;19(6):840–7.
80. Auerbach AD, Rehman S, Kleiner MT. Selective transcatheter arterial embolization of the internal iliac artery does not cause gluteal necrosis in pelvic trauma patients. J Orthop Trauma. 2012;26(5):290–5.
81. Manson TT, Perdue PW, Pollak AN, O'Toole RV. Embolization of pelvic arterial injury is a risk factor for deep infection after acetabular fracture surgery. J Orthop Trauma. 2013;27(1):11–5.

82. Chernobylsky D, Inaba K, Matsushima K, Clark D, Demetriades D, Strumwasser A. Internal iliac artery embolization versus Silastic loop ligation for control of traumatic pelvic hemorrhage. Am Surg. 2018;84(10):1696–700.
83. Shim H, Jang JY, Kim JW, Ryu H, Jung PY, Kim S, et al. Effectiveness and postoperative wound infection of preperitoneal pelvic packing in patients with hemodynamic instability caused by pelvic fracture. PLoS One. 2018;13(11):e0206991.
84. Li Q, Dong J, Yang Y, Wang G, Wang Y, Liu P, et al. Retroperitoneal packing or angioembolization for haemorrhage control of pelvic fractures—quasi-randomized clinical trial of 56 haemodynamically unstable patients with injury severity score >/=33. Injury. 2016;47(2):395–401.
85. Burlew CC, Moore EE, Smith WR, Johnson JL, Biffl WL, Barnett CC, et al. Preperitoneal pelvic packing/external fixation with secondary angioembolization: optimal care for life-threatening hemorrhage from unstable pelvic fractures. J Am Coll Surg. 2011;212(4):628–35; discussion 35–37.
86. Kim TH, Yoon YC, Chung JY, Song HK. Strategies for the management of hemodynamically unstable pelvic fractures: from preperitoneal pelvic packing to definitive internal fixation. Asian J Surg. 2019;42(11):941–6.
87. Duchesne J, Costantini TW, Khan M, Taub E, Rhee P, Morse B, et al. The effect of hemorrhage control adjuncts on outcome in severe pelvic fracture: a multi-institutional study. J Trauma Acute Care Surg. 2019;87(1):117–24.
88. Joseph B, Zeeshan M, Sakran JV, Hamidi M, Kulvatunyou N, Khan M, et al. Nationwide analysis of resuscitative endovascular balloon occlusion of the aorta in civilian trauma. JAMA Surg. 2019;154(6):500–8.
89. Huh J, Stinner DJ, Burns TC, Hsu JR. Infectious complications and soft tissue injury contribute to late amputation after severe lower extremity trauma. J Trauma. 2011;71(1 Suppl):S47–51.
90. Srour M, Inaba K, Okoye O, Chan C, Skiada D, Schnuriger B, et al. Prospective evaluation of treatment of open fractures: effect of time to irrigation and debridement. JAMA Surg. 2015;150(4):332–6.
91. Lack WD, Karunakar MA, Angerame MR, Seymour RB, Sims S, Kellam JF, et al. Type III open tibia fractures: immediate antibiotic prophylaxis minimizes infection. J Orthop Trauma. 2015;29(1):1–6.
92. Cross WW 3rd, Swiontkowski MF. Treatment principles in the management of open fractures. Indian J Orthop. 2008;42(4):377–86.
93. Gustilo RB, Anderson JT. Prevention of infection in the treatment of one thousand and twenty-five open fractures of long bones: retrospective and prospective analyses. J Bone Joint Surg Am. 1976;58(4):453–8.
94. Gustilo RB, Mendoza RM, Williams DN. Problems in the management of type III (severe) open fractures: a new classification of type III open fractures. J Trauma. 1984;24(8):742–6.
95. Surgeons CIACo, editor. 10th Edition of the Advanced Trauma Life Support (ATLS) Student Course Manual. 2018.
96. Benson DR, Riggins RS, Lawrence RM, Hoeprich PD, Huston AC, Harrison JA. Treatment of open fractures: a prospective study. J Trauma. 1983;23(1):25–30.
97. Chang Y, Bhandari M, Zhu KL, Mirza RD, Ren M, Kennedy SA, et al. Antibiotic prophylaxis in the Management of Open Fractures: a systematic survey of current practice and recommendations. JBJS Rev. 2019;7(2):e1.
98. Hoff WS, Bonadies JA, Cachecho R, Dorlac WC. East practice management guidelines work group: update to practice management guidelines for prophylactic antibiotic use in open fractures. J Trauma. 2011;70(3):751–4.
99. Collinge CA, McWilliam-Ross K, Kelly KC, Dombroski D. Substantial improvement in prophylactic antibiotic administration for open fracture patients: results of a performance improvement program. J Orthop Trauma. 2014;28(11):620–5.

The Value of Microbiological Cultures: When to Perform Them and How to Read Them

19

Jan Ulrych

19.1 Introduction

Microbiology is integrated in general surgical practice, and a knowledge of basic microbiology is essential for appropriate and safe surgical practice. The cornerstones of the management of surgical infections are effective source control and appropriate antimicrobial therapy. For instance, poor antibiotic coverage, as well as inappropriate antibiotic regimens are the variables strongly associated with unfavourable outcomes. Therefore, it is often necessary to use microbiological laboratory methods to identify a specific aetiologic pathogen of surgical infections and to determine microbial susceptibility to antimicrobial agents.

Surgical infections are caused by pathogenic microorganisms, mostly bacteria are responsible for majority of surgical infections. Some surgical infections are distinctive enough to be identified clinically. However, a single clinical syndrome may result from infection with any one of many pathogens. Even despite the fact that the bacterial aetiology of many surgical infections is initially unknown, the surgeon is responsible for adequate therapy, including the administration of appropriate antibiotics. On the opposite side, medical microbiology is the discipline that identifies aetiologic microbial pathogens of disease. Unfortunately, the microbiologist has no information about the patient: no details of their clinical syndrome, prior antibiotic therapy, immunologic status and underlying conditions. Therefore, collaboration of surgeons and clinical microbiologists is crucial.

J. Ulrych (✉)
First Department of Surgery, Department of Abdominal, Thoracic Surgery and Traumatology,
First Faculty of Medicine, Charles University and General University Hospital,
Prague, Czech Republic
e-mail: Jan.Ulrych@vfn.cz

© Springer Nature Switzerland AG 2021
M. Sartelli et al. (eds.), *Infections in Surgery*, Hot Topics in Acute Care Surgery
and Trauma, https://doi.org/10.1007/978-3-030-62116-2_19

19.2 Microbiological Examination

A detailed knowledge of microbiological tests is not mandatory for surgeons. This is because the field of microbiology is extremely wide, and appropriate laboratory analysis of microbial specimens is the responsibility of the microbiological laboratory. It is the clinical microbiologist that should determine the appropriate laboratory procedures for confirming the bacterial aetiology of surgical infections. The microbiological armamentarium comprises a broad spectrum of laboratory techniques and microbiological tests.

The most rapid confirmation of bacterial aetiology of infection is provided by direct examination using a binocular microscope (microscopic examination). However, the conventional identification of bacteria consists of performing Gram stain, followed by bacterial culture and identification. Gram staining is a diagnostic test that gives an early indication of potential bacteria through visualization of the bacteria. This laboratory technique is used to differentiate between different types of bacteria based on their shape, and the type of their cell walls. Since not all bacteria can be stained by Gram stain, specialized stains are available (e.g. Ziehl-Neelson stain for mycobacteria).

In many instances, the microbial pathogen that causes an infection can be identified by culturing and isolating the microorganism. The basic methods for detection of bacteria from specimen are cultures in liquid media (broth), or on solid media (agar). The advantage of culture in liquid media is that it is more sensitive than culture on agar; however, the disadvantage is that it is not easy to determine the type of bacteria cultured. In cultures on solid media, the bacteria grow on the surface of agar and produce different characteristic colonies. The agar media can be classified into selective and non-selective ones. Agar becomes more selective by the addition of antibiotics or other inhibitory substances. Cultures may be incubated under different conditions—in air, with carbon dioxide, anaerobically, etc. The identification of bacteria is usually based on Gram stain appearance, colony morphology, growth characteristics and biochemical characteristics. Moreover, specialized techniques may be used for identification of bacteria, such as immunologic detection of microbial antigens (latex particle agglutination, enzyme-linked immunosorbent assay) and molecular technology (the polymerase chain reaction—PCR). The clinical microbiologist participates in decisions regarding the microbiologic diagnostic methods and the choice of test for bacteria culture. Bacterial identification depends on many factors, including the expertise of the clinical microbiologist. The culture results may usually be available within 24 h.

An important task of the microbiology laboratory is the performance of antimicrobial susceptibility testing. Antimicrobial susceptibility testing (AST) is a laboratory procedure used to identify which antibiotic is specifically effective for an individual patient's infection, in order to guide the appropriate antibiotic therapy. Bacterial isolates from clinical specimens are tested in vitro to determine whether they are susceptible/resistant to various antimicrobial agents. Standardly, AST is performed from single pure colonies; however, direct sensitivity test may be performed in some situations. Direct sensitivity test means that AST is performed from the specimen itself. AST should be performed only on clinically significant bacterial isolates, not on all microorganisms recovered in culture. Susceptibility testing may not be routinely performed in the following circumstances: (1) the antimicrobial susceptibility pattern of bacteria is predictable, (2) the bacterial isolates are likely to represent normal microbial flora of the body site, (3) insufficient numbers of bacterial colonies are likely to represent contamination. Antimicrobial susceptibility tests are either performed by a disk diffusion method or a dilution method. In the disk diffusion test, the zones of growth inhibition around each of the antibiotic disks are measured. In dilution method the lowest concentration of antibiotic that inhibits bacteria growth represents the minimal inhibitory concentration (MIC). The surgeon does not need to know the exact MIC or the exact diameter of zone of growth inhibition, but they do need to know which antibiotics the pathogen is susceptible, intermediate, or resistant to. Susceptible results indicate that the antibiotic concentration that inhibits the growth of bacterial isolates is usually achieved with administration of the recommended antibiotic dose. In this case, clinical efficacy of antibiotic therapy is expected. Intermediate results indicate that the MIC of the antibiotic falls within required levels, but response rates may be reduced compared with susceptible microorganisms. Clinical efficacy can be achieved when higher-than-normal doses of antibiotic can be safely administered. Resistant results indicate that the antibiotic administered at conventional doses do not inhibit the isolate's growth. Therefore, the reliable clinical efficacy of antibiotic against the bacteria has not been established. The results of AST are reported on the antibiogram.

19.3   Specimen Selection, Collection and Processing

Besides laboratory analytic processes, the reliability of microbiological diagnosis may be altered by incorrect sampling technique and the inappropriate pre-analytical specimen management processes. The collection and selection a microbiology specimen are the responsibility of the surgeon. Therefore, the surgeon should know how to perform the sampling technique in a correct way - the impact of proper specimen management on the quality of the specimen submitted for analysis is enormous. When the preanalytical specimen management is performed incorrectly, the results of analysis will be influenced, which means that their interpretation can be misleading. Surgeons should consult the laboratory to ensure that sampling technique, specimen storage before transportation and specimen transportation are managed properly.

Sampling technique A specimen should be collected prior to the administration of antibiotics. If not possible, the antibiotic used for the therapy has to be reported to microbial laboratory. This information is helpful for the interpretation of microbiological test results.

A specimen should be collected in sufficient quantity to allow complete microbiological examination. Swabbing is not the best technique for specimen collection because only extremely small volume of the specimen is obtained. Thus, microscopic examination is not feasible with a swab specimen. Moreover, it is more difficult to transfer bacteria from the swab into the culture media. So, swabbing should only be used to collect material from the skin and mucous membranes. The best type of swab (flocked swabs, cotton swabs, etc.) is determined by presumed

Fig. 19.1 Injection
syringe with a
combi-stopper

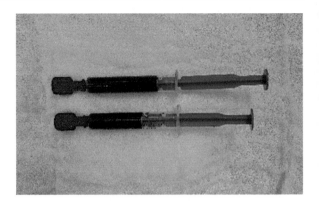

bacterial aetiology, and the choice of the most appropriate swab should be consulted with the microbiology laboratory. Biological materials including body tissues and body fluids are always specimens of choice. The number of microorganisms per millilitre or per gram of this biological material (usually from 10^3 to 10^8 colony-forming units) allow to perform full spectrum microbiological examination. Biological materials should be collected into a sterile container; test-tube or injection syringe with a combi-stopper can be used too (Fig. 19.1). Sufficient sample volume is approximately 1–2 ml of fluid or tissue.

A specimen should be representative of the disease process. This means that the specimen should contain only pathologic tissue or pathologic fluid, while contamination by commensal microorganisms is avoided. Generally, specimens may be taken from sterile sites and non-sterile sites. In the sterile sites, bacteria are not present in the absence of infection. The samples from the sterile sites are usually obtained via percutaneous route with needle under sterile conditions. A risk of contamination of the specimen can be reduced by using antiseptic agents on skin and mucosa surface before aspirating or incising a lesion. The culture of bacteria from such specimens is usually indicative of definitive infection aetiology. In the non-sterile sites, colonizing microorganisms (commensal bacteria) may be present. Skin and mucous membranes are colonized by commensal microorganisms, therefore specimens from these non-sterile sites contain commensal bacteria with no clinical relevance in addition to possible bacteria pathogens. In the case of a single large lesion, several samples should be taken from different loci of the lesion. In the case of several smaller lesions, samples from each of the lesions should be obtained. For microbiological examination of an abscess it is recommended to collect 2–5 ml of pus, as well as a sample of the abscess wall [1]. This is due to the fact that pus alone may not reveal the aetiologic pathogen, as leukocytes may destroy pathogenic bacteria.

Storage and Transport of the Specimen Nowadays, transport of microbiological specimens from healthcare facilities to a microbiological laboratory is a common feature. These biological materials must be adequately packed to prevent specimen deterioration. Correct specimen labelling is essential, as well. Every specimen should be transported immediately to a microbiological laboratory, and storage of specimens is not recommended generally. The maximum time for sample

Table 19.1 Basic principles of collection and transport of samples for microbiological examination

Diagnostic procedure used in surgical infections[a]	Optimum specimen	Collection device, temperature, and ideal transport time
Gram stain prior to culture	Tissue, fluid (peritoneal fluid), aspirate, biopsy, etc.	RT, do not refrigerate
Aerobic bacterial culture	Tissue, fluid (peritoneal fluid), aspirate, biopsy, etc.	Sterile container, RT, immediately, if >1–2 h, 4°C
	Swab (second choice); flocked swabs are recommended	Swab transport device, RT, 2 h
Aerobic and anaerobic bacterial culture	Tissue, fluid (peritoneal fluid), aspirate, biopsy, etc.	Sterile anaerobic container, RT, immediately, if >1–2 h, 4°C
	Swab (second choice); flocked swabs are effective	Anaerobic swab transport device, RT, 2 h
Fungal culture	Tissue, fluid, aspirate, biopsy, etc.	Sterile container, RT, 2 h, if >1–2 h, 4°C
	Swab (second choice)	Swab transport device, RT, 2 h
AFB stain and culture Mycobacterium	Tissue, fluid, aspirate, biopsy, etc.	Sterile container, RT, 2 h, if >1–2 h, 4°C
	Swab (second choice)	Swab transport device, RT, 2 h
Blood culture	2–3 sets blood culture bottles	Blood culture bottles, RT, <2 h

Notes: *AFB* acid-fast bacilli, *RT* room temperature
[a]Surgical infections include intra-abdominal infections, skin and soft tissue infections and surgical site infections

transportation is 1–2 h. Delays in processing may result in the overgrowth of some microorganisms or the death of other bacteria. Moreover, tissue or fluid in a syringe must be transferred in a hermetically sealed system. Before the transport, the needle is removed from the syringe and replaced with a cap. Sometimes the prompt transportation may not be feasible - in these cases, the specimens (with the exception of blood) must be placed in transport medium and should be refrigerated (4°C) until transported. Basic principles of collection and transport of microbiological specimens are summarized in Table 19.1.

19.4   The Value of Microbiological Examination

The microbiological examination may play different roles in patient care. Generally, the results of microbiological examination may be utilized for two purposes: (1) diagnosis and therapy of infection in individual patient, and, (2) support to the healthcare-associated infections prevention and control in the hospital. Every surgeon should be aware of both purposes of microbiological examination. In surgical practice, the microbiological examination is most frequently performed for diagnosis of infection disease, however, the indirect effect related to nosocomial infection prevention and control should be mentioned. If the microbiological diagnosis of infection is accurate and rapid, the patient therapy management will be adequate at the beginning of infection. This means that the period of dispersing microbial pathogens will be shorter. If the surgical infection is caused by multidrug-resistant bacteria, early barrier precautions and patient isolation will prevent the spread of multidrug-resistant bacteria to other patients.

19.4.1 Diagnostic Microbiological Cultures

As mentioned above, the surgeon is responsible for diagnosis and therapy management, including appropriate indication for microbiological examination. At an elementary level, the surgeon must answer two basic questions: Is the patient's disease caused by a microorganism? If so, do I need the identification of the microbe and antimicrobial susceptibility profile for optimal therapy? You know that some surgical infections can be treated by surgery alone, and antibiotic therapy is not necessary. For example, a lack of impact on patient outcomes by bacteriological cultures has been documented in patients with uncomplicated acute appendicitis [2]. Based on the WSES recommendation (Word Society of Emergency Surgery), in patients with uncomplicated intra-abdominal infections such as uncomplicated appendicitis and uncomplicated cholecystitis, where the source of infection is treated definitively, post-operative antibiotic therapy is not necessary [3]. Also, small uncomplicated subcutaneous abscesses may be successfully treated by surgical incision and drainage, without antibiotic therapy. In these cases, there is no change in patient's therapy management based on results of microbiological cultures. Therefore, microbiological examination has little clinical value for such cases. Initial antimicrobial therapy in patients with surgical infections is typically empirical in nature because patients often need immediate treatment. Microbiological data (results of culture and antimicrobial susceptibility) usually requires ≥ 48 h for the identification of pathogens and antibiotic susceptibility patterns. So, the selection of initial antibiotic regimen is based on presumed microbial pathogens. If it is supposed that it is not safe to predict microbial aetiology and/or the antibiotic therapy will be determined or modified according to results of antimicrobial susceptibility test, microbiological examination is fully justified. Generally, microbiological examination is mandatory for surgical infections in patients with less predictable bacterial aetiology of infection, in patients with high risk of the presence of multidrug-resistant pathogens, and in critically ill patients or in immunocompromised patients (patients with kidney failure, organ transplant patients and patients using corticosteroids). Regarding less predictable bacterial aetiology and presence of multidrug-resistant pathogens, the significant risk factor is acquisition in a healthcare setting. In the instance of intra-abdominal infections, the microbiology of postoperative peritonitis differs significantly from that of community-acquired disease. The major pathogens involved in community-acquired intra-abdominal infections are *Enterobacteriaceae* (predominantly *Escherichia coli* and *Klebsiella species*), *Streptococcus species* and certain anaerobes (particularly *Bacteroides fragilis*). In the post-operative peritonitis, *Enterococci* are significantly the most often involved pathogen, and an increased prevalence of infections caused by antibiotic-resistant pathogens, including extended-spectrum beta-lactamase (ESBL)-producing *Escherichia coli* and

Klebsiella species, vancomycin-resistant *Enterococcus species*, carbapenem-resistant *Pseudomonas aeruginosa*, has been observed [4, 5]. Moreover, emergence of multidrug-resistant bacteria is frequent and increases progressively with the number of reoperations [6]. So, in the healthcare-associated infections, the causative pathogens and the related resistance patterns are not readily predictable - therefore, nosocomial infections require further microbiological analysis. In the community-acquired surgical infections, previous antimicrobial therapy and healthcare exposure are the most important risk factors for multidrug-resistant (MDR) pathogens. Methicillin-resistant *Staphylococcus aureus* (MRSA) is the most prevalent of community-acquired MDR bacteria and the main threat on the horizon is represented by *Enterobacteriaceae* producing extended spectrum β-lactamases (ESBL) or carbapenemase [7]. The colonization of otherwise healthy hosts, and an antibiotic resistance phenotype that is stable in the absence of antibiotic pressure are a common characteristic of community-associated MDR bacteria. In critically ill patients and in immunocompromised patients, an inappropriate antimicrobial therapy may have a strong negative impact on the outcome. Therefore, the result of antimicrobial susceptibility test is essential to guide the ongoing antimicrobial therapy. On the other hand, microbiological examination in patients with uncomplicated community-acquired surgical infection rarely influences the individual patient management, as the microbial pathogens and their antimicrobial susceptibility are predictable. However, every microbiological examination provides data for microbiological surveillance and helps detect epidemiological trends in pathogen incidence, as well as antimicrobial resistance patterns at regional level. These epidemiological data are important because local epidemiology plays a key role in choice of empirical antimicrobial regimen for risk patients.

What remains a subject of discussion is the prognostic value of microbiological results for an individual patient. In patients with tertiary peritonitis, a microbial shift towards *Enterococcus ssp.*, *Enterobacter spp.*, *Pseudomonas spp.* and *Candida spp.* has been observed. Therefore, the relationship between the microbial profile of peritoneal infection and ongoing infection (tertiary peritonitis) or patient outcomes has been studied. van Ruler et al. [8] reported that microbial profiles in secondary peritonitis do not predict ongoing abdominal infection, while Montravers et al. [6] identified that presence of *Candida spp.* in surgical samples is the significant risk factor for persistent peritonitis. The inconclusive evidence can be explained by unfeasibility of distinguishing colonizing bacteria from pathogenic bacteria. Although the impact of microbial profile from the site of infection on patient outcome is questionable, the antimicrobial resistance is a significant risk factor for morbidity and mortality. Outcomes in patients infected with MDR bacteria tend to be worse as compared to patients infected with susceptible microorganisms. Based on the meta-analysis of 30 studies, infection with multidrug-resistant Gram-negative bacteria was identified as significant predictor of mortality [9]. Also, for Gram-positive infections, a significant difference in mortality between MRSA infections and methicillin-sensitive *Staphylococcus aureus* (MSSA) infections was reported [10]. However, it should be emphasized that antimicrobial resistance is a risk factor for mortality only if it is associated with inadequate antibiotic therapy.

The results of microbiological testing may have great importance for the choice of therapeutic strategy of every individual patient, in particular in the adaptation of targeted antimicrobial therapy. Obtaining microbiological results from biological specimen culture from the site of infection has two advantages: (1) it provides an opportunity to expand antimicrobial regimen if the initial choice was too narrow and (2) it also allows the de-escalation of antimicrobial therapy if the empirical regimen was too broad.

> It can be summarized that microbiological examination of biological specimens from the site of infection is always recommended for:
> - all patients with healthcare-associated surgical infections
> - patients with community-acquired surgical infections at risk for multidrug-resistant pathogens (previous antimicrobial therapy and healthcare exposure)
> - critically ill patients and immunocompromised patients with community–acquired surgical infections

> Routine microbiological examination of low-risk patients with community-acquired surgical infection is considered optional in the individual patient but may be of value in detecting epidemiological changes in the resistance patterns of pathogens.

19.4.2 Active Surveillance Cultures (Microbiological Screening)

There is no doubt that the clinical microbiology laboratory is an essential component of an effective infection control program. In terms of nosocomial infection prevention, the infection control officer is usually a medical microbiologist, and the management of microbiological surveillance is tvhe microbiologist's responsibility. Microbiological surveillance is usually defined as the ongoing and systematic collection, analysis and interpretation of microbiological data, with subsequent planning, implementation and evaluation of infection control practices and treatment strategies. Microbiological surveillance may be performed in three different levels—geographical level, institutional level and patient level.

Institutional microbiological surveillance, including the surveillance of resistance to antimicrobial agents, is very important for an antibiotic management team in hospitals. The results serve to make institutional guidelines for prophylactic and therapeutic antibiotic use with the ultimate goal to decrease resistance. Institutional microbiological surveillance is essential for recognizing of outbreaks.

Patient microbiological surveillance is more familiar practice for surgeons. Patient microbiological screening should reveal the colonization status of mucosa and skin in an individual patient. The assumptions underlying a microbiological screening in surgical patients are that (1) patient colonization status is an important characteristic for individual patient risk of infection, and (2) MDR pathogen colonization may be a threat for other patients. It has been reported repeatedly that a large proportion of healthcare-associated infections after surgery originate from the patients' own flora. Surgical site infection (SSI) is the most prevalent type of nosocomial infection in surgery. It has been demonstrated that *Staphylococcus aureus* carriers have higher rates of SSIs. Moreover, a systemic review showed a four-fold increase in the risk of infection after MRSA colonization compared with MSSA colonization [11]. Preoperative knowledge of the MRSA status in elective surgical patients allows for both—selection of adequate prophylactic antibiotics, and implementation of a preoperative decolonization. WHO recently recommended decolonization of *Staphylococcus aureus* carriers for the prevention of SSI; however, there is no recommendation concerning surgical patient population that should undergo screening for *Staphylococcus aureus* carriage [12]. Some authors advocate the screening of all surgical patients for *Staphylococcus aureus* [13]. Current guidelines recommend screening only surgical patients indicated for high-risk procedures (orthopaedic surgery and cardiothoracic surgery) or screening surgical patients based on clinical risk assessment [14]. Concerning screening for ESBL bacteria colonization and its impact on surgical antibiotic prophylaxis, no recommendation has been formulated due to the lack of evidence [12].

Early identification of patients colonized by MDR bacteria and subsequent infection control measures are believed to be a strong intervention that reduces the prevalence of nosocomial infections. These control measures include active surveillance culture (screening culture), pre-emptive isolation of patients at high risk, education of healthcare workers in hand-washing practices, decolonization therapy and contact isolation of patients colonized with MDR pathogens. Initially, mandatory microbiological screening at hospital admission has been advocated in order to identify colonized patients. However, Harbarth et al. [15] showed that an universal MRSA admission screening strategy did not reduce nosocomial MRSA infection in the surgical department. Interestingly, a comparative review published in 2014 found that screening of all hospitalized patients for MRSA carriage (universal screening) decreases the rate of nosocomial MRSA infection compared with no screening [16]. Nevertheless, the strong of evidence to support this effect was low. Concerning the method of screening, the use of rapid screening tests was not associated with a significant decrease in MRSA acquisition rate, when compared with culture screening [17, 18]. Nowadays, target microbiological screening based on patients' risk factors is preferred instead of universal screening. Active surveillance culture is recommended for patients at the time of admission to high-risk area (ICU) and for patients in populations at risk (patients in intensive care units, patients transferred from facilities known to have high MDR bacteria prevalence rates, roommates of colonized or infected persons, and patients known to have been previously infected or colonized with an MDR bacteria) [19].

Screening swabs are routinely obtained from nose, throat, axilla, groin and perineal or rectal area.

19.5   Interpretation of Microbiological Results

The proper interpretation of microbiology results is one of the most challenging and important functions of clinical microbiology laboratory. Collaborative medicine is an essential requirement for microbiology results interpretation, as they provide a basis for appropriate patient therapy. Thus, the microbiologist and the surgeon should interact directly. Valid interpretation of the microbiological results of culture can be achieved only if the specimen obtained is appropriate for processing. The responsibility of the surgeon is formulating the request properly, and providing the laboratory with complete and precise patient information. Based on the information about patient (diagnosis, patient history, antimicrobial therapy, etc.), and the specimen source (specimen specification, date and time of collection, etc.), the laboratory can determine the appropriate microbiological method for processing the specimen (appropriate type of culture media, incubation under various conditions, etc.). If the specimen is obtained from normally sterile sites, the presence of bacteria will almost always be considered a significant result. However, Gram stains and culture results of specimens from non-sterile sites must be interpreted with care. Many body sites have normal, commensal microorganisms that can easily contaminate the inappropriately collected specimen and complicate interpretation. It is sometimes difficult to identify the exact causative microorganism. The surgeon should not demand that the microbiological laboratory report "everything that grows"—this can provide irrelevant information [1]. The clinical significance of the bacteria found in the specimen depends on the clinical situation and must be thoroughly evaluated to avoid overuse of antibiotics. Antimicrobial resistance is a growing threat in both community settings and healthcare settings. Therefore, decisions regarding empirical antibiotic therapy are more complex, and the importance of routine antimicrobial susceptibility testing to guide therapeutic decisions has increased. Susceptibility testing is subject to great variability depending on the pathogen tested, media used, conditions of incubation, and the method of accessing bacterial growth. AST is an in vitro procedure and does not necessarily predict in vivo efficacy. The efficacy of antimicrobial agents depends on their capacity to achieve a MIC concentration at the site of infection. However, antibiotic concentration at the site of infection may be much lower than its serum level (e.g., abscess). The presence of foreign bodies and biofilm formation at the site of infection also affects antimicrobial activity. Biofilms are defined as organized bacterial communities embedded in an extracellular polymeric matrix attached to living or abiotic surfaces. It has been reported that the bacteria living in biofilms can tolerate up to 100–1000 times higher concentrations of antibiotics and disinfectants [20]. If the patient's clinical status is worsening and microbiological results show that an antibiotic regimen is appropriate, both microbiologist and surgeon should consider several other causes of antibiotic therapy failure. The microbiologist must re-evaluate pharmacokinetic and pharmacodynamic characteristics of the used antimicrobial therapy (e.g., appropriate dosing of antibiotics in critically ill patients or obese patients). The surgeon should recognize the non-antimicrobial therapy causes of treatment failure—inadequate surgical source control (insufficient surgical drainage and debridement), development of superinfection and host immunosuppression. The clinical microbiologist provides important guidance regarding the clinical significance of microbiological results and antimicrobial susceptibility testing.

References

1. Miller JM, Binnicker MJ, Campbell S, Carroll KC, Chapin KC, Gilligan PH, et al. A guide to utilization of the microbiology laboratory for diagnosis of infectious diseases: 2018 update by the Infectious Diseases Society of America and the American Society for Microbiology. Clin Infect Dis. 2018;67(6):813–6. https://doi.org/10.1093/cid/ciy584.
2. Foo FJ, Beckingham IJ, Ahmed I. Intra-operative culture swabs in acute appendicitis: a waste of resources. Surgeon. 2008;6(5):278–81.
3. Sartelli M, Catena F, Abu-Zidan FM, Ansaloni L, Biffl WL, Boermeester MA, et al. Management of intra-abdominal infections: recommendations by the WSES 2016 consensus conference. World J Emerg Surg. 2017;12:22. https://doi.org/10.1186/s13017-017-0132-7.
4. Sartelli M, Catena F, Ansaloni L, Coccolini F, Corbella D, Moore EE, et al. Complicated intra-abdominal infections worldwide: the definitive data of the CIAOW study. World J Emerg Surg. 2014;9:37. https://doi.org/10.1186/1749-7922-9-37.
5. Sitges-Serra A, López MJ, Girvent M, Almirall S, Sancho JJ. Postoperative enterococcal infection after treatment of complicated intra-abdominal sepsis. Br J Surg. 2002;89(3):361–7. https://doi.org/10.1046/j.0007-1323.2001.02023.x.
6. Montravers P, Dufour G, Guglielminotti J, Desmard M, Muller C, Houissa H, et al. Dynamic changes of microbial flora and therapeutic consequences in persistent peritonitis. Crit Care. 2015;19:70. https://doi.org/10.1186/s13054-015-0789-9.
7. van Duin D, Paterson DL. Multidrug-resistant bacteria in the community: trends and lessons learned. Infect Dis Clin North Am. 2016;30(2):377–90. https://doi.org/10.1016/j.idc.2016.02.004.
8. van Ruler O, Kiewiet JJ, van Ketel RJ, Boermeester MA, Dutch Peritonitis Study Group. Initial microbial spectrum in severe secondary peritonitis and relevance for treatment. Eur J Clin Microbiol Infect Dis. 2012;31(5):671–82. https://doi.org/10.1007/s10096-011-1357-0.
9. Vardakas KZ, Rafailidis PI, Konstantelias AA, Falagas ME. Predictors of mortality in patients with infections due to multi-drug resistant Gram negative bacteria: the study, the patient, the bug or the drug? J Infect. 2013;66(5):401–14. https://doi.org/10.1016/j.jinf.2012.10.028.
10. Gandra S, Tseng KK, Arora A, Bhowmik B, Robinson ML, Panigrahi B, et al. The mortality burden of multidrug-resistant pathogens in India: a retrospective observational study. Clin Infect Dis. 2019;69(4):563–70. https://doi.org/10.1093/cid/ciy955.
11. Safdar N, Bradley EA. The risk of infection after nasal colonization with Staphylococcus aureus. Am J Med. 2008;121(4):310–5. https://doi.org/10.1016/j.amjmed.2007.07.034.
12. Allegranzi B, Bischoff P, de Jonge S, Kubilay NZ, Zayed B, Gomes SM, et al. New WHO recommendations on preoperative measures for surgical site infection prevention: an evidence-based global perspective. Lancet Infect Dis. 2016;16(12):e276–87. https://doi.org/10.1016/S1473-3099(16)30398-X.
13. Kavanagh KT, Abusalem S, Calderon LE. View point: gaps in the current guidelines for the prevention of methicillin-resistant Staphylococcus aureus surgical site infections. Antimicrob Resist Infect Control. 2018;7:112. https://doi.org/10.1186/s13756-018-0407-0.

14. Anderson DJ, Podgorny K, Berríos-Torres SI, Bratzler DW, Dellinger EP, Greene L, et al. Strategies to prevent surgical site infections in acute care hospitals: 2014 update. Infect Control Hosp Epidemiol. 2014;35(6):605–27. https://doi.org/10.1086/676022.
15. Harbarth S, Fankhauser C, Schrenzel J, Christenson J, Gervaz P, Bandiera-Clerc C, et al. Universal screening for methicillin-resistant Staphylococcus aureus at hospital admission and nosocomial infection in surgical patients. JAMA. 2008;299(10):1149–57. https://doi. org/10.1001/jama.299.10.1149.
16. Glick SB, Samson DJ, Huang ES, Vats V, Aronson N, Weber SG. Screening for methicillin-resistant Staphylococcus aureus: a comparative effectiveness review. Am J Infect Control. 2014;42(2):148–55. https://doi.org/10.1016/j.ajic.2013.07.020.
17. Tacconelli E, De Angelis G, de Waure C, Cataldo MA, La Torre G, Cauda R. Rapid screening tests for meticillin-resistant Staphylococcus aureus at hospital admission: systematic review and meta-analysis. Lancet Infect Dis. 2009;9(9):546–54. https://doi.org/10.1016/ S1473-3099(09)70150-1.
18. Wu PJ, Jeyaratnam D, Tosas O, Cooper BS, French GL. Point-of-care universal screening for meticillin-resistant Staphylococcus aureus: a cluster-randomized cross-over trial. J Hosp Infect. 2017;95(3):245–52. https://doi.org/10.1016/j.jhin.2016.08.017.
19. Siegel JD, Rhinehart E, Jackson M, Chiarello L, Healthcare Infection Control Practices Advisory Committee. Management of multidrug-resistant organisms in health care settings, 2006. Am J Infect Control. 2007;35(10 Suppl 2):S165–93. https://doi.org/10.1016/j. ajic.2007.10.006.
20. Macià MD, Rojo-Molinero E, Oliver A. Antimicrobial susceptibility testing in biofilm-growing bacteria. Clin Microbiol Infect. 2014;20(10):981–90. https://doi. org/10.1111/1469-0691.12651.

Invasive Candidiasis in Surgical Patients

20

Sganga Gabriele, Fransvea Pietro, Pepe Gilda,
Di Grezia Marta, and Cozza Valerio

20.1 Epidemiology

The overall incidence of systemic fungal infections in the surgical patient and particularly in the modern surgical intensive care unit increased constantly over the last decade [1–3]. Patients at risk for invasion and dissemination are common, and are not as ill as thought previously due to several risk factors that we consider in this chapter.

At first it should be noticed that the incidence of fungal infections has globally increased worldwide. Fungal diseases kill more than 1.5 million and affect over a billion people. Recent global estimates have found 3,000,000 cases of chronic pulmonary aspergillosis, ~223,100 cases of cryptococcal meningitis complicating HIV/AIDS, ~700,000 cases of invasive candidiasis, ~500,000 cases of *Pneumocystis jirovecii* pneumonia, ~250,000 cases of invasive aspergillosis, ~100,000 cases of disseminated histoplasmosis, over 10,000,000 cases of fungal asthma and ~1,000,000 cases of fungal keratitis occur annually. Since 2013, the Leading International Fungal Education (LIFE) portal has facilitated the estimation of the burden of serious fungal infections country by country for over 5.7 billion people (>80% of the world's population) [4–6].

Furthermore isolation of mycetes, as a cause of nosocomial infections, has increased more in departments where complex and invasive procedures are performed. To determine the prevalence of nosocomial infections, the SOAP Study [7] was conducted in 2002 among European intensive care units as a 15-day

S. Gabriele (✉) · F. Pietro · P. Gilda · D. G. Marta · C. Valerio
Emergency Surgery and Trauma, Fondazione Policlinico Universitario A. Gemelli IRCCS,
Università Cattolica del Sacro Cuore, Rome, Italy
e-mail: gabriele.sganga@policlinicogemelli.it; pietro.fransvea@policlinicogemelli.it;
gilda.pepe@policlinicogemelli.it; marta.digrezia@policlinicogemelli.it;
valerio.cozza@policlinicogemelli.it

© Springer Nature Switzerland AG 2021
M. Sartelli et al. (eds.), *Infections in Surgery*, Hot Topics in Acute Care Surgery
and Trauma, https://doi.org/10.1007/978-3-030-62116-2_20

observation with 3147 included patients. In this study 37% of all ICU patients had an identified infection and almost 24% of them had their infection acquired in the ICU. Between 1980 and 1989 a remarkable increase was observed up to five times and the magnitude of this increase was observed in the surgical patient population. The incidence of nosocomial infection by Candida species has surged over the past few decades from the eight to the fourth most common cause of nosocomial blood-stream infection in the general hospital population. In the former EPIC Study which was conducted in 1992 among European intensive care units to determine the prevalence of nosocomial infections, the isolation of Candida spp. ranked fifth among isolated pathogens, reaching 17.1% of all isolated microorganisms [8]. Of all septic patients 21.4% were surgical patients. In a multicenter, prospective study conducted in 28 Spanish hospitals the incidence of candidemia was of one critical patient for every 500 intensive care admissions, confirming the incidence of systemic candidiasis (documented by positive blood culture for candida spp.) equal to about 2.2% [9]. In surgical patients the incidence of candida infection has increased from 2.5% up to 5.6% per 1000 discharges and Candida peritonitis is associated with a markedly raised mortality rate which can reach as high as 60–70% with almost half of the deaths occurring in the first week after diagnosis. Intraabdominal candidiasis (IAC), which includes peritonitis and intraabdominal abscesses, may occur in around 40% of patients following repeat gastrointestinal (GI) surgery, GI perforation, anastomotic leakage, or necrotizing pancreatitis [10, 11].

Among the various causes that led to this increase, it should be remembered that surgery, in recent years, has greatly broadened its field of action by extending the indications to patients with multiple risk factors previously considered not operable and has crossed borders until recently considered utopian as is the case of solid organ transplantation and trauma surgery. Among trauma patients, isolated candida species were reported by a few studies, with an isolated rate up to 22% in trauma patients who did not respond to antibiotic therapy while in the ICU [12–18].

Immunocompromised patients due to underlying disease (asthma, AIDS, cancer, organ transplantation), or to antineoplastic and/or anti-rejection drugs and cortison, are now more and more frequently admitted to the surgical wards. Moreover, the continuous technological and pharmacological improvements allow longer survival rate for patients who would be died in the past and who today develop multi-organ dysfunctions supported by invasive replacement therapies such as mechanical ventilation, dialysis, artificial nutrition, and prolonged use of antibiotics especially associated with use of endovascular catheters. It is very easy to recognize how the conditions listed are very frequent in the surgical patient throughout his clinical course; this list of factors becomes even more suggestive if applied to the patient subjected to solid organ transplant surgery, or to a severe trauma patient where all the factors listed can coexist simultaneously. All this has led to an increased risk of systemic fungal infections with a significant increase in morbidity and mortality.

20.2   Pathogenesis

The "gut origin of sepsis" hypothesis proposes that bacteria, which are normally resident within the lumen of the intestinal tract, translocate across the intestinal epithelial barrier and act as a source of sepsis at distant sites. Many animal studies support this concept [19–24]. The polymorphic fungus *Candida albicans* is a member of the normal human microbiome. In most individuals, *C. albicans* resides as a lifelong, harmless commensal and as part of the normal intestinal bacterial microflora [25–27].

Both alterations of immune system and damage of the gastrointestinal mucosa are risk factors for the development of experimental systemic (disseminated) candidiasis due to an increased passage of candida, bacteria, toxins and bio-products from the intestinal lumen to the peri-intestinal lymphatics, and from there to the portal blood, to the liver, to the lungs and, finally, to the systemic circulation [28, 29]. Further risk factors include central venous catheters, which allow direct access of the fungus to the bloodstream, the application of broad-spectrum antibacterials, which enable fungal overgrowth, and trauma or gastrointestinal surgery, which disrupts mucosal barriers. This microorganismic spread leads to a further trigger of cytokine production that is strictly correlated to systemic response of the organism to the septic insult [30, 31].

The upper gut and stomach are usually sterile or sparsely populated with relatively avirulent bacteria. These are most commonly Gram positive and aerobic and the most frequently isolated species are streptococci, staphylococci, lactobacilli, and various fungi. In the distal ileum Gram negative bacteria outnumber Gram positive organisms. Enterobacteriaceae predominate and anaerobic bacteria are found in substantial numbers [32, 33].

Critical illness is often associated with significant proximal gut overgrowth of enteric organisms mostly due to the use of anti-acids (which elevate the gastric pH), the nonuse of the digestive tract, and repeated hypo-perfusion phenomena resulting from shock states even clinically undetectable. Over 90% of ICU patients with infection had at least one episode of infection with an organism that was simultaneously present in the upper gastrointestinal tract. Moreover it has been seen that Candida, Pseudomonas, *Staphylococcus epidermidis*, and *Streptococcus faecalis* were the commonest organisms responsible [34]. Although there is increasing circumstantial evidence to suggest that it may play an important role in the causation of sepsis. Candida was reported to be isolated in 41% of upper gastrointestinal (GI) sites, 35% of small bowel, 12% of colorectal, and less than 5% of appendicular sites in. European studies have demonstrated a predominance of *C. albicans* isolates (ranging from 65 to 82%), followed by *C. glabrata* in intraabdominal Candida infections in surgical patients. Increased rates of non-albicans Candida isolates from abdominal samples in comparison to other studies have been reported in ICU patients by Montravers et al. (42 vs. 26%, respectively) [35]. Table 20.1 summarizes risks factor for invasive candidiasis.

Table 20.1 Risk factors for invasive candidiasis

Adult population	Neonates and children
Critical illness, with particular risk among patients with long-term ICU stay	Prematurity
Abdominal surgery, with particular risk among patients who have anastomotic leakage or have had repeat laparotomies	Low birth weight
Acute necrotizing pancreatitis	Low APGAR score
Hematologic malignant disease	Congenital malformation
Solid organ transplantation	
Solid organ tumors	
Use of broad-spectrum antibiotics	
Presence of central vascular catheter, total parenteral nutrition	
Hemodialysis	
Glucocorticoids use or chemotherapy for cancer	
Candida colonization, particularly if multifocal (colonization index >0.5)	

Certainly the clinical significance of bacterial translocation remains unclear and we cannot say that this phenomenon is the main cause of infections found in intensive care: but at the same time we can underline how even if there is no available level 1 evidence in the literature to recommend a therapeutic strategy for decreasing bacterial translocation in humans, several measures have shown some significance in modulating gut barrier function and consequently decreasing bacterial translocation in clinical practice and reduce the percentage of infections in intensive care.

Among these we can list:

- reduction of gastric cytoprotective therapy with H2-receptor blockers, resulting in a more appropriate preservation of gastric acid barrier
- the use of Selective Digestive Decontamination (SDD) with reduction, at least of nosocomial pneumonia and perhaps associated to reduction of mortality rate
- the early use of the digestive system with enteral diets with the aim of preventing acute atrophy of microvilli, maintaining the integrity of the gastroenteric mucosa to basically prevent any translocation attempts.
- last but not least, the optimization of circulating volume and splanchnic circulation, avoiding local hypoperfusion and triggering of ischemia-reperfusion mechanisms that are the basis of any mechanism of alteration of cellular and subcellular membranes and therefore at the base of trophic alterations of enterocytes which could facilitate the translocation of microorganisms.

Summing up, the gastrointestinal tract has various functions apart from digestion. It produces hormones with local and systemic effects, plays a major role in immunological function, and serves as a barrier against antigens within its lumen. Gastrointestinal dysfunction or gut failure is frequently encountered in critical care patients and is associated with bacterial translocation, which can lead to the development of sepsis, initiation of a cytokine-mediated systemic inflammatory response syndrome (SIRS), multiple organ dysfunction syndrome (MODS), and death.

Table 20.2 Risk factors for intraabdominal candidiasis (IAC)

Specific	Nonspecific
Recurrent gastrointestinal perforations	Central venous catheter
Anastomotic leakages	Prolonged ICU stay
Surgery for acute pancreatitis	Diabetes (and immunosuppression)
Splenectomy	Prolonged broad-spectrum antibiotics
Transplantation	Total parenteral nutrition (TPN)
Open abdomen techniques (abdominal compartmental syndrome, VAC therapy)	
Peritonectomy and hyperthermic intraoperative chemotherapy for peritoneal carcinomatosis	

20.3 Risk Factors

Thirty to forty percent of patients with secondary and tertiary peritonitis may develop intraabdominal candidiasis (IAC), mainly represented by, but not limited to, Candida peritonitis or intraabdominal abscesses in patients with abdominal surgery. In Table 20.2, specific and nonspecific risk factors for IAC are summarized. No specific predictors of mortality have been identified, while the overall prognosis of IAC is known to be influenced by selected site-dependent (i.e., infection extension, nonappendicular origin) and host-related factors (i.e., age, comorbidities) [36, 37].

The increased incidence of fungal infections in surgical patients is basically correlated with the combination of a series of risk factors that include among other the following conditions. Table 20.1 shows the most common risk factor for IAC.

- increased number of surgical procedures performed in extreme ages (premature and newborn on one side, elderly on the other) and fragile patient
- increased number of critical patients admitted to intensive care unit with critical underlying diseases (tumors, leukemia, organ transplants, AIDS)
- increasing numbers of complex abdominal surgical procedure
- increased incidence of re-laparotomies to control intraabdominal source of sepsis
- severe burns
- significant increase in number of immunocompromised patients due to chemotherapies, immunotherapy, chronic use of corticosteriods, etc.

Beyond these conditions several factors must be underlined as risk factors that predispose the critical-ill surgical patient in intensive care unit to fungal infections [38–41].

Some of the most important risk factors are discussed below in more detail.

20.3.1 Candida Colonization

The role of Candida colonization has been identified since the 1970s. Several factors enhance translocation of microbes across intestinal barriers. At high concentrations, yeast will pass across even intact, healthy gut, which occurs more easily when the intestinal barriers is disrupted by operation, trauma, or disuse atrophy. Once the mucosal barrier is breached, immune defects associated with host respond to severe injuries may predispose patient to disseminate infection. Solomkin et al., in particular, underlined the link between colonization and infection in the surgical patient: it was suggested that an early antifungal therapy could be effective in preventing infections in colonized patients in more than two sites [42–44]. Moreover Pittet et al. has identified a colonization index to identify patients at risk for fungal infections [45]. The endogenous origin of the fungal infection appears once again unquestionable: the increased number of critical ill patients needing prolonged antibiotic therapies shows a greater multiplication of Candida in the gastrointestinal tract and consequently a greater susceptibility to colonization and infections spreading.

20.3.2 Malnutrition

Optimal nutritional status contributes to health maintenance and the prevention of infection. It should be remembered that the periods of the most famous famines are associated with as many periods of pestilence. The function of healthy cells is maintained by the provision of adequate nutrition. When nutrient availability is disrupted, primary and secondary malnutrition develop. Malnutrition contributes to a cascade of adverse metabolic events that compromise the immune system and impair the body's ability to adapt, recover, and survive [46–47].

In the intensive care units the problem of the malnutrition can affect the patient's evolution up to 50% or more. Interpretation of nutritional status in septic patients treated in ICU poses several difficulties. It is known that nutritional status disorders have a significant impact on the results of treatment and they should be carefully monitored in the group of malnourished septic patients requiring nutrition [48–52].

At the same time, the relationship between failure to use the gastrointestinal tract (due to prolonged total parenteral feeding) and degenerative changes of the external surface of enterocytes (in particular of microvilli up to true atrophy phenomena) is well known. Malnutrition is treated by the early delivery of essential nutrients in an effective and comprehensive manner. In the face of these evidences, we must also remember some unequivocal clinical evidences, especially in a field where there are many controversies still debated:

- the gastrointestinal tract should be used for nutritional purposes as soon as possible following the aphorism "if the gut works, use it" Practice guidelines in Europe, Canada, and the US endorse enteral feeding for patients who are critically ill and hemodynamically stable. Enteral nutrition is preferred over parenteral nutrition for most ICU patients, including those with trauma, burns, head injury, major surgery, and acute pancreatitis. For ICU patients who are hemodynamically stable and have a functioning gastrointestinal tract (GI) tract, early enteral feeding (within 24–48 h of arrival in the ICU) has become a recommended standard of care. Experts identify these early hours as a window of opportunity to provide nutrition that maintains gut barrier function and support immune responses

- if it is not possible to use only the digestive tract for a complete enteral nutrition, it should be used at least in part as "minimal enteral feeding," with the aim of facilitating intestinal motility, preventing villous atrophy, promoting the hormonal activity. In this sense it should be remembered that the intestine, more than a passive organ, should be considered a true metabolically active organ with an important nutrient "processing" action
- if the patient receives total parenteral nutrition (TPN) only and cannot use the gastroenteric tract, it means that it is a particularly severe condition and therefore at greater risk for fungal infections.

Finally it should be underlined that in case of TPN, the increased incidence of fungal infections is due to a combination of factors as well as metabolic and disuse of the digestive tract, the need of central venous catheters for long periods, hyperglycemia and the use of insulin [53–55].

20.3.3 Hyperglycemia

Diabetes mellitus (DM) is a metabolic disorder that predisposes individuals to fungal infections, including those related to Candida sp., due to an immunosuppressive effect on the patient. Several mechanisms are attributed to higher Candida sp. predisposition among DM patients depending on the local or systemic infection. Among the recognized host conditions for Candida colonization and subsequent infection are yeast adhesion to epithelial cell surfaces, higher salivary glucose levels, reduced salivary flow, microvascular degeneration, and impaired candidacidal activity of neutrophils. These conditions are particularly serious in the presence of glucose, secretion of several degradative enzymes or even a generalized immunosuppression state of the patient. Moreover, it seems that in these conditions Candida expresses in excess a receptor protein of the C3 type that inhibits the phagocytic function and favors the fungal adhesion to the endothelium and to the mucosal surfaces. These factors have a major influence on the balance between host and yeasts, favoring the transition of Candida sp. from commensal to pathogen and causing infection [56–59].

20.3.4 Antibiotics Therapy

The use of antibiotics in some way allows for the growth of Candida species on mucosal surfaces. The most commonly cited explanation is that the elimination of bacterial colonization increases substrates available for fungal overgrowth, although recent evidence suggests that more subtle alterations in the nature of the mucus covering the intestinal epithelium might be involved. The number of antibiotics used and the duration of treatment appear particularly important. It has been shown that broad-spectrum antibiotics and in particular those against gram-negative anaerobic bacteria promote Candida growth in the gastrointestinal tract and facilitate fungal infections. These data suggest once again the importance a targeted and short antibiotic therapy [60–63].

20.3.5 Pre-existing Conditions

The severity of the patient's general clinical condition is one of the most important risk factors linked with incidence of fungal infections. The original definition of compromised host was restricted to patients with advanced neoplasia and leukemia and to transplant recipients. More recent studies have shown that patients suffering from malnutrition, multiple trauma, ongoing sepsis, and burns are severely immune-depressed and also at risk of developing systemic fungal infections. In the light of these it should be considered that in the surgical patient and especially in the complicated post-operative phase many of these factors coexist at the same time [64, 65].

20.3.6 Factors Associated with Intensive Care Unit Admission

Patients needing intensive care unit admission are both more critical illness and require a series of invasive therapeutic interventions to support organ functions that could interrupt the normal anatomical protection barriers and alter the normal immunological defense mechanisms against microorganisms. Severity of illness defined by APACHE II score grater then 10 has been reported as risk factor and independently predicted Candida infections in a multivariate analysis by Pittet et al. [10, 45, 66–69].

20.4   Diagnosis

The diagnosis of intraabdominal candida infections is difficult because clinical signs and laboratory findings like elevated acute phase reactants (e.g. CRP) or fever are unspecific [70–75].

In surgical patients with a sepsis, showing no response to a broad-spectrum antibiotic therapy, a fungal infection must be taken into consideration. Risk factors for intraabdominal candidiasis are shown in Table 20.2. Positive blood cultures confirm the diagnosis of a fungal origin; however, their sensitivity is just 70%. Intraoperative samples, percutaneous punctures, drainage fluids, and urine cultures could help the diagnosis of fungal infection. However, early microbiological documentation remains a major challenge. Cultures from nonsterile sites are frequently positive, but lack specificity for differentiating infection from colonization. Only histologically proven invasive fungal growth in a biopsy of sterile tissues confirms the

Table 20.3 Most frequent candida isolation related with secondary peritonitis origin

Secondary peritonitis	*Candida* spp isolates
Appendicular	<5%
Colorectal	12%
Small bowel	35%
Upper GI tract	41%

diagnosis. Table 20.3 sum-up how different types of secondary peritonitis are most frequent related with candida isolation and IAC [76]. Moreover, it is still unclear which patients could benefit from empiric antifungal treatment and which ones might be at risk of dwelling fluconazole-resistant strains. Recently updated international guidelines preferentially targeted on candidemia and not on complicated intraabdominal fungal infections [77, 78]. Only a few statements in the above-mentioned guidelines specifically targeted IAC diagnosis and management aspects, probably because of the lack of standardized diagnostic criteria. Dupont et al. developed and validated a predictive score for likelihood of Candida involvement in peritonitis; factors included were female sex, upper gastrointestinal tract origin of peritonitis, perioperative cardiovascular failure, and previous antimicrobial therapy [79, 80]. The "Candida score" developed by Leon et al. and validated in his second study is unique in combining multiple-site colonization with pathogenesis and disease severity with previous abdominal surgery in a predictive clinical tool of invasive candidiasis, not specifically addressing IAC [81, 82]. According to Calandra et al., quantitative cultures should be performed in order to characterize patients with more severe IAC. Candida spp. obtained from surgical drainage are not sufficient for diagnosis of IAC, considering the high capability of Candida to adhere to foreign bodies [83]. These results may be useful if the drainage was inserted from\24 h; otherwise it should be considered as a colonization. Samples should be obtained from different sites of the body (feces, urine, axilla, tracheal aspirates, and gastric aspirates) in order to measure the colonization index and/or establish multifocal colonization. Non-culture-based methods can be considered a useful tool for early diagnosis of invasive candidiasis. Blood test for Candida invasive infections is based on the measurement of (1-3)-beta-Dglucan (BDG): in a recent bivariate meta-analysis, sensitivity of 76% and specificity of 85% were reported. As the negative predictive value of BDG is consistently higher than its positive predictive value, the test appears more useful to exclude rather than to confirm fungal infection. False-positive results may be related to other fungal infections (i.e., Aspergillus, Fusarium, Pneumocystis), albumin use, immunoglobulins, gauze (particularly used in the setting of abdominal surgery), hemodialysis, bacteremia, or antibiotic use (especially piperacillin/tazobactam). A new tool that could help in the diagnosis of IAC is the novel T2 magnetic resonance (T2MR) nano-diagnostic panels for Candida and bacterial bloodstream infections (BSIs). T2Candida is cleared by the US FDA and EMA for the diagnosis of candidemia with a mean time to species identification of less than 5 h. T2Candida panel amplifies DNA and detects the amplified product by amplicon-induced agglomeration of supermagnetic particles and T2 Magnetic Resonance (T2MR) measurement. T2Candida detects the five most common pathogenic Candida species, which account for 95% of candidemia at most centers. In conclusion the T2MR assay can be used to detect ongoing candidemia in a more timely fashion than the traditionally used blood cultures. However, at present, the incorporation of the T2MR assay in daily practice is anticipated to pose financial challenges to the hospital budget. Both (1-3)-beta-Dglucan (BDG) and T2 magnetic resonance (T2MR) can be very useful tools if combined together and with all other diagnostic tools and clinical signs and score improving the chance of a specific diagnosis of IAC [84–87].

20.5 Treatment and Outcomes

Aggressive management is crucial for improved outcomes, as source control interventions and antifungal treatment within 5 days are independently associated with higher survival rate [88–90]. In patients with candidemia, rates of septic shock between 20 and 38% and mortality rates above 60% have been documented. Overall, mortality rates for Candida peritonitis ranging from 25% to 60% have been reported. The mortality is higher in patients admitted to ICU (38.9%) [91]. Montravers et al. showed mortality rates of 38% among patients with Candida peritonitis in ICU but no specific factors for death were detected. Nevertheless, Bassetti M et al. showed that when the mortality is analyzed in the subgroups of patients without adequate therapy or without source control, the rates increased up to 48% and above 60%, respectively. In patients with candidemia, rates of septic shock between 20 and 38% and mortality rates above 60% have been documented [92]. Septic shock was frequently associated with the absence of an initial antifungal therapy and source control representing an independent risk factor for mortality in patients with IAC. Table 20.4 sums up the most recent guideline indication treatment.

In the light of these findings, a carefully-coordinated, multidisciplinary patient care is essential to improving outcomes for IAC, with strong interactions between intensivists, surgeons, infection disease specialists, and radiologists, recognizing the need for standardized antimicrobial stewardship and source control protocols. Moreover, it is still unclear which patients could benefit from empiric antifungal treatment and which ones might be at risk of dwelling fluconazole-resistant strains [92, 93]. Recently, abdominal candidiasis has been described as a hidden reservoir for the emergence of echinocandin-resistant Candida. *C. albicans* is the most common species isolated in IAC, and *C. glabrata* is the second most common species, notable for significant associations with multiple prior abdominal surgeries and MDR Gram-negative bacterial coinfection. *C. glabrata* candidemia also has been linked to GI tract and biliary sources. Interestingly, 10% of Candida isolates were

Table 20.4 Recommended drugs according to different guidelines

Guidelines	Recomended first-line drug
IDSA 2009	Fluconazole/echinocandins
ESCMID 2012	Echinocandins
SITI/ISC 2013	Echinocandins
ITALIC 2013	Echinocandins

C. parapsilosis, a species long associated with exogenous sources such as intravenous catheters. Recently, abdominal candidiasis has been described as a hidden reservoir for the emergence of echinocandin-resistant Candida. Source control is the primary therapeutic procedure in patients with IAC. Several antifungal agents are nowadays available for empirical and targeted treatment of IAC; however, international guidelines preferentially target clinical settings such as candidemia or bacterial intraabdominal infections, without providing enough clinical support for the management of IAC patients. Based on the most recent evidences we can suggest that empirical antifungal treatment with echinocandins or lipid formulations of amphotericin B should be strongly considered in critically ill patients or those with previous exposure to azoles and suspected intraabdominal infection with at least one specific risk factor for Candida infection. In a recent study we tested the treatment with anidulafungin in a group of patients with microbiologically documented IAC, and as conclusion we found that anidulafungin provided good efficacy and tolerability, with adequate plasma concentrations, even if further studies are needed to address if anidulafungin has an adequate penetration of the peritoneum (Fig. 20.1). In patients with nonspecific risk factors, a positive mannan/antimannan or (1-3)-beta-Dglucan (BDG) or polymerase chain reaction (PCR) test result should be present to start empirical therapy. Fluconazole can be adopted for the empirical and targeted therapy of noncritically ill patients without previous exposure to azoles, unless they are known to be colonized with a Candida strain with reduced susceptibility to

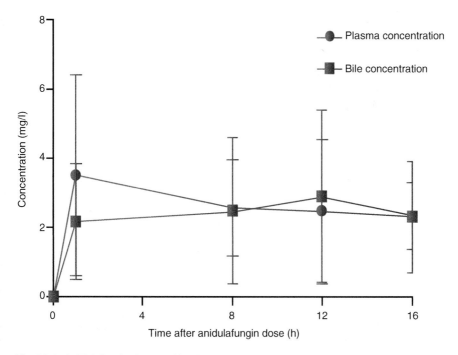

Fig. 20.1   Anidulafungin pharmacokinetic

azoles. Treatment can be simplified by stepping down to an azole (fluconazole or voriconazole) after at least 5–7 days of treatment with echinocandins or lipid formulations of amphotericin B, if the species is susceptible and the patient has clinically improved. The duration of treatment depends on the extent of organ involvement, the patient's clinical condition, and the presence or absence of positive blood cultures. Few data are available about duration of therapy in patients with IAC. After an adequate source control, as well as in candidemia, 14 days of antifungal therapy, after the first negative blood culture, should be prescribed for patients with IAC without documented organ involvement. In the study of Mortravers et al., median duration of antifungal treatment in patients with Candida peritonitis was 20 days in survivors [94–124].

References

 1. Bassetti M, Giacobbe DR, Vena A, Trucchi C, Ansaldi F, Antonelli M, Adamkova V, Alicino C, et al. Incidence and outcome of invasive candidiasis in intensive care units (ICUs) in Europe: results of the EUCANDICU project. Crit Care. 2019 Jun 14;23(1):219.
 2. Bassetti M, Righi E, Ansaldi F, Merelli M, Scarparo C, Antonelli M, Garnacho-Montero J, Diaz-Martin A, Palacios-Garcia I, et al. A multicenter multinational study of abdominal candidiasis: epidemiology, outcomes and predictors of mortality. Intensive Care Med. 2015 Sep;41(9):1601–10.
 3. Vincent JL, Anaissie E, Bruining H, Demajo W, el-Ebiary M, Haber J, Hiramatsu Y, Nitenberg G, Nyström PO, et al. Epidemiology, diagnosis and treatment of systemic Candida infection in surgical patients under intensive care. Intensive Care Med. 1998 Mar;24(3):206–16.
 4. Bongomin F, Gago S, Oladele RO, Denning DW. Global and multi-national prevalence of fungal diseases-estimate precision. J Fungi (Basel). 2017 Oct 18;3(4):pii: E57.
 5. Denning DW. Global fungal burden. Mycoses. 2013;56:13.
 6. Limper AH, Adenis A, Le T, Harrison TS. Fungal infections in HIV/AIDS. Lancet Infect Dis. 2017;17(11):e334–43.
 7. Vincent JL, Sakr Y, Sprung CL, Ranieri VM, Reinhart K, Gerlach H, Moreno R, Carlet J, Le Gall JR, Payen D. Sepsis occurrence in acutely ill patients investigators. Sepsis in European intensive care units: results of the SOAP study. Crit Care Med. 2006 Feb;34(2):344–53.
 8. Vincent JL, Bihari DJ, Suter PM, Bruining HA, White J, Nicolas-Chanoin MH, Wolff M, Spencer RC, Hemmer M. The prevalence of nosocomial infection in intensive care units in Europe. Results of the European Prevalence of Infection in Intensive Care (EPIC) study. EPIC International Advisory Committee. JAMA. 1995 Aug 23–30;274(8):639–44.
 9. Miguel N, León MA, Ibáñez J, Díaz RM, Merten A, Gahete F. Sepsis-related organ failure assessment and withholding or withdrawing life support from critically ill patients. Crit Care. 1998;2(2):61–6.
10. Aguilar G, Delgado C, Corrales I, Izquierdo A, Gracia E, Moreno T, Romero E, Ferrando C, Carbonell JA, Borrás R, Navarro D, Belda FJ. Epidemiology of invasive candidiasis in a surgical intensive care unit: an observational study. BMC Res Notes. 2015;8:491.
11. Sganga G. Clinical aspects of invasive candidiasis in the surgical patient. Drugs. 2009;69(Suppl 1):29–32.
12. Haltmeier T, Inaba K, Effron Z, Dollbaum R, Shulman IA, Benjamin E, Lam L, Demetriades D. Candida score as a predictor of worse outcomes and mortality in severely injured trauma patients with positive Candida cultures. Am Surg. 2015 Oct;81(10):1067–73.
13. Enoch DA, Yang H, Aliyu SH, Micallef C. The changing epidemiology of invasive fungal infections. Methods Mol Biol. 2017;1508:17–65. Review.

14. Blyth DM, Mende K, Weintrob AC, Beckius ML, Zera WC, Bradley W, Lu D, Tribble DR, Murray CK. Resistance patterns and clinical significance of Candida colonization and infection in combat-related injured patients from Iraq and Afghanistan. Open Forum Infect Dis. 2014 Dec 16;1(3):ofu109.

15. Manolakaki D, Velmahos G, Kourkoumpetis T, Chang Y, Alam HB, De Moya MM, Mylonakis E. Candida infection and colonization among trauma patients. Virulence. 2010 Sep–Oct;1(5):367–75.

16. Mathur P, Hasan F, Singh PK, Malhotra R, Walia K, Chowdhary A. Five-year profile of candidaemia at an Indian trauma centre: High rates of Candida auris blood stream infections. Mycoses. 2018 Sep;61(9):674–80.

17. Cruciani M, de Lalla F, Mengoli C. Prophylaxis of Candida infections in adult trauma and surgical intensive care patients: a systematic review and meta-analysis. Intensive Care Med. 2005 Nov;31(11):1479–87. Epub 2005 Sep 20. Review.

18. Guery BP, Arendrup MC, Auzinger G, Azoulay E, Borges Sá M, Johnson EM, Müller E, Putensen C, Rotstein C, Sganga G, Venditti M, Zaragoza Crespo R, Kullberg BJ. Management of invasive candidiasis and candidemia in adult non-neutropenic intensive care unit patients: Part I. Epidemiology and diagnosis. Intensive Care Med. 2009 Jan;35(1):55–62.

19. Deitch EA. Gut-origin sepsis: evolution of a concept. Surgeon. 2012 Dec;10(6):350–6.

20. MacFie J, O'Boyle C, Mitchell CJ, et al. Gut origin of sepsis: a prospective study investigating associations between bacterial translocation, gastric microflora, and septic morbidity. Gut. 1999;45:223–8.

21. Schweinburg FB, Frank HA, Frank ED, et al. Transmural migration of intestinal bacteria during peritoneal irrigation in uremic dogs. Proc Soc Exp Biol Med. 1949;71:150–3.

22. Assimakopoulos SF, Triantos C, Thomopoulos K, Fligou F, Maroulis I, Marangos M, Gogos CA. Gut-origin sepsis in the critically ill patient: pathophysiology and treatment. Infection. 2018 Dec;46(6):751–60.

23. Lu F, Inoue K, Kato J, Minamishima S, Morisaki H. Functions and regulation of lipocalin-2 in gut-origin sepsis: a narrative review. Crit Care. 2019 Aug 2;23(1):269.

24. Jiang LY, Zhang M, Zhou TE, Yang ZF, Wen LQ, Chang JX. Changes of the immunological barrier of intestinal mucosa in rats with sepsis. World J Emerg Med. 2010;1(2):138–43.

25. Orasch C, Marchetti O, Garbino J, Schrenzel J, Zimmerli S, Mühlethaler K, Pfyffer G, Ruef C, Fehr J, Zbinden R, Calandra T, Bille J. FUNGINOS. Candida species distribution and antifungal susceptibility testing according to European Committee on Antimicrobial Susceptibility Testing and new vs. old Clinical and Laboratory Standards Institute clinical breakpoints: a 6-year prospective candidaemia survey from the fungal infection network of Switzerland. Clin Microbiol Infect. 2014 Jul;20(7):698–705.

26. Lilly EA, Ikeh M, Nash EE, Fidel PL Jr, Noverr MC. Immune protection against lethal fungal-bacterial intra-abdominal infections. MBio. 2018 Jan 16;9(1):e01472–17.

27. Arendrup MC. Candida and candidaemia. Susceptibility and epidemiology. Dan Med J. 2013 Nov;60(11):B4698.

28. Amornphimoltham P, Yuen PST, Star RA, Leelahavanichkul A. Gut leakage of fungal-derived inflammatory mediators: part of a gut-liver-kidney axis in bacterial sepsis. Dig Dis Sci. 2019 Sep;64(9):2416–28.

29. Khatib R, Johnson LB, Fakih MG, Riederer K, Briski L. Current trends in candidemia and species distribution among adults: Candida glabrata surpasses C. albicans in diabetic patients and abdominal sources. Mycoses. 2016 Dec;59(12):781–6.

30. Albac S, Schmitz A, Lopez-Alayon C, d'Enfert C, Sautour M, Ducreux A, Labruère-Chazal C, Laue M, Holland G, Bonnin A, Dalle F. Candida albicans is able to use M cells as a portal of entry across the intestinal barrier in vitro. Cell Microbiol. 2016 Feb;18(2):195–210.

31. Cheng S, Clancy CJ, Xu W, Schneider F, Hao B, Mitchell AP, Nguyen MH. Profiling of Candida albicans gene expression during intra-abdominal candidiasis identifies biologic processes involved in pathogenesis. J Infect Dis. 2013 Nov 1;208(9):1529–37.

32. Kronen R, Liang SY, Bochicchio G, Bochicchio K, Powderly WG, Spec A. Invasive fungal infections secondary to traumatic injury. Int J Infect Dis. 2017 Sep;62:102–11.

33. Rasilainen SK, Juhani MP, Kalevi LA. Microbial colonization of open abdomen in critically ill surgical patients. World J Emerg Surg. 2015 Jun 25;10:25.
34. Jabra-Rizk MA, Kong EF, Tsui C, Nguyen MH, Clancy CJ, Fidel PL Jr, Noverr M. Candida albicans pathogenesis: fitting within the host-microbe damage response framework. Infect Immun. 2016 Sep 19;84(10):2724–39.
35. Montravers P, Blot S, Dimopoulos G, Eckmann C, Eggimann P, Guirao X, Paiva JA, Sganga G, De Waele J. Therapeutic management of peritonitis: a comprehensive guide for intensivists. Intensive Care Med. 2016 Aug;42(8):1234–47.
36. Blumberg HM, Jarvis WR, Soucie JM, Edwards JE, Patterson JE, Pfaller MA, Rangel-Frausto MS, Rinaldi MG, Saiman L, Wiblin RT, Wenzel RP. National Epidemiology of Mycoses Survey (NEMIS) study group: risk factors for candidal bloodstream infections in surgical intensive care unit patients: the NEMIS prospective multicenter study. The National Epidemiology of Mycosis Survey. Clin Infect Dis. 2001;33:177–86.
37. Rajendran R, Sherry L, Deshpande A, Johnson EM, Hanson MF, Williams C, Munro CA, Jones BL, Ramage G. A prospective surveillance study of candidaemia: epidemiology, risk factors, antifungal treatment and outcome in hospitalized patients. Front Microbiol. 2016 Jun 16;7:915.
38. Eggimann P, Bille J, Marchetti O. Diagnosis of invasive candidiasis in the ICU. Ann Intensive Care. 2011 Sep 1;1:37.
39. Sandven P, Qvist H, Skovlund E, Giercksky KE. NORGAS Group and the Norwegian Yeast Study Group. Significance of Candida recovered from intraoperative specimens in patients with intra-abdominal perforations. Crit Care Med. 2002 Mar;30(3):541–7.
40. de Ruiter J, Weel J, Manusama E, Kingma WP, van der Voort PH. The epidemiology of intra-abdominal flora in critically ill patients with secondary and tertiary abdominal sepsis. Infection. 2009 Dec;37(6):522–7.
41. León C, Alvarez-Lerma F, Ruiz-Santana S, León MA, Nolla J, Jordá R, Saavedra P, Palomar M, EPCAN Study Group. Fungal colonization and/or infection in non-neutropenic critically ill patients: results of the EPCAN observational study. Eur J Clin Microbiol Infect Dis. 2009 Mar;28(3):233–42.
42. Solomkin JS, Mazuski JE, Bradley JS, Rodvold KA, Goldstein EJ, Baron EJ, O'Neill PJ, Chow AW, Dellinger EP, Eachempati SR, Gorbach S, Hilfiker M, May AK, Nathens AB, Sawyer RG, Bartlett JG. Diagnosis and management of complicated intra-abdominal infection in adults and children: guidelines by the Surgical Infection Society and the Infectious Diseases Society of America. Clin Infect Dis. 2010 Jan 15;50(2):133–64.
43. Solomkin JS. Pathogenesis and management of Candida infection syndromes in non-neutropenic patients. New Horiz. 1993 May;1(2):202–13. Review.
44. Solomkin JS, Flohr AB, Quie PG, Simmons RL. The role of Candida in intraperitoneal infections. Surgery. 1980 Oct;88(4):524–30.
45. Eggimann P, Pittet D. Candida colonization index and subsequent infection in critically ill surgical patients: 20 years later. Intensive Care Med. 2014 Oct;40(10):1429–48.
46. Khanna K, Yi PH, Sing DC, Geiger E, Metz LN. Hypoalbuminemia is associated with septic revisions after primary surgery and postoperative infection after revision surgery. Spine (Phila Pa 1976). 2018 Mar 15;43(6):454–60.
47. de Luis DA, Culebras JM, Aller R, Eiros-Bouza JM. Surgical infection and malnutrition. Nutr Hosp. 2014 Sep 1;30(3):509–13.
48. McCall ME, Adamo A, Latko K, Rieder AK, Durand N, Nathanson T. Maximizing nutrition support practice and measuring adherence to nutrition support guidelines in a Canadian tertiary care ICU. J Intensive Care Med. 2018 Mar;33(3):209–17.
49. Cahill NE, Dhaliwal R, Day AG, Jiang X, Heyland DK. Nutrition therapy in the critical care setting: what is "best achievable" practice? An international multicenter observational study. Crit Care Med. 2010 Feb;38(2):395–401.
50. Kizilarslanoglu MC, Kuyumcu ME, Yesil Y, Halil M. Sarcopenia in critically ill patients. J Anesth. 2016 Oct;30(5):884–90.

51. Weimann A, Braga M, Carli F, Higashiguchi T, Hübner M, Klek S, Laviano A, Ljungqvist O, Lobo DN, Martindale R, Waitzberg DL, Bischoff SC, Singer P. ESPEN guideline: clinical nutrition in surgery. Clin Nutr. 2017 Jun;36(3):623–50.
52. Braga M, Ljungqvist O, Soeters P, Fearon K, Weimann A, Bozzetti F. ESPEN guidelines on parenteral nutrition: surgery. Clin Nutr. 2009 Aug;28(4):378–86.
53. Livingston A, Seamons C, Dalton T. If the gut works use it. Nurs Manage. 2000 May;31(5):39–42.
54. Yamashiro Y. Gut microbiota in health and disease. Ann Nutr Metab. 2017;71(3–4):242–6.
55. Sam QH, Chang MW, Chai LY. The fungal mycobiome and its interaction with gut bacteria in the host. Int J Mol Sci. 2017 Feb 4;18(2):330.
56. Hostetter MK. Handicaps to host defense. Effects of hyperglycemia on C3 and Candida albicans. Diabetes. 1990 Mar;39(3):271–5. Review.
57. Bader MS, Hinthorn D, Lai SM, Ellerbeck EF. Hyperglycaemia and mortality of diabetic patients with candidaemia. Diabet Med. 2005 Sep;22(9):1252–7.
58. Bader MS, Lai SM, Kumar V, Hinthorn D. Candidemia in patients with diabetes mellitus: epidemiology and predictors of mortality. Scand J Infect Dis. 2004;36(11–12):860–4.
59. Rodrigues CF, Rodrigues ME, Henriques M. Candida sp. infections in patients with diabetes mellitus. J Clin Med. 2019 Jan 10;8(1):76.
60. Shahin J, Allen EJ, Patel K, Muskett H, Harvey SE, Edgeworth J, Kibbler CC, Barnes RA, Biswas S, Soni N, Rowan KM, Harrison DA. FIRE study investigators. Predicting invasive fungal disease due to Candida species in non-neutropenic, critically ill, adult patients in United Kingdom critical care units. BMC Infect Dis. 2016 Sep 9;16:480.
61. Sganga G, Bianco G, Fiori B, Nure E, Spanu T, Lirosi MC, Frongillo F, Agnes S. Surveillance of bacterial and fungal infections in the postoperative period following liver transplantation: a series from 2005–2011. Transplant Proc. 2013 Sep;45(7):2718–21.
62. Muskett H, Shahin J, Eyres G, Harvey S, Rowan K, Harrison D. Risk factors for invasive fungal disease in critically ill adult patients: a systematic review. Crit Care. 2011;15(6):R287.
63. Leroy O, Gangneux JP, Montravers P, Mira JP, Gouin F, Sollet JP, Carlet J, Reynes J, Rosenheim M, Regnier B, Lortholary O, AmarCand Study Group. Epidemiology, management, and risk factors for death of invasive Candida infections in critical care: a multicenter, prospective, observational study in France (2005–2006). Crit Care Med. 2009 May;37(5):1612–8.
64. Sganga G, Bianco G, Frongillo F, Lirosi MC, Nure E, Agnes S. Fungal infections after liver transplantation: incidence and outcome. Transplant Proc. 2014 Sep;46(7):2314–8.
65. Bassetti M, Peghin M, Carnelutti A, Righi E, Merelli M, Ansaldi F, Trucchi C, Alicino C, Sartor A, Wauters J, Lagrou K, Tascini C, Menichetti F, Mesini A, De Rosa FG, Lagunes L, Rello J, Colombo AL, Vena A, Munoz P, Tumbarello M, Sganga G, Martin-Loeches I, Viscoli C. Invasive candida infections in liver transplant recipients: clinical features and risk factors for mortality. Transplant Direct. 2017 Apr 18;3(5):e156.
66. Yang Y, Guo F, Kang Y, Zang B, Cui W, Qin B, Qin Y, Fang Q, Qin T, Jiang D, Cai B, Li R, Qiu H, China-SCAN Team. Epidemiology, clinical characteristics, and risk factors for mortality of early- and late-onset invasive candidiasis in intensive care units in China. Medicine (Baltimore). 2017 Oct;96(42):e7830.
67. Massou S, Ahid S, Azendour H, Bensghir M, Mounir K, Iken M, Lmimouni BE, Balkhi H, Drissi Kamili N, Haimeur C. Systemic candidiasis in medical intensive care unit: analysis of risk factors and the contribution of colonization index. Pathol Biol (Paris). 2013 Jun;61(3):108–12.
68. Playford EG, Lipman J, Jones M, Lau AF, Kabir M, Chen SC, Marriott DJ, Seppelt I, Gottlieb T, Cheung W, Iredell JR, McBryde ES, Sorrell TC. Problematic dichotomization of risk for Intensive Care Unit (ICU)-acquired invasive candidiasis: results using a risk-predictive model to categorize 3 levels of risk from a multicenter prospective cohort of Australian ICU patients. Clin Infect Dis. 2016 Dec 1;63(11):1463–9.
69. Guo F, Yang Y, Kang Y, Zang B, Cui W, Qin B, Qin Y, Fang Q, Qin T, Jiang D, Li W, Gu Q, Zhao H, Liu D, Guan X, Li J, Ma X, Yu K, Chan D, Yan J, Tang Y, Liu W, Li R, Qiu

H. China-SCAN team invasive candidiasis in intensive care units in China: a multicentre prospective observational study. J Antimicrob Chemother. 2013 Jul;68(7):1660–8.

70. Clancy CJ, Nguyen MH. Diagnosing invasive candidiasis. J Clin Microbiol. 2018 Apr 25;56(5):e01909–17.

71. Clancy CJ, Nguyen MH. Non-culture diagnostics for invasive candidiasis: promise and unintended consequences. J Fungi (Basel). 2018 Feb 19;4(1):27.

72. McCarty TP, Pappas PG. Invasive candidiasis. Infect Dis Clin North Am. 2016 Mar;30(1):103–24.

73. Antinori S, Milazzo L, Sollima S, Galli M, Corbellino M. Candidemia and invasive candidiasis in adults: a narrative review. Eur J Intern Med. 2016 Oct;34:21–8.

74. Pitarch A, Nombela C, Gil C. Diagnosis of invasive candidiasis: from gold standard methods to promising leading-edge technologies. Curr Top Med Chem. 2018;18(16):1375–92.

75. Backx M, White PL, Barnes RA. New fungal diagnostics. Br J Hosp Med (Lond). 2014 May;75(5):271–6.

76. Pagès A, Iriart X, Molinier L, Georges B, Berry A, Massip P, Juillard-Condat B. Cost effectiveness of candida polymerase chain reaction detection and empirical antifungal treatment among patients with suspected fungal peritonitis in the intensive care unit. Value Health. 2017 Dec;20(10):1319–28.

77. Pappas PG, Kauffman CA, Andes DR, Clancy CJ, Marr KA, Ostrosky-Zeichner L, Reboli AC, Schuster MG, Vazquez JA, Walsh TJ, Zaoutis TE, Sobel JD. Clinical practice guideline for the management of candidiasis: 2016 update by the Infectious Diseases Society of America. Clin Infect Dis. 2016 Feb 15;62(4):e1–50.

78. Cornely OA, Bassetti M, Calandra T, Garbino J, Kullberg BJ, Lortholary O, Meersseman W, Akova M, Arendrup MC, Arikan-Akdagli S, Bille J, Castagnola E, Cuenca-Estrella M, Donnelly JP, Groll AH, Herbrecht R, Hope WW, Jensen HE, Lass-Flörl C, Petrikkos G, Richardson MD, Roilides E, Verweij PE, Viscoli C, Ullmann AJ, ESCMID Fungal Infection Study Group. ESCMID guideline for the diagnosis and management of Candida diseases 2012: non-neutropenic adult patients. Clin Microbiol Infect. 2012 Dec;18(Suppl 7):19–37.

79. Dupont H, Paugam-Burtz C, Muller-Serieys C, Fierobe L, Chosidow D, Marmuse JP, Mantz J, Desmonts JM. Predictive factors of mortality due to polymicrobial peritonitis with Candida isolation in peritoneal fluid in critically ill patients. Arch Surg. 2002 Dec;137(12):1341–6.

80. Dupont H, Mahjoub Y, Chouaki T, Lorne E, Zogheib E. Antifungal prevention of systemic candidiasis in immunocompetent ICU adults: systematic review and meta-analysis of clinical trials. Crit Care Med. 2017 Nov;45(11):1937–45.

81. León C, Ruiz-Santana S, Saavedra P, Almirante B, Nolla-Salas J, Alvarez-Lerma F, Garnacho-Montero J, León MA, EPCAN Study Group. A bedside scoring system ("Candida score") for early antifungal treatment in nonneutropenic critically ill patients with Candida colonization. Crit Care Med. 2006 Mar;34(3):730–7.

82. León C, Ruiz-Santana S, Saavedra P, Galván B, Blanco A, Castro C, Balasini C, Utande-Vázquez A, González de Molina FJ, Blasco-Navalproto MA, López MJ, Charles PE, Martín E, Hernández-Viera MA, Cava Study Group. Usefulness of the "Candida score" for discriminating between Candida colonization and invasive candidiasis in non-neutropenic critically ill patients: a prospective multicenter study. Crit Care Med. 2009 May;37(5):1624–33.

83. Calandra T, Roberts JA, Antonelli M, Bassetti M, Vincent JL. Diagnosis and management of invasive candidiasis in the ICU: an updated approach to an old enemy. Crit Care. 2016 May 27;20(1):125.

84. Novy E, Laithier FX, Machouart MC, Albuisson E, Guerci P, Losser MR. Determination of 1,3-β-D-glucan in the peritoneal fluid for the diagnosis of intra-abdominal candidiasis in critically ill patients: a pilot study. Minerva Anestesiol. 2018 Dec;84(12):1369–76.

85. León C, Ruiz-Santana S, Saavedra P, Castro C, Loza A, Zakariya I, Úbeda A, Parra M, Macías D, Tomás JI, Rezusta A, Rodríguez A, Gómez F, Martín-Mazuelos E, Cava Trem Study Group. Contribution of Candida biomarkers and DNA detection for the diagnosis of invasive candidiasis in ICU patients with severe abdominal conditions. Crit Care. 2016 May 16;20(1):149.

86. Nguyen MH, Wissel MC, Shields RK, Salomoni MA, Hao B, Press EG, Shields RM, Cheng S, Mitsani D, Vadnerkar A, Silveira FP, Kleiboeker SB, Clancy CJ. Performance of Candida real-time polymerase chain reaction, β-D-glucan assay, and blood cultures in the diagnosis of invasive candidiasis. Clin Infect Dis. 2012 May;54(9):1240–8.

87. Alam FF, Mustafa AS, Khan ZU. Comparative evaluation of (1, 3)-beta-D-glucan, mannan and anti-mannan antibodies, and Candida species-specific snPCR in patients with candidemia. BMC Infect Dis. 2007 Sep 4;7:103.

88. Sartelli M, Chichom-Mefire A, Labricciosa FM, Hardcastle T, Abu-Zidan FM, Adesunkanmi AK, Ansaloni L, et al. The management of intra-abdominal infections from a global perspective: 2017 WSES guidelines for management of intra-abdominal infections. World J Emerg Surg. 2017 Jul 10;12:29.

89. Scudeller L, Viscoli C, Menichetti F, del Bono V, Cristini F, Tascini C, Bassetti M, Viale P, ITALIC Group. An Italian consensus for invasive candidiasis management (ITALIC). Infection. 2014 Apr;42(2):263–79.

90. Sartelli M, Weber DG, Ruppé E, Bassetti M, Wright BJ, Ansaloni L, Catena F, Coccolini F, et al. Antimicrobials: a global alliance for optimizing their rational use in intra-abdominal infections (AGORA). World J Emerg Surg. 2016 Jul 15;11:33.

91. Vergidis P, Clancy CJ, Shields RK, Park SY, Wildfeuer BN, Simmons RL, Nguyen MH. Intra-abdominal candidiasis: the importance of early source control and antifungal treatment. PLoS One. 2016 Apr 28;11(4):e0153247.

92. Bassetti M, Marchetti M, Chakrabarti A, Colizza S, Garnacho-Montero J, Kett DH, Munoz P, Cristini F, Andoniadou A, Viale P, Rocca GD, Roilides E, Sganga G, Walsh TJ, Tascini C, Tumbarello M, Menichetti F, Righi E, Eckmann C, Viscoli C, Shorr AF, Leroy O, Petrikos G, De Rosa FG. A research agenda on the management of intra-abdominal candidiasis: results from a consensus of multinational experts. Intensive Care Med. 2013 Dec;39(12):2092–106.

93. Lagunes L, Borgatta B, Martín-Gomez MT, Rey-Pérez A, Antonelli M, Righi E, Merelli M, Brugnaro P, Dimopoulos G, Garnacho-Montero J, Colombo AL, Luzzati R, Menichetti F, Muñoz P, Nucci M, Scotton G, Viscoli C, Tumbarello M, Bassetti M, Rello J, IAC Study Investigators. Predictors of choice of initial antifungal treatment in intraabdominal candidiasis. Clin Microbiol Infect. 2016 Aug;22(8):719–24.

94. Benoist H, Rodier S, de La Blanchardière A, Bonhomme J, Cormier H, Thibon P, Saint-Lorant G. Appropriate use of antifungals: impact of an antifungal stewardship program on the clinical outcome of candidaemia in a French University Hospital. Infection. 2019 Jun;47(3):435–40.

95. O'Leary RA, Einav S, Leone M, Madách K, Martin C, Martin-Loeches I. Management of invasive candidiasis and candidaemia in critically ill adults: expert opinion of the European Society of Anaesthesia Intensive Care Scientific Subcommittee. J Hosp Infect. 2018 Apr;98(4):382–90.

96. Sganga G, Wang M, Capparella MR, Tawadrous M, Yan JL, Aram JA, Montravers P. Evaluation of anidulafungin in the treatment of intra-abdominal candidiasis: a pooled analysis of patient-level data from 5 prospective studies. Eur J Clin Microbiol Infect Dis. 2019 Jul 6;38(10):1849–56.

97. Pappas PG, Kauffman CA, Andes DR, Clancy CJ, Marr KA, Ostrosky-Zeichner L, Reboli AC, Schuster MG, Vazquez JA, Walsh TJ, Zaoutis TE, Sobel JD. Clinical practice guideline for the management of candidiasis: 2016 update by the Infectious Diseases Society of America. Clin Infect Dis. 2016 Feb 15;62(4):e1–50.

98. Guery BP, Arendrup MC, Auzinger G, Azoulay E, Borges Sá M, Johnson EM, Müller E, Putensen C, Rotstein C, Sganga G, Venditti M, Zaragoza Crespo R, Kullberg BJ. Management of invasive candidiasis and candidemia in adult non-neutropenic intensive care unit patients: Part II. Treat Intensive Care Med. 2009 Feb;35(2):206–14.

99. Zaragoza R, Pemán J, Salavert M, Viudes A, Solé A, Jarque I, Monte E, Romá E, Cantón E. Multidisciplinary approach to the treatment of invasive fungal infections in adult patients. Prophylaxis, empirical, preemptive or targeted therapy, which is the best in the different hosts? Ther Clin Risk Manag. 2008 Dec;4(6):1261–80.

100. Montagna T, Lovero G, Coretti C, Martinelli D, De Giglio O, Iatta R, Balbino S, Rosato A, Caggiano G. Susceptibility to echinocandins of Candida spp. strains isolated in Italy assessed by European Committee for Antimicrobial Susceptibility Testing and Clinical Laboratory Standards Institute broth microdilution methods. Montagna BMC Microbiol. 2015 May 20;15:106.

101. Occhionorelli S, Zese M, Cultrera R, Lacavalla D, Albanese M, Vasquez G. Open abdomen management and candida infections: a very likely link. Gastroenterol Res Pract. 2017;2017:5187620.

102. Zilberberg M, Yu HT, Chaudhari P, Emons MF, Khandelwal N, Shorr AF. Relationship of fluconazole prophylaxis with fungal microbiology in hospitalized intra-abdominal surgery patients: a descriptive cohort study. Crit Care. 2014 Oct 29;18(5):590.

103. Lima WG, Alves-Nascimento LA, Andrade JT, Vieira L, de Azambuja Ribeiro RIM, Thomé RG, Dos Santos HB, Ferreira JMS, Soares AC. Are the statins promising antifungal agents against invasive candidiasis? Biomed Pharmacother. 2019 Mar;111:270–81.

104. Maseda E, Rodríguez-Manzaneque M, Dominguez D, González-Serrano M, Mouriz L, Álvarez-Escudero J, Ojeda N, Sánchez-Zamora P, Granizo JJ, Giménez MJ, Peri-Operative Infection Working Group of the Spanish Society of Anesthesiology and Critical Care (GTIPO-SEDAR). Intraabdominal candidiasis in surgical ICU patients treated with anidula-fungin: a multicenter retrospective study. Rev Esp Quimioter. 2016 Feb;29(1):32–9.

105. Pea F, Righi E, Cojutti P, Carnelutti A, Baccarani U, Soardo G, Bassetti M. Intra-abdominal penetration and pharmacodynamic exposure to fluconazole in three liver transplant patients with deep-seated candidiasis. J Antimicrob Chemother. 2014 Sep;69(9):2585–6.

106. Vincent JL. Microbial resistance: lessons from the EPIC study. European Prevalence of Infection. Intensive Care Med. 2000;26(Suppl 1):S3–8.

107. Olaechea PM, Palomar M, León-Gil C, Alvarez-Lerma F, Jordá R, Nolla-Salas J, León-Regidor MA. EPCAN Study Group Economic impact of Candida colonization and Candida infection in the critically ill patient. Eur J Clin Microbiol Infect Dis. 2004 Apr;23(4):323–30.

108. Knitsch W, Vincent JL, Utzolino S, François B, Dinya T, Dimopoulos G, Özgüneş İ, Valía JC, Eggimann P, León C, Montravers P, Phillips S, Tweddle L, Karas A, Brown M, Cornely OA. A randomized, placebo-controlled trial of preemptive antifungal therapy for the prevention of invasive candidiasis following gastrointestinal surgery for intra-abdominal infections. Clin Infect Dis. 2015 Dec 1;61(11):1671–8.

109. Shields RK, Nguyen MH, Press EG, Clancy CJ. Abdominal candidiasis is a hidden reservoir of echinocandin resistance. Antimicrob Agents Chemother. 2014 Dec;58(12):7601–5.

110. Dimopoulos G, Paiva JA, Meersseman W, Pachl J, Grigoras I, Sganga G, Montravers P, Auzinger G, Sá MB, Miller PJ, Marček T, Kantecki M, Ruhnke M. Efficacy and safety of anidulafungin in elderly, critically ill patients with invasive Candida infections: a post hoc analysis. Int J Antimicrob Agents. 2012 Dec;40(6):521–6.

111. Sganga G, Pepe G, Cozza V, Nure E, Lirosi MC, Frongillo F, Grossi U, Bianco G, Agnes S. Anidulafungin—a new therapeutic option for Candida infections in liver transplantation. Transplant Proc. 2012 Sep;44(7):1982–5.

112. Ruhnke M, Paiva JA, Meersseman W, Pachl J, Grigoras I, Sganga G, Menichetti F, Montravers P, Auzinger G, Dimopoulos G, Borges Sá M, Miller PJ, Marček T, Kantecki M. Anidulafungin for the treatment of candidaemia/invasive candidiasis in selected critically ill patients. Clin Microbiol Infect. 2012 Jul;18(7):680–7.

113. Xie GH, Fang XM, Fang Q, Wu XM, Jin YH, Wang JL, Guo QL, Gu MN, Xu QP, Wang DX, Yao SL, Yuan SY, Du ZH, Sun YB, Wang HH, Wu SJ, Cheng BL. Impact of invasive fungal infection on outcomes of severe sepsis: a multicenter matched cohort study in critically ill surgical patients. Crit Care. 2008;12(1):R5.

114. Almirante B, Rodríguez D, Park BJ, Cuenca-Estrella M, Planes AM, Almela M, Mensa J, Sanchez F, Ayats J, Gimenez M, Saballs P, Fridkin SK, Morgan J, Rodriguez-Tudela JL, Warnock DW, Pahissa A. Barcelona Candidemia Project Study Group: Epidemiology and predictors of mortality in cases of Candida bloodstream infection: results from population-based surveillance, barcelona, Spain, from 2002 to 2003. J Clin Microbiol. 2005;43:1829–235.

115. Raymond DP, Pelletier SJ, Crabtree TD, Gleason TG, Pruett TL, Sawyer RG. Impact of bloodstream infection on outcomes among infected surgical inpatients. Ann Surg. 2001;233:549–55.

116. Maseda E, Rodríguez-Manzaneque M, Dominguez D, González-Serrano M, Mouriz L, Álvarez-Escudero J, Ojeda N, Sánchez-Zamora P, Granizo JJ, Giménez MJ, Peri-Operative Infection Working Group of the Spanish Society of Anesthesiology and Critical Care (GTIPO-SEDAR). Intraabdominal candidiasis in surgical ICU patients treated with anidulafungin: a multicenter retrospective study. Rev Esp Quimioter. 2016 Feb;29(1):32–9.

117. Choi H, Kim JH, Seong H, Lee W, Jeong W, Ahn JY, Jeong SJ, Ku NS, Yeom JS, Kim YK, Kim HY, Song YG, Kim JM, Choi JY. Changes in the utilization patterns of antifungal agents, medical cost and clinical outcomes of candidemia from the health-care benefit expansion to include newer antifungal agents. Int J Infect Dis. 2019 Jun;83:49–55.

118. Heimann SM, Cornely OA, Wisplinghoff H, Kochanek M, Stippel D, Padosch SA, Langebartels G, Reuter H, Reiner M, Vierzig A, Seifert H, Vehreschild MJ, Glossmann J, Franke B, Vehreschild JJ. Candidemia in the intensive care unit: analysis of direct treatment costs and clinical outcome in patients treated with echinocandins or fluconazole. Eur J Clin Microbiol Infect Dis. 2015 Feb;34(2):331–8.

119. Lortholary O, Renaudat C, Sitbon K, Madec Y, Denoeud-Ndam L, Wolff M, Fontanet A, Bretagne S, Dromer F, French Mycosis Study Group. Worrisome trends in incidence and mortality of candidemia in intensive care units (Paris area, 2002–2010). Intensive Care Med. 2014 Sep;40(9):1303–12.

120. Puig-Asensio M, Pemán J, Zaragoza R, Garnacho-Montero J, Martín-Mazuelos E, Cuenca-Estrella M, Almirante B, Prospective Population Study on Candidemia in Spain (CANDIPOP) Project, Hospital Infection Study Group (GEIH), Medical Mycology Study Group (GEMICOMED) of the Spanish Society of Infectious Diseases and Clinical Microbiology (SEIMC), Spanish Network for Research in Infectious Diseases. Impact of therapeutic strategies on the prognosis of candidemia in the ICU. Crit Care Med. 2014 Jun;42(6):1423–32.

121. Auzinger G, Playford EG, Graham CN, Knox HN, Weinstein D, Kantecki M, Schlamm H, Charbonneau C. Cost-effectiveness analysis of anidulafungin for the treatment of candidemia and other forms of invasive candidiasis. BMC Infect Dis. 2015 Oct 26;15:463.

122. Murri R, Scoppettuolo G, Ventura G, Fabbiani M, Giovannenze F, Taccari F, Milozzi E, Posteraro B, Sanguinetti M, Cauda R, Fantoni M. Initial antifungal strategy does not correlate with mortality in patients with candidemia. Eur J Clin Microbiol Infect Dis. 2016 Feb;35(2):187–93.

123. Tadec L, Talarmin JP, Gastinne T, Bretonnière C, Miegeville M, Le Pape P, Morio F. Epidemiology, risk factor, species distribution, antifungal resistance and outcome of candidemia at a single French hospital: a 7-year study. Mycoses. 2016 May;59(5):296–303.

124. Garnacho-Montero J, Díaz-Martín A, Cantón-Bulnes L, Ramírez P, Sierra R, Arias-Verdú D, Rodríguez-Delgado M, Loza-Vázquez A, Rodriguez-Gomez J, Gordón M, Estella Á, García-Garmendia JL. Initial antifungal strategy reduces mortality in critically ill patients with candidemia: a propensity score-adjusted analysis of a multicenter study. Crit Care Med. 2018 Mar;46(3):384–93.

The Role of Antimicrobial Stewardship Programs to Optimize Antibiotics Use in the Surgical Departments

21

Gina Riggi and Lilian M. Abbo

21.1 Introduction

Antimicrobial stewardship strategies in surgical patients are of high importance, surgical patients receive antibiotics both as perioperative prophylaxis and for the management of surgical site infections [1]. Many of the most common surgical conditions are infectious including appendicitis, cholecystitis, and diverticulitis [2]. Hospitalized surgical patients are also at high risk for prolonged hospitalizations and sometimes acquire healthcare-associated infections including surgical site infections, ventilator-associated pneumonia, central line and urinary catheter-associated infections.

Timely and appropriate antimicrobial administration is a key element in the management of surgical-related infections. Often these infections are treated for longer than necessary and lead to further complications. There is concern that overuse of antimicrobials will result in the emergence of resistance or possibly the occurrence *Clostridium difficile* infections, both of which could be avoided with more judicious antimicrobial treatment [2]. The global increase in multidrug-resistant organisms causing serious infections is a growing concern and highlights the need for antimicrobial stewardship multidisciplinary teams in surgery [1].

Although antimicrobial stewardship is essential to limiting antibiotic exposure and the emergence of resistance, there is very little literature that evaluates these principles in the surgical population. An opportunity has been identified in surgical antibiotic prescribing patterns, specifically to follow evidence-based practices [2]. Many surgical opinion papers describe that surgical antimicrobial prescribing patterns do not always

G. Riggi
Jackson Health System, Miami, FL, USA
e-mail: Gina.riggi@jhsmiami.org

L. M. Abbo (✉)
Jackson Health System, Miami, FL, USA

University of Miami Miller School of Medicine, Miami, FL, USA
e-mail: LAbbo@med.miami.edu

© Springer Nature Switzerland AG 2021
M. Sartelli et al. (eds.), *Infections in Surgery*, Hot Topics in Acute Care Surgery and Trauma, https://doi.org/10.1007/978-3-030-62116-2_21

adhere to evidence-based practices [2]. Even at medical centers that have a strong stewardship team, surgeons have been found to deviate from recommended antimicrobial guidance algorithms [2]. Appropriateness of antimicrobials should be reviewed daily and surgeons should include antimicrobial stewardship practices into their daily routine [2]. Understanding the local culture and hierarchy of decision making in surgical teams is extremely imprtant in order to implement successful and long lasting interventions. Charani et al., [3] analyzed antimicrobial prescribing strategies in medical vs. surgical teams, and reported that in some hospitals surgical teams prioritized their activities between 3 settings: operating room, outpatient clinic, and ward. Senior surgeons are often absent from the ward, leave junior staff to make complex medical decisions. This results in defensive antibiotic decision-making, leading to prolonged and inappropriate antibiotic use. In this chapter, we discuss several stewardship strategies that can be implemented specifically in the areas of surgery and trauma to overcome barriers, help ensure appropriate antimicrobial therapy. These measures should result in improved patient outcomes and a reduction in the emergence of resistance [1].

21.2   Personnel Involved

In 2016, the global alliance for infections in surgery performed an international web-based cross sectional survey to define a model for antimicrobial stewardship [4], respondents included experts in surgery, infection control and antimicrobial stewardship. The goal of the study was to evaluate structures and personnel of antimicrobial stewardship programs around the world; 156 (98.7%) participants stated that they had a multidisciplinary team, 85.4% of participants had at least one surgeon with an interest or skills in surgical infections within their department and a surgeon was more likely to be involved in university hospitals stewardship programs. Educational materials, expert approval, audit and feedback, and educational outreach were the most common types of stewardship interventions in surgical departments. Only 55.8% respondents had both an infectious diseases specialist and a hospital pharmacist on their stewardship team. The results of this survey emphasize the critical need for a multidisciplinary approach to collaborate against the emergence of resistant bacteria and optimize patient outcomes in surgery.

There is lacking consensus on the best practice for ASP teams to model, instead most strategies rely on local practice patterns based on resources, patient population and hospital capacity with local epidemiology. To promote continuous improvement in antimicrobial usage there are several core stewardship strategies that can be done at the local level by the stewardship team. These include clinical decision support, performance feedback, and surgical engagement in antimicrobial stewardship activities including bedside multidisciplinary rounds and measuring antibiotic use and patient outcomes [2].

21.3   Core Stewardship Strategies

The surgeon can play a pivotal role in antimicrobial stewardship and has the unique position of identifying disease states or surgical issues that are noninfectious and do not require antimicrobials. In 2011, Dortch et al. [5], described their experience

Fig. 21.1 Core stewardship strategies to address the gaps in antibiotic prescribing. Prospective audit and feedback and preauthorization have been identified as the two most effective interventions for inpatient stewardship teams [6]

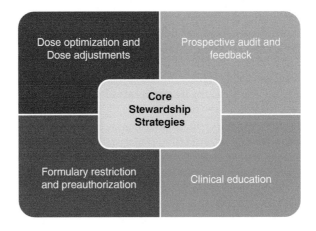

implementing a combined infection reduction and antibiotic stewardship protocols in the trauma and surgical intensive care units in one tertiary care institution. Over an eight-year period 1794 Gram negative isolates were cultured and identified from healthcare-associated infections (HAIs). In that study, the antimicrobial stewardship program included a protocol specific empiric and therapeutic antibiotics for HAIs, standardized surgical antibiotic prophylaxis protocols, and quarterly rotation/limitation of dual antibiotic classes. There was a significant reduction in the rates of infections caused by gram negative multidrug-resistant bacteria from 37.4 to 8.5% at the end of the study period. Additionally, the amount of patients with pan-sensitive infections increased from 34.1 to 53.2%. The authors concluded that antimicrobial stewardship strategies had a huge impact on the rates of multidrug-resistant gram negative infections and the utilization of broad spectrum agents in the ICU setting. In addition to the stewardship activities included in the noted study, there are core stewardship processes that continuously evaluate appropriateness of antimicrobial therapy and provide continued education on the most recent evidence-based practices as seen in Fig. 21.1.

21.3.1 Prospective Audit and Feedback

This is an external review of antimicrobial appropriateness performed by an expert in antibiotic use. This strategy is highly effective in critically ill patients when broad spectrum therapy is being used [6, 7]. A daily review would be optimal; however, even an external review of antimicrobials a few times a week can have a large impact on patient outcomes. This information should be communicated to the providers taking care of the patient with the key outcome being reduction of inappropriate antimicrobial use. The strategy requires resources, leadership support, expertise, and time commitment to review prescribing patterns and provide feedback to the end-users. In the case of surgical teams, this strategy requires buy-in from the surgical and critical care teams. Understanding the local epidemiology and patterns of antimicrobial resistance, focusing on the appropriate empiric selection of antibiotics, de-escalation or escalation of appropriate therapy once cultures are available, selecting the right dose and duration of therapy are all important components of this strategy [6, 7].

21.3.2 Formulary Restriction and Preauthorization

Some facilities use the approach of preauthorization of broad spectrum therapy with the hopes of limiting antimicrobial use of certain agents to patients that meet criteria for use (e.g. high risk for toxicity, collateral damage, cost, or broad spectrum). This intervention must be completed in a timely manner with an expert in antibiotic use. The purpose of this intervention is to ensure that providers consult with the antimicrobial stewardship team to ensure the selection of the appropriate antimicrobial agent and avoid the misuse of antibiotics. This requires less resources and time commitment than the prospective audit and feedback strategy but still requires persuasion and education to convey the rationale for approving or denying the antibiotic requests. Most effective programs use a combination of both strategies and not a single one in order to be most effective.

21.3.3 Clinical Education

This is a core element to the sustained success of influencing prescribing patterns and long-term change in resistance patterns. Education can be achieved in many different forums including presentations, clinical pathways in electronic medical records, and prospective audit and feedback. There are virtual learning platforms at no cost to the users in antimicrobial stewardship such as the British Society of Antimicrobial Chemotherapy massive online learning courses (MOOC) in antimicrobial stewardship, management of resistant Gram negative infections, management of wound infections and many other relevant topics available at: http://www.bsac-vle.com [8]. Many others such as the Infectious Diseases Society of America (IDSA) the Society of Healthcare Epidemiology of America (SHEA) and the European Society of Clinical Microbiology and Infectious Diseases (ESCMID) have electronic tools and educational resources. See Table 21.1 for a list of some of the available antimicrobial stewardship resources worldwide.

21.3.4 Dose Optimization

Pharmacokinetics and pharmacodynamics parameters should be considered when dosing antibiotic therapy. Patients that are septic, for example, have a high volume of distribution, and many antibiotics require dose adjustments to ensure adequate drug levels. Patients that are obese may also require dose adjustments to meet adequate drug levels.

Table 21.1 List of some of the available resources for antimicrobial stewardship recommendations and activities

Antimicrobial stewardship resources		
Society	Available resources	Website information
European Society of Clinical Microbiology and Infectious Diseases 2019	Educational courses	https://www.escmid.org/escmid_publications/
British Society for Antimicrobial Chemotherapy	Open online course on antimicrobial stewardship	http://www.bsac-vle.com
Centers for Disease Control and Prevention	Core elements of antimicrobial stewardship	https://www.cdc.gov/antibiotic-use/core-elements/index.html
Infectious Diseases Society of America	Implementing an Antibiotic Stewardship Program: Guidelines by the Infectious Diseases Society of America and the Society for Healthcare Epidemiology of America	https://www.idsociety.org/practice-guideline/implementing-an-ASP/
Society of Healthcare Epidemiology of America	Antimicrobial stewardship implementation tools and resources	https://www.shea-online.org/index.php/practice-resources/priority-topics/antimicrobial-stewardship/implementation-tools-resources

21.3.5 Dose Adjustments

Many antimicrobials have dose adjustment requirements in the setting of organ dysfunction. Drug interaction evaluation and renal dosing adjustment are also important activities. Many surgical patients have changes in the volume of distribution; others might be on continuous renal replacement or extra-corporeal membrane oxygenation. It is extremely important to understand the need to adjust antimicrobial doses accordingly to maximize the efficacy of the antibiotics and optimize the management of the infections.

21.4   Prophylaxis

The strength of data for antimicrobial surgical prophylaxis lies in the 24-h postoperative period. Longer durations of therapy are thought to increase the rates of multidrug resistance in subsequent infections. There have now been several studies in the past few years that describe an increase in multidrug-resistant organisms as a result of extended duration of unnecessary antimicrobials. In 2019, Branch et al. [9], published a study evaluating antimicrobial-associated adverse events with antimicrobial prophylaxis in surgical patients. About 79,000 patients that underwent various surgical procedures in a multicentered retrospective study were evaluated. The exposure of antimicrobials was broken into the following categories: <24 h, 24–48 h,

48–72 h and greater than 72 h. The results showed that there were increased odds of acute kidney injury and *C difficile* infections with increased durations of antimicrobial prophylaxis in this surgical population. Additionally, longer durations of antimicrobial prophylaxis were not associated with decreases in surgical site infections. The authors also concluded that the results suggested that only pre-incision intraoperative antimicrobial dosing have the biggest impact on decreasing surgical site infections while minimizing adverse effects.

Multidrug resistance has also been evaluated specifically in trauma patients that develop ventilator-associated pneumonia [10]. This study examined the changing sensitivity patterns for *Acinetobacter spp* and *Pseudomonas spp* over time and consistently identified prophylactic antibiotics as an independent risk factor for multidrug-resistant ventilator-associated pneumonia. Limiting prophylactic antibiotics days is a modifiable risk factor that can impact the rates of resistance in subsequent infections [10].

21.5   Intraoperative Prophylaxis

Antimicrobial prophylaxis is only appropriate for indications that have shown to be beneficial to the patients. Joint guidelines published in 2013 with recommendations for antimicrobial prophylaxis from several different societies including the American Society of Health-System Pharmacists, Infectious Diseases Society of America, Surgical Infection Society and SHEA [11]. Their recommendations for antimicrobial surgical prophylaxis included surgical procedures where there is a high risk of surgical site infections including clean contaminated procedures and contaminated cases. They additionally made recommendations for prophylaxis for patients that have comorbid conditions that increase surgical site infection risk.

While there is a large amount of data supporting the use of prophylaxis antimicrobials intraoperatively, the strength of evidence is with the need for prophylaxis. Selection, dose and duration of antimicrobial prophylaxis are not as well defined. Antimicrobial stewardship teams can play a vital role in these areas based on recent evidence-based literature to help decrease inappropriate use [1].

The goal of antimicrobial prophylaxis in this setting is to provide sufficient drug therapy to prevent infections without adverse events or increased resistance from the agent selection. Selection should include the consideration of the most common organisms at the affected site. When there is skin incision, coverage for gram positive infections on the skin should always be covered. Additionally the surgical site microorganisms should be considered and narrowest appropriate coverage should be added. The most important dose is the initial dose of surgical prophylaxis that should be given within 60 min of surgical incision time. Vancomycin and fluoroquinolones should be administered within 120 min of incision time to account for longer infusion times. Within the surgical prophylaxis category, selection and dosing of the prophylactic agent are equally important to the timing of administration [11].

As we gain a better understanding of the relationship between antimicrobial drug levels and increased bacterial suppression, dose optimization may lead to shorter lengths of therapy in addition to decreased exposure to the patient [1]. Perioperative surgical prophylaxis protocols can optimize drug dosing and redosing of antimicrobials appropriately based on the length of the procedure. Institutional protocols should be created for redosing antimicrobials based on the length of the procedure. Additionally, a reminder system may help improve compliance with redosing prophylactic antibiotics intraoperatively. The Department of Anesthesiology and the Antimicrobial Stewardship Program at one institution created a real-time reminder page based on the timing of the initial preoperative antimicrobial administration, the specific antimicrobial dosing requirements and the duration of the procedure. The real-time electronic alerts combined with updated hospital-wide antimicrobial surgical prophylaxis standardized protocol and education to the anesthesiology and surgical staff resulted in significantly increased compliance with redosing [12]. Weight-based dosing should also be considered for obese patients since this patent population has an increased risk of surgical site infections [11].

21.6   Prophylaxis in Trauma

21.6.1 Open Fractures

Open fractures are common after blunt or penetrating traumatic injuries. There is a large amount of data to support the use of prophylactic antibiotics for patients with open fractures. Open fractures are commonly categorized by the Gustilo-anderson classification based on the size of the wound, degree of contamination, and degree of soft tissue injury. Antibiotic prophylaxis therapy is recommended within the first six hours of presentation based on the trauma quality improvement standards. Therapy is tailored to the most common species encountered. For type I and type II fractures, cefazolin is appropriate for prophylaxis. Several recent studies have evaluated the use of ceftriaxone as prophylaxis for type III open fractures in place of regimens that include an aminoglycoside in the regimen. Ceftriaxone will cover more resistant gram negative Enterobacteriaceae infections associated with type-III open fractures without exposing patients to the higher adverse event profile and drug level monitoring associated with aminoglycoside therapy [13]. Duration of therapy should be for 24 h post soft tissue closure or for 72 h post injury whichever duration is shorter. Longer durations of antibiotics for open fractures are not associated with better outcomes [14]. Antibiotic prophylaxis is not warranted for closed fractures.

21.6.2 Facial Fractures

The use of antibiotics in the management of facial fractures is currently widely debated and highly variable in clinical practice. Currently, there are no guidelines for use of antibiotics in facial fractures. In 2015 [15], a systematic review concluded that the use of postoperative antibiotics was not supported in facial fractures based on available literature. Despite this finding, the results of the survey showed that 64.7% of practitioners reported that they administer postoperative antibiotics for an average of 4.6 days postoperatively [15]. Although an ideal duration is not clearly defined, several more recent studies have evaluated the use of shorter durations of antibiotic prophylaxis for facial fractures. The types of facial fractures with the highest risk of infections are mandibular fractures. The more recent available literature supports the use of short courses of antimicrobial prophylaxis [16]. Shorter courses of antibiotics have not been found to be associated with higher rates of infections. Antimicrobial stewardship team members can play a role in limiting antibiotic exposure in this patient population.

21.7   Intraabdominal Prophylaxis

There is very little guidance and literature to guide surgeons on the use of antimicrobials for patients with open abdomens. More than 24 h of antibiotics postoperatively is not recommended or needed similar to other surgical antimicrobial prophylaxis. There is literature to suggest that patients with open abdomens have an increased rate of intraabdominal infections if they are exposed to extended periods of antimicrobial prophylaxis [17].

Abdominal washout procedures are commonly performed to reduce the risk of infections and minimize inflammatory factors. These washout procedures can be performed with normal saline solutions or antibiotic solutions. Data in favor of antibiotic irrigation solutions are limited and outdated, with the potential negative impact of increasing resistance rates. As a result the joint guidelines from ASHP/IDSA/SHEA/SIS for surgical antimicrobial prophylaxis do not recommend the practice of antibiotic irrigations due to the lack of high-quality evidence [11].

21.8   Intraabdominal Infections

Management of intraabdominal infections includes diagnosis, initial resuscitation, source control, and antimicrobial therapy [18]. Source control is summarized in the surgical infection society guidelines as definitive measures to control contamination and restore normal gastrointestinal function. This may include the drainage of infected fluid collections and the debridement of necrotic infected tissue. Delays in achieving source control may lead to a higher mortality [18].

Appropriate empiric antimicrobial regimens for intraabdominal infections are associated with improved outcomes for patients [19, 20]. In general, empiric antimicrobial therapy should cover gram-negative Enterobacteriaceae, aerobic streptococci, and enteric anaerobic organisms. Studies have shown an increased rate of treatment failure in hospitalized adults with complicated intra-abdominal infections and has been associated with longer hospitalization, higher hospital charges, and a higher mortality rate [19]. Antimicrobial stewardship teams can guide empiric antimicrobial therapy based on patients' risk factors [19]. Patients at risk for infections with a resistant gram negative infection include patients who have received broad spectrum antimicrobial therapy, prolonged hospitalization, multiple invasive interventions, and patients known to be colonized or treated for a previous resistant gram negative infection. These risk factors should help prescribers select an agent with more broad coverage of gram negative pathogens including extended spectrum beta-lactamases (ESBL), Ambler Class-C (amp-C) resistance, and *Pseudomonas spp* resistance [18, 19].

21.9 Shorter Antibiotic Courses

There are several recent studies that have evaluated the use of shorter courses of antibiotic therapy for intraabdominal infections (IAI). The Study to Optimize Peritoneal Infection Therapy (STOP-IT) trial [21] was an open-label study on patients in the United States and Canada evaluating a fixed course for 4 days after source control versus continuation of therapy for resolution of WBC, fever, and ileus with a maximum of 10 days of treatment. One-third of the patients had infections that originated in the colon or rectum. The primary endpoint was a composite of surgical site infections (SSI), recurrent IAI, or death. There was no difference in the primary outcome between the two groups. The acuity of these patients was questioned, but further subgroup analysis showed no difference in outcomes in patients that specifically had sepsis [22].

Expert opinion is that if the patient does not have resolution of symptoms then a further workup for infection should be completed after the fixed course of antibiotics is completed. Prolonged antibiotic therapy cannot replace source control; a prolonged course of antimicrobials does not translate to better patient outcomes. Patients who do not have resolution of these signs and symptoms may have ongoing or recurrent IAI [18]. The short-course antibiotic therapy for critically ill patients treated for complicated postoperative intraabdominal infection (DURAPOP) study [23] also evaluated a shorter course of antibiotics for patients with postoperative IAI. This trial enrolled patients with successful source control to receive 8 versus 15 days of antibiotics postoperatively. The primary endpoint was the number of antibiotic-free days from days 8 to 28. Patients in this trial had a higher acuity compared to the STOP-IT trial, with about 40% of the patients having infections in the colon or rectum and about half of the infections being the result of GI perforation. The shorter course of antibiotics helped to reduce antibiotic exposure and did not result in recurrent infections, clinical failure, or reoperation [23].

21.10 Antimicrobial Selection

Time to initial appropriate antibiotic administration is a critical component to patient outcomes. Appropriate empiric antibiotics are essential after the suspicion or diagnosis of infection [24]. Antibiograms can help guide therapy based on local resistance patterns and susceptibility data. Unit specific data is even more helpful in the guidance of antimicrobial therapy for hospital acquired infections. Depending on the patient populations within one health-system, there can be large variations in resistance patterns from one hospital unit to another. Guidelines are available for the development of antibiograms. While unit specific antibiograms are very helpful, one study evaluated a population specific antibiogram for transplant patients and found it may be more useful for appropriate empiric antibiotic section [25].

Empiric agents should be based on unit-specific data, or if that is not available use hospital-specific data. Empiric therapy should also include the least number of agents and classes to effectively reduce antibiotic exposure. When culture and sensitivity data is available, the antibiotic with the narrowest spectrum of activity with proven efficacy should be selected when de-escalating.

The duration of treatment should be driven by patient's clinical status and response to antimicrobial therapy. Shorter durations of antimicrobial courses of therapy for active infections decrease exposure and resistance to subsequent infections.

21.11 Antifungal Stewardship

Antifungal stewardship can be described as optimizing the selection, dosing and duration of antifungal treatment [26]. Practitioners in general have more experience treating bacterial infections since they are much more common than antifungal infections.

Surgical patients, however, are at risk for invasive fungal infections. Risk factors identified for hospital acquired infections based on patients with candidemia include previous surgical procedures, history of broad spectrum antimicrobial therapy, pancreatitis, use of parenteral nutrition, presence of invasive catheters, and presence of medical comorbidities [18]. There are also studies that have identified specific risk factors for *Candida* peritonitis including recurrent gastrointestinal perforations, upper gastrointestinal perforations, surgically treated pancreatitis, and previous antimicrobial administration. Echinocandins are recommended as empiric therapy for critically ill patients including patients with hospital acquired intraabdominal infections. The echinocandins have activity against all *Candida* species making them a good empiric choice. Amphotericin was historically the first-choice empiric agent because of its spectrum of activity against yeast, but its use has declined due to its adverse effect profile. Some *Candida* species have variable resistance and inherent resistance to azole therapy including *C. glabrta* and *C. kruseii*, respectively. Still, fluconazole has been used extensively as empiric therapy for high-risk surgical patients. Antifungal stewardship interventions can have a big impact on selection, dose optimization, the identification of drug–drug interactions, and duration of therapy [18].

21.12 Dosing Strategies

Dosing strategies are equally critical to patient outcomes when treating infections, considerations for dosing are summarized in Fig. 21.2. Critically ill patients, specifically patients with sepsis, infection, and severe trauma can experience augmented renal clearance. Augmented renal clearance (ARC) is described as increased creatinine clearance greater than 130 mL/min and is associated with sub therapeutic antibiotic concentrations and worse patient outcomes when standard antibiotic dosing is administered [27]. The cockcroft-gault equation does not adequately measure clearance in this patient population. Some experts recommend screening ICU patients for ARC using a continuous urine collection. Empiric dosing regimens for these patients should be evaluated on a case-by-case basis taking into account pharmacokinetics- and pharmacodynamics-specific criteria. Patients' ARC should be continued to be monitored as their status improves during their ICU admission and dosing regimens should be adjusted as necessary [28].

One study [29] evaluated beta-lactam drug levels in critically ill patients in a multicenter study including patients from 68 ICUs. Two levels were evaluated at the middle and the end of the dosing interval to evaluate if the drug concentration levels were above the minimum inhibitory concentration. The study results showed that 20% of patients did not achieve a minimum conservative pharmacokinetic/pharmacodynamics goal. Insufficient antibiotic exposure with beta-lactam antibiotics in the critically ill population is very concerning and may lead to worse outcomes [29].

Fig. 21.2 Factors that influence antimicrobial dosing in surgery and critical care

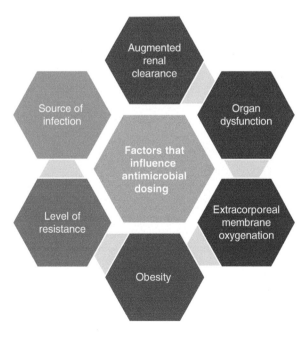

Another population that demonstrates altered kinetics in the acute phase is burn injury patients. These patients have altered physiology including increased cardiac output, increased blood flow to the kidneys, and decreased albumin concentrations [30]. These changes often result in an increased drug clearance, higher volumes of distribution and changes in total drug exposure that will also impact antimicrobial dosing recommendations [30].

Antimicrobial stewardship interventions should include dosing strategies to optimize dosing, specifically dosing for the beta-lactam class. For example, patients with ARC should receive higher than traditional antibiotic doses of piperacillin-tazobactam, cefepime, and meropenem. Another strategy is extended and continuous dosing strategies of beta-lactams. These antibiotic infusion strategies are another way to maximize antibacterial effects and possibly improve the coverage of bacteria that may be initially classified as resistant [31].

21.13 Rapid Diagnostics Testing

Rapid diagnostic testing may be helpful for clinicians to target infections with appropriate antimicrobial therapy faster. Currently microbiological results take up to 72 h for most bacteria and sometimes even longer for other slow growing bacteria and yeast. This means that patients may stay on broad coverage without the available information to de-escalate therapy leading to more antibiotic exposure [32]. While these rapid diagnostic tests do not provide drug susceptibility data, they do identify pathogens quickly. For example, if methicillin-resistant *Staphylococcus aureus* or vancomycin-resistant Enterococcus is isolated based on genetic identification, practitioners can tailor drug therapy and dosing in a timely manner which would most likely translate into better patient outcomes. As more rapid diagnostic testing becomes available, it is important for antimicrobial stewardship teams to develop processes to guide prescribers on how to interpret and intervene based on these results [24].

21.14 Conclusion

Antimicrobial therapy is vital to the management of most surgical infections. Exposure to antimicrobial therapy for longer than necessary exposes the patients to potentially adverse effects and the emergence of antimicrobial-resistant organisms. There are several key antimicrobial stewardship activities to incorporate into surgical clinical practice including daily assessment of antimicrobial appropriateness, dosing considerations, and optimizing duration of therapy. Organized efforts can have a substantial impact on the use of broad spectrum antimicrobial agents and the rates of multidrug-resistant organisms. The strategies described in this chapter can be implemented in healthcare systems to improve clinical prescribing of antimicrobials in the surgical patient population. Multidisciplinary collaborations between surgeons, clinical pharmacists, and infectious diseases specialists are critical to the success of effective antimicrobial stewardship teams with impactful and long-standing successful interventions. Everyone should be an antimicrobial steward in surgery.

References

1. Tarchini G, Liau K, Solomkin J. Antimicrobial stewardship in surgery: challenges and opportunities. Clin Infect Dis. 2017;64(S2):S112–4.
2. Leeds I, Fabrizio A, Cosgrove S, Wick E. Treating wisely: the surgeon's role in antibiotic stewardship. Ann Surg. 2017;265:871–3.
3. Charani E, Ahmad R, Rawson TM, Castro-Sanchèz E, Tarrant C, et al. The differences in antibiotic decision-making between acute surgical and acute medical teams: an ethnographic study of culture and team dynamics. Clin Infect Dis. 2019;69(1):12–20.
4. Sartelli M, Labricciosa F, Barbadoro P, Pagani L, et al. The global alliance for infections in surgery: defining a model for antimicrobial stewardship-results from an international cross-sectional survey. World J Emerg Surg. 2017;12:34.
5. Dortch M, Fleming S, Kauffmann R, Dossett L, Talbot T, et al. Infections reduction strategies including antibiotic stewardship protocols in surgical and trauma intensive care units are associated with reduces resistant gram-negative healthcare-associated infections. Surg Infect (Larchmt). 2011;12(1):15–25.
6. CDC. Core elements of hospital antibiotic stewardship programs. Atlanta, GA. US Department of Health and Human Services, CDC. 2019. http://www.cdc.gov/getsmart/healthcare/implementation/core-elements.html.
7. CDC. Core elements of hospital antibiotic stewardship programs. Atlanta, GA. US Department of Health and Human Services, CDC. 2014. http://www.cdc.gov/getsmart/healthcare/implementation/core-elements.html.
8. British Society for Antimicrobial Chemotherapy. 2019. http://www.bsac-vle.com/. Accessed Nov 2019.
9. Branch-Elliman W, O'Brien W, Strymish J, Itani K, Wyatt C, et al. Association of duration and type of surgical prophylaxis with antimicrobial-associated adverse events. JAMA Surg. 2019;154(7):590–8.
10. Lewis R, Sharpe J, Swanson J, Fabian T, Croce M, et al. Reinventing the wheel: impact of prolonged antibiotic exposure on multi-drug resistant ventilator associated pneumonia in trauma patients. J Trauma Acute Care Surg. 2018;85:256–62.
11. Bratzler D, Dellinger P, Olsen K, Perl T, Auwaerter P, et al. Clinical practice guidelines for antimicrobial prophylaxis in surgery. Am J Health Sys Phar. 2013;70:195–283.
12. Riggi G, Castillo M, Fernandez M, Wawrzyniak A, et al. Improving compliance with timely intraoperative redosing of antimicrobials in surgical prophylaxis. Infect Control Hosp Epidemiol. 2014;35(10):1236–40.
13. Rodriguez L, Jung H, Goulet J, et al. Evidence-based protocol for prophylactic antibiotics in open fractures: improved antibiotic stewardship with no increase in infection rates. J Trauma Acute Care Surg. 2014;77:400–7.
14. Dunkel N, Pittet D, Tovmirzaeva L, Suva D, et al. Short duration of antibiotic prophylaxis in open fractures does not enhance risk of subsequent infection. Bone Joint J. 2013;95-B(6):831–7.
15. Mundinger G, Borsuk D, Okhah Z, Christy M, et al. Antibiotics and facial fractures: evidence-based recommendations compared with experience-based practice. Craniomaxillofac Trauma Reconstr. 2015;8:64–78.
16. Zosa B, Elliot C, Kurlander D, Johnson F, Ho V, et al. Facing the facts on prophylactic antibiotics for facial fractures. J Trauma Acute Care Surg. 2018;85:444–50.

17. Goldberg S, Henning J, Wolfe L, et al. Practice patterns for the use of antibiotic agents in damage control laparotomy and its impact on outcomes. Surg Infect. 2017;18:282–6.
18. Mazuski J, Tessier J, May A, Sawyer R, Nadler E, et al. The surgical infection society revised guidelines on the management of intra-abdominal infections. Surg Infect (Larchmt). 2017;18:1–55.
19. Sartelli M, Duane T, Catena F, Tessier J, Coccolini F, et al. Antimicrobial stewardship: a call to surgeons. Surg Infect (Larchmt). 2016;17:625–31.
20. Edelsberg J, Berger A, Schell S, et al. Economic consequences of failure of initial antibiotic therapy in hospitalized adults with complicated intra-abdominal infections. Surg Infect (Larchmt). 2008;9:335–47.
21. Sawyer R, Claridge J, Nathens A, Rotstein O, et al. Trial of short-course antimicrobial therapy for intraabdominal infection. N Engl J Med. 2015;372:1996–2005.
22. Rattan R, Allen C, Sawyer R, Askari R. Patients with complicated intra-abdominal infection presenting with sepsis do not require longer duration of antimicrobial therapy. J Am Coll Surg. 2016;222:440–6.
23. Montravers P, Tubach F, Lescot T, Veber B, et al. Short-course antibiotic therapy for critically ill patients treated for postoperative intra-abdominal infection; the DURAPOP randomized clinical trial. Intensive Care Med. 2018;44:300–10.
24. Barlam T, Cosgrove S, Abbo L, MacDougall C, Schuetz A, et al. Implementing an antibiotic stewardship program: guidelines by the Infectious Diseases Society of America and the Society for Healthcare Epidemiology of America. Clin Infect Dis. 2016;62(10):e51–77.
25. Rosa R, Simkins J, Camargo JF, Martinez O, Abbo L. Solid organ transplant antibiograms: an opportunity for antimicrobial stewardship. Diagn Microbiol Infect Dis. 2016;86(4):460–3.
26. Enoch D, Whitney L. Chapter 21: Antifungal stewardship. British Society for antimicrobial chemotherapy. In: Antimicrobial stewardship: from principles to practice. 2018.
27. Hobbs A, Shea K, Roberts K, Daley M. Implications of augmented renal clearance on drug dosing in critically ill patients: a focus on antibiotics. Pharmacotherapy. 2015;35(11):1063–75.
28. Cook A, Hatton-Kolpek J. Augmented renal clearance. Pharmacotherapy. 2019;39(3):346–54.
29. Roberts J, Paul S, Akova M, Bassetti M, et al. DALI: defining antibiotic levels in intensive care unit patients: are current β-lactam antibiotic doses sufficient for critically ill patients? Clin Infect Dis. 2014;58(8):1072–83.
30. Ortwine J, Pogue J, Faris J. Pharmacokinetics and pharmacodynamics of antibacterial and antifungal agents in adult patients with thermal injury: a review of the current literature. J Burn Care Res. 2015;36:e72–84.
31. MacGowan A, Baxter M. Chapter 8: Optimising stewardship through better PK-PD. British Society for antimicrobial chemotherapy. In: Antimicrobial stewardship: from principles to practice. 2018.
32. Brown N. Chapter 7: The role of laboratory and rapid diagnostics/biomarkers in stewardship. British Society for antimicrobial chemotherapy. In: Antimicrobial stewardship: from principles to practice. 2018.

What Healthcare Workers Should Know About the "One Health Approach" and the Global Impact of Antimicrobial Resistance

Leonardo Pagani, Giada Fasani, and Richard Aschbacher

22.1 Introduction

The twenty-first century is being shaped by technology and innovation, but the whole world could soon find itself in an era where simple infections might once again kill millions every year. Antimicrobial resistance (AMR) is indeed one of the most complex global health challenges today: the world has long ignored warnings that antibiotics were losing their effectiveness after decades of overuse and misuse in human medicine, animal health, agriculture, and dispersion into the environment [1].

Antibiotics are the foundation of modern medicine: the medical world relies on the possibility to treat infections to relentlessly progress. Without safe and effective antibiotics, extensive abdominal surgery, solid organ- or bone marrow transplantation, cancer chemotherapy, or high-dose corticosteroid treatments, the whole edifice of modern medicine itself will crumble. Even common illnesses such as pneumonia, postoperative infections, diarrheal and sexually transmitted diseases are becoming untreatable because of the spread of AMR.

In 2014, the UK Prime Minister commissioned an independent review to evaluate the potential impact of AMR on the world health. In May 2016, the conclusive report estimated that at least 700,000 people die each year from antimicrobial-resistant infections and that number could rise up to 10 million deaths by 2050 [2], though some conclusions about these figures have been questioned thereafter [3]. Four months after the report was released, the United Nations General Assembly deliberated on AMR and issued a declaration reaffirming the World Health Organization's global action plan as the key framework for tackling the problem.

Several interconnected human, animal, and environmental habitats can contribute to the emergence, evolution, and spread of AMR; the expansion of resistant clones and antibiotic resistance determinants among human-associated,

L. Pagani (✉) · G. Fasani · R. Aschbacher
Antimicrobial Stewardship Program, Bolzano Central Hospital, Bolzano, Italy

© Springer Nature Switzerland AG 2021
M. Sartelli et al. (eds.), *Infections in Surgery*, Hot Topics in Acute Care Surgery and Trauma, https://doi.org/10.1007/978-3-030-62116-2_22

animal-associated, and environmental microbiomes have the potential to alter bacterial population genetics at local and global levels, thereby modifying the structure of microbiomes where antibiotic-resistant bacteria can expand.

Better managing this problem includes taking steps to preserve the continued effectiveness of existing antimicrobials such as trying to eliminate their inappropriate use, particularly where they are used in high volumes. Examples are the mass medication of animals with critically important antimicrobials for humans, such as third generation cephalosporins and fluoroquinolones, and the long term, in-feed use of antimicrobials, such colistin, tetracyclines, and macrolides, for growth promotion. In humans, it is essential to better prevent infections, reduce over-prescribing and over-use of antimicrobials and stop resistant bacteria from spreading by improving hygiene and infection control, drinking water, and sanitation. Pollution from inadequate treatment of industrial, residential, and farm waste is expanding the resistome in the environment. Numerous countries and several international agencies have now included a One Health Approach within their action plans to address AMR. Necessary actions include improvements in antimicrobial use, better regulation and policy, as well as improved surveillance, stewardship, infection control, sanitation, animal husbandry, and alternatives, if any, to antimicrobials.

It is essential to recognize that the health of people is connected to the health of animals and the environment. AMR has clear links to each of these three domains. The contribution of animal production, both terrestrial livestock and aquaculture, to the global AMR crisis is sometimes questioned because we do not see so many animal-associated infections in humans [4]. While this may be true, because of the way that many antibiotics are used in animal production, in sub-therapeutic doses and with long exposure periods, these production systems create ideal conditions for bacteria to fix genes that confer resistance. These genes can subsequently be transmitted to human-adapted pathogens or to human gut microbiota via people, contaminated food, or the environment. They also provide ideal conditions for the amplification of genes that may have arisen in people or the environment [5]. The fact that the antibiotics used in human and animal health largely comprise the same or very similar molecules would be expected to drive the transmission of resistance between animals and people, either directly or via the environment.

One Health is defined as a concept and approach to "designing and implementing programs, policies, legislation and research in which multiple sectors communicate and work together to achieve better public health outcomes. The areas of work in which a One Health approach is particularly relevant include food safety, the control of zoonoses and combatting antibiotic resistance." It needs to involve the "collaborative effort of multiple health science professions, together with their related disciplines and institutions—working locally, nationally, and globally—to attain optimal health for people, domestic animals, wildlife, plants, and our environment" [5]. The declaration also stated that a One Health approach is essential for developing comprehensive and integrative measures to address AMR, recognizing that human, animal, and environmental health are strictly linked. This One Health approach should include surveillance of microbes in humans, animals, and environments to better understand AMR, and to develop effective preventive and control strategies [4]. One Health recognizes that human and animal health are interconnected, that diseases are transmitted from humans to animals and vice versa, and must therefore be tackled in both. Such an approach also encompasses the environment, another link between humans and animals and likewise a potential source of new resistant microorganisms. This term is now globally recognized, having been widely used in the EU and in the 2016 United Nations Political Declaration on AMR [6].

22.2   AMR in Clinical Settings

AMR is one of the greatest challenges of the twenty-first century. One major global driver for the development of AMR is the misuse or overuse of antimicrobials. A variety of factors can result in the misuse or overuse of antimicrobials in healthcare settings including: a lack of knowledge or up-to-date information on prescription of antimicrobials, lack of treatment guidelines, lack of laboratory capacity to identify the organism and its antimicrobial susceptibility, unreliable or absent surveillance data on AMR and antimicrobial usage, unregulated over-the-counter availability and use, and poor antimicrobial stewardship (AMS). In addition, patient and public expectation and pressure to prescribe antibiotics, or situations that allow for financial benefit from the supply of medicines, can also drive inappropriate antimicrobial prescribing. Inadequate adherence to infection prevention and control (IPC) measures in healthcare facilities and poor hygiene and sanitation in communities exacerbate the spread of infections and increase the use of antimicrobial agents. This situation is made worse in many settings around the world by gaps that are known to still exist in knowledge and awareness of AMR, as well as the availability of quality teaching resources to address education on AMR.

AMR mechanisms encoded by genes have a greater impact on transfer than mutations. Depending on how the resistance mechanism is transferred, the power of dissemination is different. By vertical transfer of the resistance gene, whatever its origin, will be transmitted to the following generations. In the case of horizontal transfer, the resistance gene moves to neighboring bacteria and therefore the range of resistance can be even greater [7, 8].

Genetically determined acquired AMR is widespread in Gram-positive and Gram-negative bacteria, and the following resistance phenotypes have a significant clinical public health impact: methicillin-resistant *Staphylococcus aureus* (MRSA), vancomycin-resistant enterococci (VRE), extended-spectrum β-lactamase (ESBL), and high-level AmpC producing *Enterobacteriaceae* and carbapenemase producing *Enterobacteriaceae, Pseudomonas aeruginosa*, and *Acinetobacter baumannii* [9]. Generally, the above-mentioned phenotypes are associated, besides β-lactam antibiotics, with resistance to various other antibiotic classes, and give rise to multidrug resistance (MDR). Moreover, many resistance genes are located on mobile genetic elements, able to move within or between DNA molecules, which include transposons and gene cassettes/integrons, or are able to horizontally transfer between bacterial cells, such as plasmids and integrative conjugative elements [10]. Healthcare institutions like hospitals, nursing homes, and rehabilitation facilities are hotbeds for MDR bacteria, but some MDR organisms have become quite prevalent causes of community-acquired infections (e.g. ESBL-producing *E. coli*, CA-MRSA); the spread of MDR bacteria into the community is a crucial development, and is associated with increased morbidity, mortality, healthcare costs and, once again, antibiotic use [11].

MRSA expresses an alternative penicillin-binding protein (PBP-2a or PBP-2c), encoded by a resistance gene (*mecA* or *mecC*), located on a genomic island (*SCCmec*) inserted at a specific locus on the bacterial chromosome [12]. Most MRSA infections in hospitalized patients or residents of long-term care and rehabilitation facilities in Europe are caused by various genotypes of healthcare-associated MRSA (HA-MRSA), but community-associated MRSA (CA-MRSA), especially expressing the Panton-Valentine Leukocidin (PVL) toxin, are an emerging cause of skin and soft tissue infections in Europe (see also below).

VRE are *Enterococcus faecalis* or *Enterococcus faecium* isolates resistant to the glycopeptide vancomycin and frequently also to teicoplanin [13]. The mechanism of resistance involves the alteration of the peptidoglycan synthesis pathway; the D-alanyl-D-alanyl sidechain antibiotic target is enzymatically modified to D-alanyl-D-lactate or D-alanyl-D-serine. Enterococci live mainly in our gut, as part of the normal microbiota, but they can also cause serious infections, such as urinary tract-, wound infections, or endocarditis.

Enterobacteriaceae can produce extended-spectrum β-lactamase (ESBLs) enzymes, such as TEM, SHV, and CTX-M, which confer resistance to most β-lactam antibiotics, including penicillins, cephalosporins (except cephamycins cefoxitin and cefotetan) and the monobactam aztreonam, but, in the absence of outer membrane porin loss or overexpression of efflux pumps, they cannot hydrolyze carbapenems (ertapenem, meropenem, and imipenem) [14]. ESBLs are generally inhibited by clavulanic acid, sulbactam, and tazobactam, which are indeed called β-lactamase inhibitors.

AmpC β-lactamases in *Enterobacteriaceae* mediate resistance to all cephalosporins (including cephamycins), except fourth-generation cephalosporins (cefepime), and β-lactamase inhibitor/β-lactam combinations [15]. In many *Enterobacteriaceae* (*Enterobacter cloacae*, *Enterobacter aerogenes*, *Citrobacter freundii*, *Providencia stuartii*, *Morganella morganii*, *Serratia marcescens*, and *Hafnia alvei*), AmpC enzymes are inducible but can be expressed at high levels by mutational derepression; this overexpression confers resistance to broad-spectrum cephalosporins including cefotaxime, ceftriaxone, and ceftazidime. Horizontal transfer and hence acquisition of a plasmidic AmpC gene by enterobacterial species without constitutive chromosomal AmpC gene, such as *Klebsiella pneumoniae*, *Klebsiella oxytoca*, *Proteus mirabilis*, *Proteus vulgaris*, and *Salmonella* spp., gives rise to a similar resistance phenotype.

Carbapenemase-producing *Enterobacteriaceae* (CPE) are among the most worrying MDR Gram-negative bacteria and their incidence is increasing worldwide [16]. CPE are resistant, besides other β-lactams, also to carbapenems. Carbapenemases of the *Klebsiella pneumoniae* carbapenemase (KPC),

OXA-48-like, Verona integron-encoded metallo-β-lactamase (VIM), New Delhi metallo-β-lactamase (NDM), and imipenemase (IMP) types are variably spread across Europe and other continents. Metallo-β-lactamases cause resistance to all β-lactam antibiotics except the monobactam aztreonam, whereas KPCs are resistant to all β-lactams except the combination of ceftazidime plus avibactam; OXA-48-like carbapenemases do not hydrolyze the extended spectrum cephalosporins cefotaxime, ceftriaxone, and ceftazidime.

Carbapenemases in *P. aeruginosa* (mainly VIM or IMP types), and in *A. baumannii* (mainly OXA-23, OXA-24, OXA-51, OXA-58), give rise, together with other resistance mechanisms for different antibiotic classes, to hard-to-treat MDR phenotypes [17].

Evaluation of the public health burden of AMR, which is needed to drive policy interventions, is done through estimates of clinical benchmarks (mainly morbidity and crude mortality) and economic indicators (direct costs, use of resources, and drug expenditures). Most of these estimates are restricted to high-income countries and retrieve data to fit the computation models from national surveillance of clinical samples, prevalence or incidence surveys, and retrospective cohorts [18].

However, the threats posed by AMR are of increasing concern even in low- and middle-income countries (LMICs), as their rates of antibiotic use increase. An understanding of the burden of resistance is rather lacking in LMICs, particularly for MDR pathogens. Gandra et al. recently conducted a retrospective, 10-hospital study on the relationship between MDR pathogens and mortality in India. Patient-level antimicrobial susceptibility test (AST) results for the most important hospital pathogens were analyzed for their association with patient mortality outcomes [19]. The authors observed that patients who acquire MDR bacterial infections, as opposed to similar drug-susceptible infections, have greater odds of mortality. Interestingly, they also observed higher odds of mortality among patients with MDR and XDR infections whose isolates were obtained outside the ICU. The overall mortality rate of patients was 13.1% ($n = 581$), and there was a significant relationship between MDR and mortality. Infections with MDR and extensively drug resistant (XDR) *E. coli*, XDR *K. pneumoniae*, and MDR *A. baumannii* were associated with 2–3 times higher mortality [19].

Beyond the geographical area or the continent evaluated, it is undoubted that AMR spread affects not only the national budgets or gross domestic product (GDP) of countries, but also the attributable mortality or related disabilities. However, estimating the incidence, complications, and attributable mortality of infections caused by resistant pathogens may be challenging. Cassini et al. [20], through a population-level modeling analysis, estimated the burden of infections caused by antibiotic-resistant bacteria in countries of the EU and European Economic Area (EEA) in 2015, measured in number of cases, attributable deaths, and disability adjusted life-years (DALYs). They estimated around 672,000 infections due to antibiotic-resistant pathogens, of which 63.5% were associated with or attributable to health care. Moreover, these infections accounted for an estimated >33,000 attributable deaths and likely 875,000 DALYs. This modeled analysis was limited to one year only (2015), but to understand the ominous burden and the practical meaning of such results it may be sufficient to figure that the burden of infections by antibiotic-resistant pathogens is similar to the cumulative burden of tuberculosis, influenza, and HIV [20].

One important conclusion that can be drawn from this study is that most of the estimated burden was in hospitals or other healthcare settings, thus suggesting the urgent need to address AMR as a patient safety issue and the need for alternative treatment options for patients with such infections.

22.3 AMR in the Food Chain and in Food-Producing Animals

The health concerns linked to AMR in the food chain encompass both the pathogenic and nonpathogenic microorganisms as both can have serious health consequences [21].

There are also two major determinants of such concerns about food and human health: I. the safety of food chain, which is the issue of preventing food to be contaminated by pathogenic strains, and II. The concerns about the emergence and spread of AMR in livestock, intensive poultry farming or aquaculture, with consequent transfer of AMR sequences or genes to consumers. This is mostly related to the massive use of antibiotics in food animals worldwide [22, 23].

The first one is the potential unsafety of food linked to contaminated water, preparation, or poor hygiene [24–26]; the impact on microbial quality of water and consequent food safety and the presence and persistence of *Salmonella* in waters have been recently reviewed [27–29]; these strains may harbor multiple AMR mechanisms [30]. Vegetables and mussels contaminated with gram-negative carriers of ESBL or KPC-3 carbapenemase in retail markets in North Africa, or imported seafood and raw dog food with the presence of *mcr-1* positive *E. coli* isolates in Norway, have been recently reported, thus highlighting new potential pathways to transfer AMR genes to "low prevalence" countries [31–35].

Antimicrobials have been and are still widely used for disease prevention and growth promotion in food animals. Expanding human population ever demands more animal-based protein, which in turn leads to more industrialized methods of food animal production, including sub-therapeutic antibiotics for growth promotion and disease prevention [36, 37]. This means that animal bacteria may become resistant under selective pressure; bacteria then travel from farms to stores, and then they may cause hard-to-treat infections in the final consumer as a consequence [38–40]. The relationship between massive use of antibiotics to treat or prevent illnesses or for growth purposes and the consequent emergence of several AMR mechanisms in food animals has been clearly highlighted in several reports [41–50]. There is another concern related to the arising of meat production set in the next years to match the ever-increasing demand that should be taken into account: even more antibiotics will be used to prophylactically prevent diseases in livestock to meet this demand.

As remarked by Clifford et al., the high proportion of poor-quality veterinary medicine for therapeutic use in livestock exacerbates the problem of antibiotic overuse or misuse, particularly in LMICs [51]. Poor-quality medicines that provide sub-therapeutic doses of active pharmaceutical ingredient, whether due to inadequate amounts of pharmaceutical, ineffective release, presence of impurities, or degradation of compounds, are believed to contribute to AMR by exposing microbes to a level of antibiotic that will not effectively kill the whole microbial population [51].

Ionophores can be another matter of concern: ionophores are the second most widely used class of antibiotics in agriculture, with over 4 million kilograms sold in the United States in 2016. Because ionophores are not used in humans, it is widely assumed that their agricultural use will not impact human health. Consequently, these drugs have not been subject to the same regulations as medically important antibiotics [52]. While they are not used in humans due to toxicity, the use of ionophores may still carry risk, owing to the possibility of cross-resistance or co-selection; several ionophores, indeed, including lasalocid, monensin, narasin, and salinomycin, are routinely administered to cattle and/or pigs for growth promotion; the same drugs, as well as maduramicin, are used for the prevention of coccidiosis in poultry and other farm animals. At last, few studies have examined cross-resistance between ionophores and antimicrobials with human interest, but there is, evidence of an emerging association between narasin resistance and vancomycin resistance in Swedish broiler chickens, with a putative narasin resistance ABC transporter located on the same plasmid as a *vanA* gene cluster, which confers vancomycin resistance in VRE [53]. This finding raises the possibility that vancomycin resistance could be maintained in animal populations not because of treatment with vancomycin or related compounds but because of ionophore use.

Intensive farming is also a stress factor for animals due to crowding and lack of hygiene, causing illnesses and increased shedding. Antibiotics consumed by animals can be excreted in urine and feces into the surrounding environment, potentially inducing or selecting for the development and maintenance of antibiotic resistance genes (ARGs) into the environment [54–56]. Infection control and prevention procedures and sanitation are concepts still not fully developed in animal farming both in very intensive ones in Western countries and in poor-resource or developing countries, and big efforts are requested at national level in any country to tackle the spread of AMR into the environment.

Aquaculture is a highly diverse activity with more than 600 different freshwater and marine animal species farmed in quite different production system [57, 58]. In 2014 only, China produced over 45 million metric tons of fish, crustaceans, and mollusks by aquaculture with more than 50% of this production exported [59]. As suggested by Cabello et al., the heavy use of colistin and other antimicrobials in this industry in China may have generated plasmid-mediated colistin-resistance genes *mcr*-1 and *mcr*-2 through the facilitation of the capture and dissemination of potential colistin resistance genes from aquatic bacteria, such as *Aeromonas* and *Shewanella*, which can be naturally resistant to colistin [59]. This hypothesis seems to be confirmed by a recent work from Chinese researchers, who explored the molecular characteristics and relationships of *mcr*-1 positive *Escherichia coli* through whole-genome sequencing (WGS) and concluded that these strains were highly prevalent in the aquaculture supply chain and resistant to most antibiotics; and that *mcr*-1 could be transferred to humans via the aquatic food chain [60].

The higher the amount of antibiotics used in animals, whatever the reason, the higher the AMR rates are anticipated [39]. However, a clear direct relationship between these facts has been demonstrated also in either sense: broad antibiotic restrictions in food animals decrease rates of resistance. When the glycopeptide avoparcin was banned across the European Union in the 1990s, the prevalence of vancomycin-resistant enterococci from both poultry and humans decreased [61]; likewise, researchers in Canada recently compared the effect of various methods of antibiotic restriction in food animals on rates of antibiotic resistance. They found that single antibiotic and single class restrictions were not associated with reductions in resistance, while complete antibiotic restrictions were linked to a 15% reduction in resistance. Restriction approaches that allowed therapeutic antibiotic use were also effective, and were linked to a 9–30% reduction in antibiotic resistance [62].

22.4 The Case of *Staphylococcus aureus*

Is methicillin-resistant *Staphylococcus aureus* (MRSA), or *Staphylococcus aureus* "*tout court*," a foodborne pathogen? *S. aureus* is a well-known major human pathogen associated with a wide spectrum of diseases, up to necrotizing pneumonia, endocarditis, and toxic shock syndromes; in addition, *S. aureus* is a pathogen also for important livestock animals, such as cows, sheep, goats, poultry, and rabbits [63]. Although most *S. aureus* strains are host-specific, an MRSA clone (ST398) has recently emerged in livestock and humans exposed to livestock, already referred to as livestock-associated MRSA (LA-MRSA), and it has been isolated from pig and pig farmers in European countries and North America [64]; MRSA has been isolated from different foods (milk, beef, chicken, and pork) [40, 65], and therefore the handling and consumption of contaminated food is considered a potential source of colonization or infection for humans [63, 66, 67]. Remarkably, an important role is played by the air-borne transmission of LA-MRSA in animal production environment, because it could be present in the dust potentially inhaled by the workers in the food animal chain [66]. Another potential health risk for consumers is the presence of *S. aureus* harboring the Panton-Valentine leucocidin (PVL), which is associated with high mortality rates because of its necrotizing properties, recently isolated and characterized in retail food in China [68].

Close to these above-mentioned concerns, there is also a potential professional threat to acquire resistance strains; Danish and Belgian veterinarians in contact with livestock were found to be at higher risk of acquiring MRSA ST398 [69], whereas veterinary hospital staff and students in UK were found to be heavily colonized by MDR- and ESBL-producing gram negatives in rectal surveillance swabs [70]. If people working in veterinary hospitals are at high risk for carriage of MDR pathogens, then it is vital that veterinary hospitals implement strict infection control and prevention procedures to avoid transmission of such pathogens between patients and staff.

22.5   The Importance of Integrated Surveillance

Building blocks of integrated surveillance between human and veterinary medicine is of paramount importance to detect and track emerging threats: very recently, linezolid-resistant coagulase-negative Staphylococci have been isolated and genetically characterized in apparently healthy turkeys in Egypt analyzing their AMR evolution, to provide a major example [71]. An integrated surveillance system data/information for action may help: (1) monitor prevalence of AMR in different reservoirs; (2) monitor AMR trends over time; (3) monitor association between AMR and use of antimicrobial agents; (4) guide evidence-based policies and guidelines to control antimicrobial use in humans and animals; and *v*. identify and evaluate the effectiveness of interventions to contain the emergence and spread of resistant bacteria.

A systematic review has been recently published by European experts on AMR surveillance programs in livestock with special focus on human consequences [72].

Three main synergistically acting surveillance levels can be prospected to improve health outcomes:

1. Locally. Allow healthcare professionals to make better informed clinical decisions to ensure better patients outcomes.
2. Nationally. Guide policy and ensure appropriate and timely public health interventions.
3. Globally. Provide early warnings of emerging threats and data to identify and act on long-term trends.

WGS has revolutionized molecular epidemiology and laboratory surveillance of infections caused by pathogens commonly transmitted though food providing public health researchers with a tool of unprecedented precision and discrimination for subtyping. Additionally, WGS may easily provide a wealth of information such as species identification, serotype, pathotype, virulence profile, AMR, and plasmid content. Using WGS, public health scientists typically detect outbreaks by looking for tight clusters of infections caused by specific pathogens in time and space [73]. However, outbreaks linked to animals and environmental sources can be challenging to recognize by laboratory surveillance by WGS because they are often polyclonal and more diverse than observed in typical point source outbreaks. All the potential advantages of this tool and the steps forward still to do to improve results have been clearly reviewed by Gerner-Smidt et al. [73].

However, it has been recently highlighted that an integration of different surveillance systems for animal and human health, or among different countries, is still lacking, and therefore great efforts should be invested in this fundamental branch of One Health [74].

The last aspect to be considered in the strict interplay between humans and animals about AMR is the relationship of humans with pets, companion animals, or animals living close to humans for work or recreational activities. Dogs are not only potential carriers of MRSA, but also can they be colonized by plasmid-mediated quinolone resistance genes to some extent, and even more frequently by different ESBL-producing *Enterobacterales* [75–77]: Ortega-Paredes et al. showed a high prevalence of multidrug resistant *E. coli* isolated from canine feces in a public park in Quito (Ecuador), where the most relevant AMR mechanisms recovered from samples were ESBL, plasmid-mediated AmpC β-lactamases, carbapenemases, and *mcr*-1 gene [78].

As epidemiological data on general equine population are limited, Kaspar et al. evaluated the carriage of MRSA and drug-resistant gram-negatives in nonhospitalized horses living in private farms in a rural area of Northwest Germany, and they found 4% colonized by ESBL *E. coli*, and this carriage was associated with prior antibiotic treatment and veterinary examinations [79]. Overall, these studies highlight also the importance of rising awareness in patients and healthcare workers: even if pets or companion animals may be very helpful for some "frail" patients for their social activities, nevertheless they must be trained to optimal animal waste disposal and contact precautions, ideally by "trained trainers" among healthcare workers; this would avoid patient colonization with MDR pathogens that may be relevant once accessing healthcare services.

22.6 Resistance in the Environment

AMR develops in and is maintained and transmitted across humans, animals, and the natural environment. The natural environment presents a transmission route and a reservoir for resistant microorganisms. Resistance is an ancient and naturally occurring phenomenon. Antibiotic producing microorganisms can protect themselves from the toxic effect of the drug using different strategies: one of the most common involves the modification of the antibiotic's target site. Fabbretti et al. very recently analyzed the molecular mechanism devised by the soil microorganism *Streptomyces* sp. strain AM-2504 to protect itself from the activity of the peptide antibiotic dityromycin, and in a very detailed analysis they demonstrated that this mechanism can be reproduced in *E. coli*, thereby eliciting antibiotic resistance in this human commensal [80]. As a matter of fact, the impact of environmental microbes as reservoir of resistance factors and the impact of the spread of drug-resistant bacteria into the environment was not considered until recently. However, it is well known that such bacteria and antibiotic resistance genes (ARGs) are ubiquitous in nature: they can indeed be found in high concentrations in clinical, industrial, and urban wastewater, as well as in animal husbandry [81]; moreover, these environments frequently contain very high levels of antibiotics and pharmaceuticals [82, 83]. As an example, Lübbert et al. sampled different sites and wastewaters in an urban Indian territory where a major production area is settled for the global bulk drug market: they found that all environmental sampling sites were contaminated with very high concentrations of antimicrobials, in particular moxifloxacin, voriconazole, and fluconazole; and that microbiological analyses revealed an extensive presence of ESBL, CPE, and nonfermenters in more than 95% of the samples [83]. Likewise, Marathe et al. highlighted the impact of uncontrolled discharge of partially treated or untreated wastewater on the structure of bacterial communities and resistome of sediments collected in some Indian districts using shotgun metagenomics [84]: they found a wide array of horizontally transferable ARGs, including carbapenemases such as NDM, VIM, KPC, OXA-48, and IMP types. The relative abundance of total ARGs was 30-fold higher in river sediments within the city compared to upstream sites. In addition to ARGs, higher abundances of various mobile genetic elements were found in city samples, as well as some biocide/metal resistance genes. *Acinetobacter*, which is often associated with MDR and nosocomial infections, comprised up to 29% of the 16S rRNA reads, and a strong correlation was found between the abundance of *Acinetobacter* and the OXA-58 carbapenemase gene [84]. Other experiences from India confirm these worrying data, and integrated plans to protect water seem now of utmost importance [85–87].

However, these concerns no longer apply only to LMICs, where hygiene and sanitation may be lower: Czekalski et al. showed increased levels of MDR bacteria and resistance genes after wastewater treatment and dissemination into Lake Geneva, in Switzerland [81], whereas Caltagirone et al. screened 11 wells, 5 streams and 4 wastewater treatment plants for the presence of third-generation cephalosporin-resistant Gram-negative bacteria in the Oltrepò region, in Northern Italy: during a one-year period, CTX-M-, SHV-, DHA-, KPC-type producing *Enterobacteriaceae* were identified. High levels of bacterial contamination and CTX-resistance rates were constantly observed in wastewater treatment plants, while seasonal changes—with highest values in spring—were recorded from stream samples [88]; very recently, Suzuki et al. confirmed these results in Japan [89].

Finally, it must be reminded that healthcare settings themselves may act as a potential reservoir for environmental pollution with MDR or even hospital-acquired outbreaks with MDR pathogens [90, 91].

22.7   Water as Common Denominator

Water is undoubtedly the common denominator of AMR across human and animal health and environment, where direct or indirect human inputs are responsible for extensive dispersal of AMR into the environment and remain a critical and pressing challenge: focused and expensive efforts to minimize pollution from agricultural sources may only provide virtuous benefits to the management of AMR across complex landscapes; those landscape features, season, and water quality variables that influence AMR dynamics [92].

The counterpoint of any human activities potentially releasing whatever ARG in the environment is that MDR bacteria or even pathogens excreted or eliminated via effluents and sewage can recontaminate humans and animals [93] even during recreational activities, and this must be taken into account when frail or immunosuppressed patients get in close contact with these environments. Hammerl et al. identified seven different VCC-1 carbapenemase-producing *Vibrio cholerae* through WGS at different locations on the coastline of Germany [94]; Akanbi et al. collected 249 samples from beach sand and coastal sea water from 10 beaches in Eastern Cape Province of South Africa and found a very high prevalence of resistance mechanisms in *S. aureus* isolates, concluding that beach water and sand from that region may be potential reservoirs of antibiotic-resistant *S. aureus*, which can be transmitted to exposed humans and animals [95]. Moreover, a recent experience showed how some thermotolerant ESBL-producing *E. coli* strains recovered from a river whose water was retained in artificial basins were then able to survive the artificial snow production process [96].

Surprisingly, even remote or uncommon environments may host AMR genes or plasmids: this is the case for the Berlenga Natural Reserve in Portugal [97], or for the sponge microbiota, hosting diverse and novel resistance genes that may be harnessed by phylogenetically distinct bacteria and may act as a reservoir of functional resistance genes [98]. As a matter of fact, the occurrence of MDR bacteria in wildlife is clearly influenced by many and different factors which have not yet been fully understood [99, 100], but it is certainly a matter of concern if Ahlstrom et al. repeatedly detected carbapenemase-producing *E. coli* in gulls inhabiting different sites in Alaska, confirming the potential for a successful interspecies transmission between wildlife, humans, and companion animals [101]; or the presence of *Salmonella* and *Campylobacter* carrying AMR in wild Bonelli's eagles nestlings in Eastern Spain [100]; or, again, the discovery of novel antibiotic resistance determinant in forest and grassland soil metagenomes [102], keeping in mind that rain falling on the earth is the same water we were talking about.

22.8   Conclusions

At last, there is a tangible and widespread shift in attitudes towards the use of antibiotics in both human and veterinary medicine. We have seen a growing understanding that AMR jeopardizes animals and humans alike, is present in different medical, environmental, and societal contexts across the globe, and crosses borders by land, water, and air. The One Health concept stresses the ecological relationships between human, animal, and environmental health [103]: since AMR is found in bacteria from animals and humans, it is a problem that cannot be solved by looking at either in isolation. And since AMR exists in a wide variety of countries and different cultures, we need to find solutions that fit best in any given environment. The AMR problem will not be solved by imposing actions that are not relevant, practical, or acceptable in a situation, even if the same interventions may be successful in a different one or in a different country. In 2018, WHO issued a public document whose target is to improve awareness and to educate any kind of healthcare worker to tackle AMR [104]: we should start acting rapidly to protect our whole world from the threat of AMR in every setting of our life.

References

1. Singer AC, Shaw H, Rhodes V, Hart A. Review of antimicrobial resistance in the environment and its relevance to environmental regulators. Front Microbiol. 2016; https://doi.org/10.3389/fmicb.2016.01728
2. O'Neill J. Tackling drug-resistant infections globally: final report and recommendations. 2016.
3. de Kraker MEA, Stewardson AJ, Harbarth S. Will 10 million people die a year due to antimicrobial resistance by 2050? PLoS Med. 2016;13:e1002184.
4. Kahn LH. Antimicrobial resistance: a one health perspective. Trans R Soc Trop Med Hyg. 2017;111:255–60.
5. Collignon P, McEwen S. One health – its importance in helping to better control antimicrobial resistance. Trop Med Infect Dis. 2019;4:22.
6. European Commission A European One Health Action Plan against Antimicrobial Resistance (AMR). 2017.
7. Florez-Cuadrado D, Moreno MA, Ugarte-Ruíz M, Domínguez L. Antimicrobial resistance in the food chain in the European Union. Adv. Food Nutr. Res. 2018;86(Elsevier):115–36.
8. Carroll LM, Gaballa A, Guldimann C, Sullivan G, Henderson LO, Wiedmann M. Identification of novel mobilized Colistin resistance gene *mcr-9* in a multidrug-resistant, Colistin-susceptible *Salmonella enterica* serotype typhimurium isolate. MBio. 2019; https://doi.org/10.1128/mBio.00853-19
9. Santajit S, Indrawattana N. Mechanisms of antimicrobial resistance in ESKAPE pathogens. Biomed Res Int. 2016;2016:2475067.
10. Partridge SR, Kwong SM, Firth N, Jensen SO. Mobile genetic elements associated with antimicrobial resistance. Clin Microbiol Rev. 2018; https://doi.org/10.1128/CMR.00088-17
11. van Duin D, Paterson DL. Multidrug-resistant bacteria in the community. Trends and Lessons Learned Infect Dis Clin North Am. 2016;30:377–90.
12. Lakhundi S, Zhang K. Methicillin-resistant Staphylococcus aureus: molecular characterization, evolution, and epidemiology. Clin Microbiol Rev. 2018; https://doi.org/10.1128/CMR.00020-18
13. Ahmed MO, Baptiste KE. Vancomycin-resistant enterococci: a review of antimicrobial resistance mechanisms and perspectives of human and animal health. Microb Drug Resist Larchmt N. 2018;24:590–606.
14. Pitout JDD, Laupland KB. Extended-spectrum beta-lactamase-producing Enterobacteriaceae: an emerging public-health concern. Lancet Infect Dis. 2008;8:159–66.
15. Jacoby GA. AmpC beta-lactamases. Clin Microbiol Rev. 2009;22:161–82, Table of Contents
16. Suay-García B, Pérez-Gracia MT. Present and future of Carbapenem-resistant Enterobacteriaceae (CRE) infections. Antibiot Basel Switz. 2019; https://doi.org/10.3390/antibiotics8030122
17. Codjoe FS, Donkor ES. Carbapenem resistance: a review. Med Sci Basel Switz. 2017; https://doi.org/10.3390/medsci6010001
18. Tacconelli E, Pezzani MD. Public health burden of antimicrobial resistance in Europe. Lancet Infect Dis. 2019;19:4–6.
19. Gandra S, Tseng KK, Arora A, Bhowmik B, Robinson ML, Panigrahi B, Laxminarayan R, Klein EY. The mortality burden of multidrug-resistant pathogens in India: a retrospective, observational study. Clin Infect Dis. 2019;69:563–70.
20. Cassini A, Högberg LD, Plachouras D, et al. Attributable deaths and disability-adjusted life-years caused by infections with antibiotic-resistant bacteria in the EU and the European economic area in 2015: a population-level modelling analysis. Lancet Infect Dis. 2019;19:56–66.
21. George A. Antimicrobial resistance (AMR) in the food chain: trade, one health and codex. Trop Med Infect Dis. 2019;4:54.

22. Pérez-Rodríguez F, Mercanoglu Taban B. A state-of-art review on multi-drug resistant pathogens in foods of animal origin: risk factors and mitigation strategies. Front Microbiol. 2019;10:2091.

23. Rhouma M, Beaudry F, Thériault W, Letellier A. Colistin in pig production: chemistry, mechanism of antibacterial action, microbial resistance emergence, and one health perspectives. Front Microbiol. 2016; https://doi.org/10.3389/fmicb.2016.01789

24. Richterman A, Azman AS, Constant G, Ivers LC. The inverse relationship between national food security and annual cholera incidence: a 30-country analysis. BMJ Glob Health. 2019;4:e001755.

25. Baschera M, Cernela N, Stevens MJA, Liljander A, Jores J, Corman VM, Nüesch-Inderbinen M, Stephan R. Shiga toxin-producing Escherichia coli (STEC) isolated from fecal samples of African dromedary camels. One Health. 2019;7:100087.

26. Stewardson AJ, Renzi G, Maury N, et al. Extended-spectrum β-lactamase-producing Enterobacteriaceae in hospital food: a risk assessment. Infect Control Hosp Epidemiol. 2014;35:375–83.

27. Liu H, Whitehouse CA, Li B. Presence and persistence of salmonella in water: the impact on microbial quality of water and food safety. Front Public Health. 2018; https://doi.org/10.3389/fpubh.2018.00159

28. Gauld JS, Olgemoeller F, Nkhata R, et al. Domestic River water use and risk of typhoid. Fever: Results From a Case-control Study in Blantyre, Malawi. Clin Infect Dis; 2019. https://doi.org/10.1093/cid/ciz405

29. Troeger C, Blacker BF, Khalil IA, et al. Estimates of the global, regional, and national morbidity, mortality, and aetiologies of diarrhoea in 195 countries: a systematic analysis for the global burden of disease study 2016. Lancet Infect Dis. 2018;18:1211–28.

30. Wang X, Biswas S, Paudyal N, Pan H, Li X, Fang W, Yue M. Antibiotic resistance in salmonella typhimurium isolates recovered from the food chain through National Antimicrobial Resistance Monitoring System between 1996 and 2016. Front Microbiol. 2019; https://doi.org/10.3389/fmicb.2019.00985

31. Mesbah Zekar F, Granier SA, Marault M, Yaici L, Gassilloud B, Manceau C, Touati A, Millemann Y. From farms to markets: gram-negative bacteria resistant to third-generation Cephalosporins in fruits and vegetables in a region of North Africa. Front Microbiol. 2017; https://doi.org/10.3389/fmicb.2017.01569

32. Mani Y, Mansour W, Mammeri H, Denamur E, Saras E, Boujâafar N, Bouallègue O, Madec J-Y, Haenni M. KPC-3-producing ST167 Escherichia coli from mussels bought at a retail market in Tunisia. J Antimicrob Chemother. 2017;72:2403–4.

33. Slettemeås JS, Urdahl A-M, Mo SS, Johannessen GS, Grave K, Norström M, Steinbakk M, Sunde M. Imported food and feed as contributors to the introduction of plasmid-mediated colistin-resistant Enterobacteriaceae to a 'low prevalence' country. J Antimicrob Chemother. 2017;72:2675–7.

34. Li H, Stegger M, Dalsgaard A, Leisner JJ. Bacterial content and characterization of antibiotic resistant Staphylococcus aureus in Danish sushi products and association with food inspector rankings. Int J Food Microbiol. 2019;305:108244.

35. Silva V, Nunes J, Gomes A, Capita R, Alonso-Calleja C, Pereira JE, Torres C, Igrejas G, Poeta P. Detection of antibiotic resistance in Escherichia coli strains: can fish commonly used in raw preparations such as sushi and sashimi constitute a public health problem? J Food Prot. 2019;82:1130–4.

36. Van Boeckel TP, Brower C, Gilbert M, Grenfell BT, Levin SA, Robinson TP, Teillant A, Laxminarayan R. Global trends in antimicrobial use in food animals. Proc Natl Acad Sci. 2015;112:5649–54.

37. Price LB, Koch BJ, Hungate BA. Ominous projections for global antibiotic use in food-animal production. Proc Natl Acad Sci. 2015;112:5554–5.

38. Founou LL, Founou RC, Essack SY. Antibiotic resistance in the food chain: a developing country-perspective. Front Microbiol. 2016; https://doi.org/10.3389/fmicb.2016.01881

39. Hao H, Sander P, Iqbal Z, Wang Y, Cheng G, Yuan Z. The risk of some veterinary antimicrobial agents on public health associated with antimicrobial resistance and their molecular basis. Front Microbiol. 2016; https://doi.org/10.3389/fmicb.2016.01626
40. Amoako DG, Somboro AM, Abia ALK, Molechan C, Perrett K, Bester LA, Essack SY. Antibiotic resistance in Staphylococcus aureus from poultry and poultry products in uMgungundlovu district, South Africa, using the "farm to fork" approach. Microb Drug Resist Larchmt N. 2019; https://doi.org/10.1089/mdr.2019.0201
41. AbuOun M, Stubberfield EJ, Duggett NA, et al. mcr-1 and mcr-2 (mcr-6.1) variant genes identified in Moraxella species isolated from pigs in Great Britain from 2014 to 2015. J Antimicrob Chemother. 2017;72:2745–9.
42. Zhang L, Fu Y, Xiong Z, Ma Y, Wei Y, Qu X, Zhang H, Zhang J, Liao M. Highly prevalent multidrug-resistant salmonella from chicken and pork meat at retail Markets in Guangdong, China. Front Microbiol. 2018; https://doi.org/10.3389/fmicb.2018.02104
43. Castellanos LR, Donado-Godoy P, León M, Clavijo V, Arevalo A, Bernal JF, Timmerman AJ, Mevius DJ, Wagenaar JA, Hordijk J. High heterogeneity of Escherichia coli sequence types harbouring ESBL/AmpC genes on Incl1 plasmids in the Colombian poultry chain. PLoS One. 2017;12:e0170777.
44. O'Dea M, Sahibzada S, Jordan D, et al. Genomic, antimicrobial resistance, and public health insights into Enterococcus spp. from Australian chickens. J Clin Microbiol. 2019; https://doi.org/10.1128/JCM.00319-19
45. Anbazhagan PV, Thavitiki PR, Varra M, Annamalai L, Putturu R, Lakkineni VR, Pesingi PK. Evaluation of efflux pump activity of multidrug-resistant salmonella typhimurium isolated from poultry wet markets in India. Infect Drug Resist. 2019;12:1081–8.
46. Chen M, Cheng J, Zhang J, et al. Isolation, potential virulence, and population diversity of Listeria monocytogenes from meat and meat products in China. Front Microbiol. 2019; https://doi.org/10.3389/fmicb.2019.00946
47. Chabou S, Leulmi H, Rolain J-M. Emergence of mcr-1-mediated colistin resistance in Escherichia coli isolates from poultry in Algeria. J Glob Antimicrob Resist. 2019;16:115–6.
48. Ghafur A, Shankar C, GnanaSoundari P, Venkatesan M, Mani D, Thirunarayanan MA, Veeraraghavan B. Detection of chromosomal and plasmid-mediated mechanisms of colistin resistance in Escherichia coli and Klebsiella pneumoniae from Indian food samples. J Glob Antimicrob Resist. 2019;16:48–52.
49. Galetti R, Antonio Casarin Penha Filho R, Ferreira JC, M. Varani A, Costa Darini AL. Antibiotic resistance and heavy metal tolerance plasmids: the antimicrobial bulletproof properties of Escherichia fergusonii isolated from poultry. Infect Drug Resist Volume. 2019;12:1029–33.
50. Delannoy S, Le Devendec L, Jouy E, Fach P, Drider D, Kempf I. Characterization of Colistin-resistant Escherichia coli isolated from diseased pigs in France. Front Microbiol. 2017; https://doi.org/10.3389/fmicb.2017.02278
51. Clifford K, Desai D, Prazeres da Costa C, Meyer H, Klohe K, Winkler A, Rahman T, Islam T, Zaman MH. Antimicrobial resistance in livestock and poor quality veterinary medicines. Bull World Health Organ. 2018;96:662–4.
52. Wong A. Unknown risk on the farm: does agricultural use of Ionophores contribute to the burden of antimicrobial resistance? mSphere. 2019; https://doi.org/10.1128/mSphere.00433-19
53. Nilsson O, Myrenås M, Ågren J. Transferable genes putatively conferring elevated minimum inhibitory concentrations of narasin in Enterococcus faecium from Swedish broilers. Vet Microbiol. 2016;184:80–3.
54. Li J, Shi X, Yin W, Wang Y, Shen Z, Ding S, Wang S. A multiplex SYBR green real-time PCR assay for the detection of three Colistin resistance genes from cultured bacteria, Feces, and environment samples. Front Microbiol. 2017; https://doi.org/10.3389/fmicb.2017.02078
55. Seiffert SN, Carattoli A, Schwendener S, Collaud A, Endimiani A, Perreten V. Plasmids Carrying blaCMY -2/4 in Escherichia coli from Poultry, Poultry Meat, and Humans Belong to a Novel IncK Subgroup Designated IncK2. Front Microbiol. 2017; https://doi.org/10.3389/fmicb.2017.00407

56. Xia X, Wang Z, Fu Y, et al. Association of colistin residues and manure treatment with the abundance of mcr-1 gene in swine feedlots. Environ Int. 2019;127:361–70.
57. Henriksson PJG, Troell M, Rico A. Antimicrobial use in aquaculture: some complementing facts. Proc Natl Acad Sci. 2015;112:E3317–E3317.
58. Troell M, Naylor RL, Metian M, et al. Does aquaculture add resilience to the global food system? Proc Natl Acad Sci USA. 2014;111:13257–63.
59. Cabello FC, Tomova A, Ivanova L, Godfrey HP. Aquaculture and mcr Colistin resistance determinants. MBio. 2017; https://doi.org/10.1128/mBio.01229-17
60. Shen Y, Lv Z, Yang L, et al. Integrated aquaculture contributes to the transfer of mcr-1 between animals and humans via the aquaculture supply chain. Environ Int. 2019;130:104708.
61. Klare I, Badstübner D, Konstabel C, Böhme G, Claus H, Witte W. Decreased incidence of VanA-type vancomycin-resistant enterococci isolated from poultry meat and from Fecal samples of humans in the community after discontinuation of Avoparcin usage in animal husbandry. Microb Drug Resist. 1999;5:45–52.
62. Tang KL, Caffrey NP, Nóbrega DB, et al. Comparison of different approaches to antibiotic restriction in food-producing animals: stratified results from a systematic review and meta-analysis. BMJ Glob Health. 2019;4:e001710.
63. Fitzgerald JR. Livestock-associated Staphylococcus aureus: origin, evolution and public health threat. Trends Microbiol. 2012;20:192–8.
64. Chuang Y-Y, Huang Y-C. Livestock-associated meticillin-resistant Staphylococcus aureus in Asia: an emerging issue? Int J Antimicrob Agents. 2015;45:334–40.
65. Ge B, Mukherjee S, Hsu C-H, et al. MRSA and multidrug-resistant Staphylococcus aureus in U.S. retail meats, 2010–2011. Food Microbiol. 2017;62:289–97.
66. Parisi A, Caruso M, Normanno G, Latorre L, Miccolupo A, Fraccalvieri R, Intini F, Manginelli T, Santagada G. MRSA in swine, farmers and abattoir workers in southern Italy. Food Microbiol. 2019;82:287–93.
67. Quijada NM, Hernández M, Oniciuc E-A, Eiros JM, Fernández-Natal I, Wagner M, Rodríguez-Lázaro D. Oxacillin-susceptible mecA-positive Staphylococcus aureus associated with processed food in Europe. Food Microbiol. 2019;82:107–10.
68. Wu S, Zhang F, Huang J, et al. Phenotypic and genotypic characterization of PVL-positive Staphylococcus aureus isolated from retail foods in China. Int J Food Microbiol. 2019;304:119–26.
69. Garcia-Graells C, Antoine J, Larsen J, Catry B, Skov R, Denis O. Livestock veterinarians at high risk of acquiring methicillin-resistant Staphylococcus aureus ST398. Epidemiol Infect. 2012;140:383–9.
70. Royden A, Ormandy E, Pinchbeck G, Pascoe B, Hitchings MD, Sheppard SK, Williams NJ. Prevalence of faecal carriage of extended-spectrum β-lactamase (ESBL)-producing Escherichia coli in veterinary hospital staff and students. Vet Rec Open. 2019;6:e000307.
71. Moawad AA, Hotzel H, Awad O, Roesler U, Hafez HM, Tomaso H, Neubauer H, El-Adawy H. Evolution of antibiotic resistance of coagulase-negative staphylococci isolated from healthy turkeys in Egypt: first report of linezolid resistance. Microorganisms. 2019;7:476.
72. Schrijver R, Stijntjes M, Rodríguez-Baño J, Tacconelli E, Babu Rajendran N, Voss A. Review of antimicrobial resistance surveillance programmes in livestock and meat in EU with focus on humans. Clin Microbiol Infect. 2018;24:577–90.
73. Gerner-Smidt P, Besser J, Concepción-Acevedo J, Folster JP, Huffman J, Joseph LA, Kucerova Z, Nichols MC, Schwensohn CA, Tolar B. Whole genome sequencing: bridging one-health surveillance of foodborne diseases. Front Public Health. 2019; https://doi.org/10.3389/fpubh.2019.00172
74. Queenan K, Häsler B, Rushton J. A one health approach to antimicrobial resistance surveillance: is there a business case for it? Int J Antimicrob Agents. 2016;48:422–7.
75. Liu X, Liu H, Li Y, Hao C. High prevalence of β-lactamase and plasmid-mediated quinolone resistance genes in extended-Spectrum cephalosporin-resistant Escherichia coli from dogs in Shaanxi, China. Front Microbiol. 2016; https://doi.org/10.3389/fmicb.2016.01843

76. Hong JS, Song W, Park H-M, Oh J-Y, Chae J-C, Shin S, Jeong SH. Clonal spread of extended-Spectrum cephalosporin-resistant Enterobacteriaceae between companion animals and humans in South Korea. Front Microbiol. 2019; https://doi.org/10.3389/fmicb.2019.01371

77. Silva MM, Fernandes MR, Sellera FP, Cerdeira L, Medeiros LKG, Garino F, Azevedo SS, Lincopan N. Multidrug-resistant CTX-M-15-producing Klebsiella pneumoniae ST231 associated with infection and persistent colonization of dog. Diagn Microbiol Infect Dis. 2018;92:259–61.

78. Ortega-Paredes D, Haro M, Leoro-Garzón P, Barba P, Loaiza K, Mora F, Fors M, Vinueza-Burgos C, Fernández-Moreira E. Multidrug-resistant Escherichia coli isolated from canine faeces in a public park in Quito, Ecuador. J Glob Antimicrob Resist. 2019;18:263–8.

79. Kaspar U, von Lützau K, Schlattmann A, Rösler U, Köck R, Becker K. Zoonotic multidrug-resistant microorganisms among non-hospitalized horses from Germany. One Health. 2019;7:100091.

80. Fabbretti A, Çapuni R, Giuliodori AM, Cimarelli L, Miano A, Napolioni V, La Teana A, Spurio R. Characterization of the self-resistance mechanism to Dityromycin in the *Streptomyces* producer strain. mSphere. 2019; https://doi.org/10.1128/mSphere.00554-19

81. Czekalski N, Berthold T, Caucci S, Egli A, Bürgmann H. Increased levels of multiresistant bacteria and resistance genes after wastewater treatment and their dissemination into Lake Geneva, Switzerland. Front Microbiol. 2012; https://doi.org/10.3389/fmicb.2012.00106

82. Waseem H, Williams MR, Stedtfeld RD, Hashsham SA. Antimicrobial resistance in the environment. Water Environ Res. 2017;89:921–41.

83. Lübbert C, Baars C, Dayakar A, Lippmann N, Rodloff AC, Kinzig M, Sörgel F. Environmental pollution with antimicrobial agents from bulk drug manufacturing industries in Hyderabad, South India, is associated with dissemination of extended-spectrum beta-lactamase and carbapenemase-producing pathogens. Infection. 2017;45:479–91.

84. Marathe NP, Pal C, Gaikwad SS, Jonsson V, Kristiansson E, Larsson DGJ. Untreated urban waste contaminates Indian river sediments with resistance genes to last resort antibiotics. Water Res. 2017;124:388–90.

85. Bengtsson-Palme J, Boulund F, Fick J, Kristiansson E, Larsson DGJ. Shotgun metagenomics reveals a wide array of antibiotic resistance genes and mobile elements in a polluted lake in India. Front Microbiol. 2014; https://doi.org/10.3389/fmicb.2014.00648

86. Paulshus E, Thorell K, Guzman-Otazo J, Joffre E, Colque P, Kühn I, Möllby R, Sørum H, Sjöling Å. Repeated isolation of extended-Spectrum-β-lactamase-positive *Escherichia coli* sequence types 648 and 131 from community wastewater indicates that sewage systems are important sources of emerging clones of antibiotic-resistant bacteria. Antimicrob Agents Chemother. 2019; https://doi.org/10.1128/AAC.00823-19

87. Kwikiriza S, Stewart AG, Mutahunga B, Dobson AE, Wilkinson E. A whole systems approach to hospital waste management in rural Uganda. Front Public Health. 2019; https://doi.org/10.3389/fpubh.2019.00136

88. Caltagirone M, Nucleo E, Spalla M, et al. Occurrence of extended Spectrum β-lactamases, KPC-type, and MCR-1.2-producing Enterobacteriaceae from Wells, river water, and wastewater treatment plants in Oltrepò Pavese area, northern Italy. Front Microbiol. 2017; https://doi.org/10.3389/fmicb.2017.02232

89. Suzuki Y, Ida M, Kubota H, Ariyoshi T, Murakami K, Kobayashi M, Kato R, Hirai A, Suzuki J, Sadamasu K. Multiple β-lactam resistance gene-carrying plasmid Harbored by *Klebsiella quasipneumoniae* isolated from urban sewage in Japan. mSphere. 2019; https://doi.org/10.1128/mSphere.00391-19

90. Marathe NP, Berglund F, Razavi M, Pal C, Dröge J, Samant S, Kristiansson E, Larsson DGJ. Sewage effluent from an Indian hospital harbors novel carbapenemases and integron-borne antibiotic resistance genes. Microbiome. 2019; https://doi.org/10.1186/s40168-019-0710-x

91. Carling PC. Wastewater drains: epidemiology and interventions in 23 carbapenem-resistant organism outbreaks. Infect Control Hosp Epidemiol. 2018;39:972–9.

92. Sanderson CE, Fox JT, Dougherty ER, Cameron ADS, Alexander KA. The changing face of water: a dynamic reflection of antibiotic resistance across landscapes. Front Microbiol. 2018; https://doi.org/10.3389/fmicb.2018.01894

93. Jørgensen SB, Søraas AV, Arnesen LS, Leegaard TM, Sundsfjord A, Jenum PA. A comparison of extended spectrum β-lactamase producing Escherichia coli from clinical, recreational water and wastewater samples associated in time and location. PLoS One. 2017;12:e0186576.

94. Hammerl JA, Jäckel C, Bortolaia V, Schwartz K, Bier N, Hendriksen RS, Guerra B, Strauch E. Carbapenemase VCC-1–producing Vibrio cholerae in coastal waters of Germany. Emerg Infect Dis. 2017;23:1735–7.

95. Akanbi OE, Njom HA, Fri J, Otigbu AC, Clarke AM. Antimicrobial susceptibility of Staphylococcus aureus isolated from recreational waters and beach sand in Eastern Cape Province of South Africa. Int J Environ Res Public Health. 2017;14:1001.

96. Lenart-Boroń A, Prajsnar J, Boroń P. Survival and antibiotic resistance of bacteria in artificial snow produced from contaminated water. Water Environ Res. 2017;89:2059–69.

97. Alves MS, Pereira A, AraÃojo SM, Castro BB, Correia ACM, Henriques I. Seawater is a reservoir of multi-resistant Escherichia coli, including strains hosting plasmid-mediated quinolones resistance and extended-spectrum beta-lactamases genes. Front Microbiol. 2014; https://doi.org/10.3389/fmicb.2014.00426

98. Versluis D, Rodriguez de Evgrafov M, Sommer MOA, Sipkema D, Smidt H, van Passel MWJ. Sponge microbiota are a reservoir of functional antibiotic resistance genes. Front Microbiol. 2016; https://doi.org/10.3389/fmicb.2016.01848

99. Dolejska M, Literak I. Wildlife is overlooked in the epidemiology of medically important antibiotic-resistant bacteria. Antimicrob Agents Chemother. 2019; https://doi.org/10.1128/AAC.01167-19

100. Martín-Maldonado B, Montoro-Dasi L, Pérez-Gracia MT, Jordá J, Vega S, Marco-Jiménez F, Marin C. Wild Bonelli's eagles (Aquila fasciata) as carrier of antimicrobial resistant Salmonella and Campylobacter in Eastern Spain. Comp Immunol Microbiol Infect Dis. 2019;67:101372.

101. Ahlstrom CA, Ramey AM, Woksepp H, Bonnedahl J. Repeated detection of Carbapenemase-producing Escherichia coli in gulls inhabiting Alaska. Antimicrob Agents Chemother. 2019; https://doi.org/10.1128/AAC.00758-19

102. Willms IM, Kamran A, Aßmann NF, Krone D, Bolz SH, Fiedler F, Nacke H. Discovery of novel antibiotic resistance determinants in Forest and grassland soil metagenomes. Front Microbiol. 2019; https://doi.org/10.3389/fmicb.2019.00460

103. Trinh P, Zaneveld JR, Safranek S, Rabinowitz PM. One health relationships between human, animal, and environmental microbiomes: a mini-review. Front Public Health. 2018; https://doi.org/10.3389/fpubh.2018.00235

104. WHO. WHO competency framework for health workers' education and training on antimicrobial resistance. 2018.

Printed by Printforce, United Kingdom